The Adult Baby Identity

The Complete Collection

By

Dylan Lewis

Title: The Adult Baby Identity

Author: Dylan Lewis

Editor: Michael and Rosalie Bent

Foreword: Michael Bent

Publisher: AB Discovery

© 2019

www.abdiscovery.com.au

Other Books from Dylan Lewis

Six Misfits
Six Misfits – A man and his dog
The Six Misfits – the seventh misfit
The Adult Baby Identity – coming out as ABDL
The Adult Baby Identity – Healing Childhood Wounds
Living with Chrissie – my life as an Adult Baby
The Adult Baby Identity – a self-help guide
The Adult Baby Identity – the dissociation spectrum
Becoming Me – The Journey of Self-acceptance
Living happily as an Adult Baby
Adult Babies and Diaper Lovers – a guidebook

Other Books from AB Discovery

There's still a baby in my bed!
So, Your teenager is wearing diapers!
Where Big Babies Live
Home Detention
Adult Babies: Psychology and Practices
Coffee with Rosie
Being an Adult Baby
The Three Chambers
A Brother for Samantha
Mummy's Diary
The Hypnotist
Chosen
The Snoop
The Washing Line

NOTES:

This remarkable collection contains the four books Dylan Lewis has written on the Adult Baby Identity. They are also published as individual books. They are:

The Adult Baby Identity: Coming out as an Adult Baby

The Adult Baby Identity: Healing Childhood Wounds

The Adult Baby Identity: A Self-help Guide

The Adult Baby Identity: An Identity on the Dissociation Spectrum

Contents

14

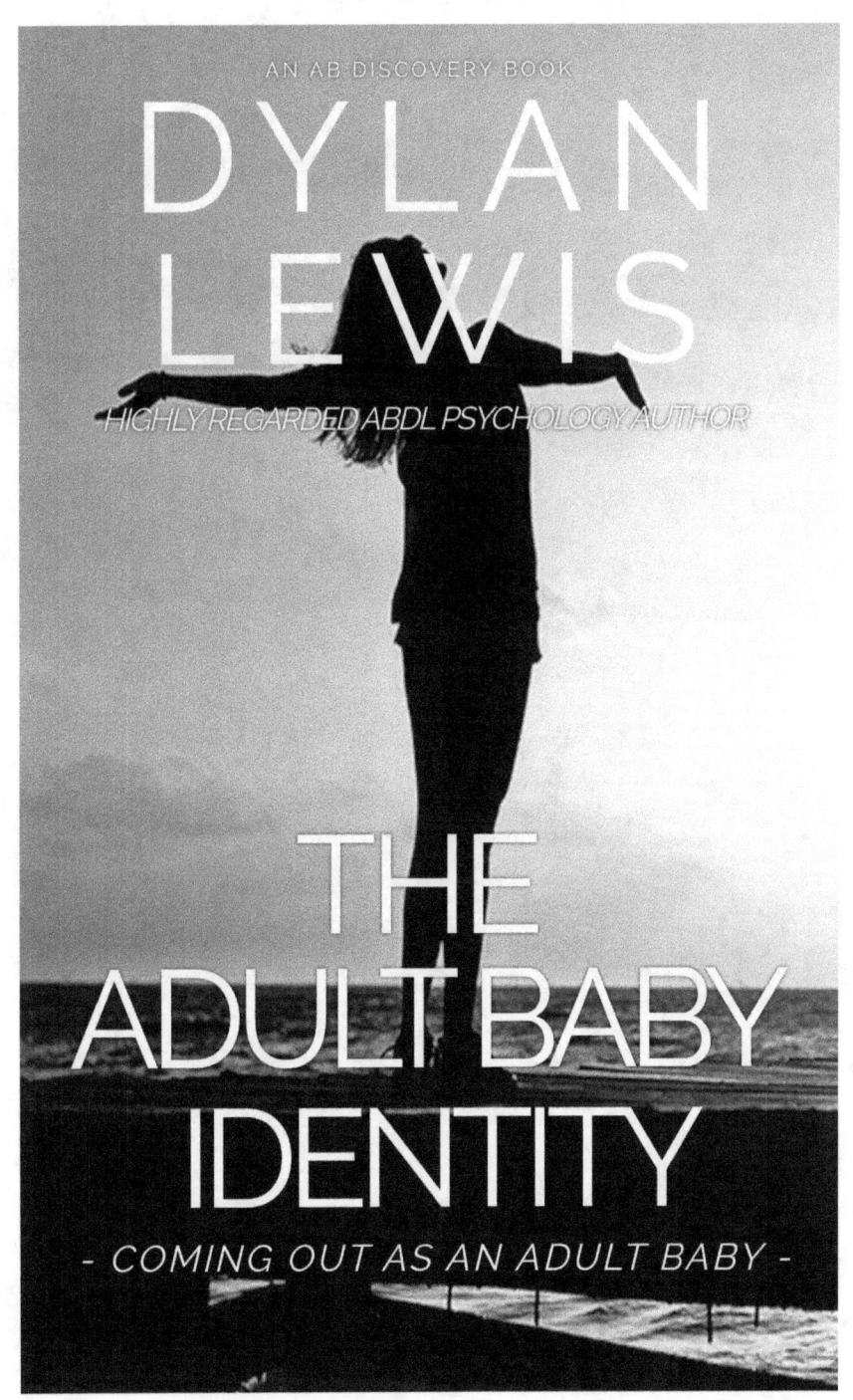

AN AB DISCOVERY BOOK

DYLAN LEWIS

HIGHLY REGARDED ABDL PSYCHOLOGY AUTHOR

THE ADULT BABY IDENTITY

- COMING OUT AS AN ADULT BABY -

The Adult Baby Identity

Coming out as an Adult Baby

© 2019

Dylan Lewis

Foreword

"There is no bigger struggle in our lives than to understand who we are – not just externally or physically, but internally. Being a human being is an immeasurably complex experience and it juxtaposes both beauty and wonder with pain and suffering. We can, at the same time, both understand something and yet be totally mystified by it.

Being an Adult Baby adds another layer of intricacy to our personal makeup. I wish I could say that it is all positive, but anyone who has been AB in a world that knows little to nothing about it, already knows that it can be far from an entirely positive experience.

In so many ways, Adult Babies are alone; sometimes grouped together, but still very much separate individuals trying to make sense of the morass of conflicts, fears and pleasures that assail us constantly. We know that our friends, family, neighbours both do not, nor ever will, fully understand us.

For decades, I struggled to find my own identity, just as thousands like me have struggled. Until relatively recently, there was very little material out there about the psychology of Adult Infants and what was there, was usually very wrong, sometimes horrifically so.

It is in this light, that I highly recommend this book. It explores the AB identity and what makes us who we are and the stages of its development. Many of you will read these pages and identify strongly with it.

I trust you will read this book and understand that you really are an Adult Baby. You are not a bad person nor a good person. You are just an Adult Baby.

Being AB can be either a curse or an astonishingly wonderful experience that very few will ever experience. As humans, we are often encouraged to metaphorically 'embrace our inner child'. We have the amazing ability to do just that, but literally so. Our 'inner child' has a name, a gender and a personality who we know and understand well.

It is who we are.

We are Adult Babies. And proudly so."

Michael Bent

1 Introduction

Being an Adult Baby is a personal identity.

It is a stable, healthy identity - when internal conflict and fear of harm from prejudice are removed. It is a minority personal identity akin to, but not the same as, LGBTQ (Lesbian, Gay, Bisexual, Transgender, Queer) identities.

This is not how most other people regard being an AB.

This is not how most health professionals regard being an AB.

This is not how many conflicted ABs themselves regard being an AB.

It *is,* however, the best way to think about being an AB.

I am an Adult Baby. I wrote this book after 'coming out' to myself. I realized that 'coming out' was an experience I shared with other people with minority identities. I realized that being an AB is a personal identity.

The alternative is to see being an Adult Baby as an addiction, a sexual fetish, a psychosexual disorder, a paraphilia – in short as a pathological condition.

That's how society and medical professionals used to think of being LGBTQ. Arguably, especially in the dark ages of public ignorance and prejudice, that's even how some conflicted LGBTQ people thought about themselves. We don't think that way about being LGBTQ anymore because we understand it's ignorant, inaccurate and hateful.

As a society, I believe that we are on the journey to understanding that being AB is a healthy minority identity. We are just several decades behind our understanding and acceptance of LGBTQ identities.

Conflicted ABs have behaviours and thoughts that are unhealthy. So do conflicted people with LGBTQ identities. That doesn't make an LGBTQ identity unhealthy. Nor does it make the AB identity unhealthy. In both cases, it is a call to resolve the conflicts driving unhealthy thoughts and behaviours and to open the door to self-acceptance and a healthy, stable minority identity.

The purpose of this book is to think about being an AB as a personal identity.

What makes it a personal identity? *(Hint: It isn't nappies!)*

What difference does that make?

What is the way forward?

Importantly, we can apply an understanding of 'coming out' to being AB. This allows ABs to understand that their struggles and conflicts are part of the process of identity formation. They can take reassurance and strength from knowing that they share this process with other people with a minority identity, including LGBTQ people. Other courageous people with minority identities have gone before us and trodden the same path to self-acceptance, full lives, and eventually public acceptance - without sacrificing their sense of self.

The key audience for the book are ABs and those who love them. This book is my best attempt to understand our shared identity. Some will disagree with my views. I do not intend to disparage any who's views are different from mine. Take what is useful or helpful from the book and leave the rest behind. Or even better, make a reasoned case for a different but constructive view of our identity and the way forward.

Another important audience is health professionals. The book makes the case for discarding offensive and empirically invalid pathological definitions of the AB identity.

This book is based on the pioneering work of Rosalie Bent and Michael Bent in identifying and understanding adult babies as a personal identity. I recommend their books and website abdiscovery.com.au. I refer to their insights and understanding throughout the book.

By Adult Baby I exclude role players and exclusively diaper lovers for whom diapers, baby clothes or baby activities are an optional extra they can freely live without, and fetishists for whom these things are confined exclusively to sexual expression.

This book is a companion to my other book, 'Becoming Me'. The latter deals principally with self-acceptance, the intra-psychic dimension of identity formation, and the childhood origin of the identity.

2 The Adult Baby Identity

A minority personal identity, such as being LGBTQ, can be expected to have the following characteristics–

   a.   it is a fundamental feature of the person's psyche – it is not transitory or ephemeral, and it reflects a compelling and non-conforming sense of self which pervades and animates the psyche - this may or may not include a non-heterosexual sexual orientation

b.   it is psychologically healthy (when internal conflict and fear of external detriment is resolved), meaning that it is intrinsically a source of positive traits and supports other positive aspects of the self

c.   it is a sustainable expression of the person's psyche – meaning a person sustains this identity by and for themselves

Being an AB (Adult Baby) meets these characteristics. It is not transitory or ephemeral. Many ABs can trace their first consciousness of the identity back to recollections in early childhood. This is usually way before puberty and didn't start out as a sexual fetish. The feelings associated with being AB never go away. They cannot be 'cured' away by psychology or religious faith. They can be denied and repressed only at the cost of an increasing level of psychic energy and eventually, pain and turmoil.

The LGBTQ identities include those based on –

1.   sexual orientation (e.g. lesbian, gay, bisexual)

2.   a non-conforming experience of self (e.g. transgender) which may be combined with one or other sexual orientations.

Being an AB fits falls into the second category – it reflects a non-conforming experience of self. You can be AB and any sexual orientation - heterosexual, lesbian, gay, bisexual or asexual. Cross-dressers and transvestites who have an experience of self as female would also fit into this second category.

The non-conflicted AB identity is psychologically healthy.

Adult babies have a baby or child persona or sub-personality. That co-exists with their functional adult self. Balanced ABs are as capable as anyone else of being a responsible, loving and creative adult. The healthy baby or child persona gives the AB access to child-like innocent happiness, contentment, security and wonder. As with other valid personal identities, self-acceptance enhances the person's confidence, resilience and creativity.

Being a non-conflicted AB is a sustainable identity. ABs can share their identity with a partner or friend(s) but it remains their identity.

So what is the AB identity? What is the compelling, non-conforming sense of self that pervades and animates the psyche of an Adult Baby?

For non-ABs, do not be distracted by the sometimes confronting images of adults wearing nappies and sucking pacifiers. For ABs, look past our obsession and our fetish with nappies. These perspectives no more fully define the AB identity than the mechanics of gay sex fully define the gay personal identity.

Being AB is essentially about having a subjectively real baby or child persona as part of your psyche.

At its core, it's that simple. Yes, the baby/child persona is the source of unconventional behaviours, but it's the existence of the persona which is the fundamental, defining characteristic of the identity. The AB's nappies, baby clothes and baby play can best be understood as a concrete affirmation *to the self* of the existence of the baby/child persona.

That persona -

a.   is a subjectively real part of the psyche

b.   has feelings and needs distinct from the person's adult persona, although those feelings and needs are ultimately those of the self

c.   has feelings which need to be recognized, and needs for comfort, safety and play which need to be met on a regular basis, for the person to function optimally

d.   is capable of acting as an almost-autonomous personality, driving compulsive behaviour, if their needs for comfort and safety are not acknowledged and met

e.   is commonly ever-present in the person's consciousness, but may move between the background and the foreground

f.   may be of a different gender from the adult self

g.   may range in age from infant to older child

h.   is a construct, both conscious and unconscious, which commonly does not accurately replicate the attributes and behaviours of a real biological child of a specified age

i.   has been present since early childhood (whether consciously recognized or not).

This formulation was first outlined in Rosalie Bent's 2012 landmark book *'There's a Baby in My Bed: Learning to Live with the Adult Baby in Your Relationship'*. It may still be controversial in that some ABs do not recognize that the source of their child-like feelings, needs and behaviours is a subjectively real baby or child persona.

In my experience, accepting the existence of such a persona is the most confronting aspect of the AB identity. For everyone, ABs and non-ABs, it is a deeply ingrained disposition to think of ourselves as having a unitary mind or consciousness. Our culture and education do little or nothing to prepare us to think in terms of a multiplicity of mind or consciousness. It is commonly linked to insanity. For anyone to contemplate a multiplicity of consciousness is confronting. For ABs, it is especially so. We have been living most of lives with compulsive behaviours at odds with our adolescent or adult character. We already fear ourselves to be weird, damaged or perverted. If we contemplate the existence of a subjectively real baby/child persona within our psyche, will we have to fear being crazy as well?

For ABs, it is paradoxically easier to live with the fear that you're a weirdo or pervert than it is to accept that you share your consciousness with an innocent baby/child persona. I believe that, for much of the identity formation process, ABs' preoccupation with nappies and the fetish side is a distraction from this deeper and more confronting reality.

Yet the idea of such personas or sub-personalities is becoming more accepted. Since the 1980s a school of psychology has emerged which views having multiple personas as normal – applicable to all. Internal Family Systems Therapy (IFS) was developed by Richard Schwartz based on his work with bulimic clients *(see the book of the same name, published in 1995)*. It posits that we all have multiple personas (termed 'parts') lead by a unifying self. The book *Subpersonalities: The People Inside Us* by psychotherapist John Rowan cites an extensive and respectable pedigree for multiplicity models of mind and consciousness.

An AB with a baby/child persona is not insane; they are not 'possessed'; they do not 'hear voices'.

On a regular basis, they experience child-like feelings, and needs for comfort, security and play. Those feelings and needs are their own, but they come from a different source than their adult personality. The feelings and needs are very real. They persist over the AB's lifetime. If they are denied or ignored, the AB finds themselves subject to compulsive behaviours which express those child-like feelings and needs (sulks or tantrums with partners, wearing nappies etcetera) in a disruptive way, which are at odds with the personality and wishes of the adult self.

Psychological health comes through accepting the existence of the baby/child persona, recognizing their feelings, and meeting their needs in a managed way. A non-conflicted AB in an accepting environment does that in a way that doesn't interfere with their adult life and responsibilities. Both the adult self and baby/child persona are functional (loving, happy, resilient) as a result.

I suspect that many non-conflicted ABs integrate their baby/child persona into their daily lives by literally 'sleeping like a baby', going to bed at night dressed like a baby with comfort objects. I do exactly that. In the morning we get up to our adult lives. If you're a non-AB you've probably at some time sat next to an AB on the bus or train, or in the next office/cubicle, who woke that morning as their baby persona. They won't necessarily be the one you would expect. As ABs, we are very good at concealing our inner identity.

In my view, the baby/child persona is the only credible explanation of why an adult would want or enjoy – outside of sexual expression - infantile things such as nappies, a pacifier or baby clothes. It's not the adult that wants or enjoys these things. It's a subjectively real baby/child persona seeking comfort and security the same way a biological baby/child does.

People most associate the existence of sub-personalities or personas with Dissociative Identity Disorder (DID), formerly known as Multiple Personality Disorder (MPD). That is an association some ABs resist for fear of being linked to insanity. However, I believe that there is a **benign** parallel between being AB and DID. I understand genuine cases of DID are very rare. I have a relative in my extended family who has DID. It was our experience with them that prompted my wife and myself to consider that I may have a child persona and to seek a counsellor experienced in such matters.

A person with DID has multiple personas or 'parts'. In an unhealthy state, the parts are autonomous, acting separately. Unhealthy DID can be a debilitating condition where the person can wake up with gaps in their recent memory, because for those periods an autonomous personality was in control of their consciousness and actions. However, with therapy and self-management, the parts work cooperatively and there is a healthy sense of self. In the absence of dysfunction, the person has a *minority identity*, not a disorder.

I believe that ABs and people with DID are at different ends of the same continuum. Both have discrete personas or sub-personalities. For both, psychological health lies in accepting the existence of those personas, meeting their valid needs and having a cooperative relationship with the self. The differences are the extent of the autonomy of the personas in the unhealthy state, and the extent of the dissociation in the origin of the personas – in both cases high for DID and moderate for ABs.

The 'parts' of people with DID are commonly borne out of deep trauma or abuse where the personality 'splits' to find refuge from great fear or danger. There is a high degree of dissociation. That is where the painful memory of the trauma, and resulting persona, has been deeply suppressed to enable the self to function. It can take a long time, and a lot of therapeutic effort, for a person with DID to identify and accept their parts.

Dissociation is a continuum. It can range from benign, mild everyday examples such as daydreaming, all the way through to psychosis. For many ABs, I believe that there is a significant element of dissociation in the origin of their child persona. I think the persona commonly emerged within the psyche during a time of distress. For ABs, the distress does not commonly relate to abuse or neglect, but rather to the usual fears and frights of childhood, such as a temporary separation from the nurturing figure. As with DID the painful memory of that distress, and resulting persona (particularly the latter), has been repressed. It often takes a long time for an AB to identify and accept that they have a baby/child persona as the source of a lifetime of compulsive child-like behaviour.

Being a non-conflicted AB is a conscious recognition of a genuine need for nurturing by the Inner Child/baby persona. As with anyone, an unmet need for nurturing can be psychologically harmful. ABs show admirable courage in not turning away from the need for nurturing, despite the seemingly confronting way that need presents itself. When internal conflicts are resolved, self-acceptance allows self-nurturing, which in turn strengthens self-acceptance in a virtuous cycle. The original childhood wounds to the psyche are unmasked and healed.

Another parallel between DID and being AB is that the latter's child persona can be a different gender from the adult self. It is not uncommon for male ABs to have a female baby/child persona. In most cases, the male adult self and the baby/little girl persona happily coexist, each in their own space, there is no sexual dysphoria as for a transgender person. A further parallel is with a non-conflicted (male) cross-dresser with a female persona as a subjectively real healthy part of the psyche.

With this understanding of the identity, it has to be admitted that the term *'Adult Baby'* is not ideal, and even counter-productive. In AB, *baby* is the noun and *adult* is an adjective. This is misleading and unhelpful in that it suggests the primary identity is the baby or child. It suggests an indulgent or neurotic renunciation of adulthood. For non-conflicted ABs, this is the reverse of reality. As Michael Bent indicates, the adult self is the primary personality and the baby or child persona is a sub-personality *(see 'The Identity Conflicts of the Adult Baby' in the book 'Being an Adult Baby').* In preference to the term AB, Rosalie and Michael Bent use the term Adult Infantile Regression (AIR). I prefer to say that I am an adult with a child persona. That said the term AB is now so widely used that I doubt it is amenable to change. It is still important to be clear about the real nature of the identity. Given the issue with the term 'Adult Baby' I prefer to use the abbreviation AB.

While it might not be pathological, being an AB is regressive, surely? Maybe. The traditional view of child and personality development is a linear model. Everyone goes through the same sequential stages in childhood, in the same order. Personality disorders in adulthood are thought to be patterned on a personality structure that is normal at some stage of childhood. Adult dysfunction arises because the person has got stuck at that stage and returns to it in stress or crisis. This view originated with the non-empirically based theories of Freud and the first schools of psychoanalysis. It has been carried into psychology more generally. It lends itself to a view that there is a single, majority pattern of personality development and any departure from that is pathological, or at least suspect. When being gay was still considered a disorder, some psychiatrists and psychologists conceived of that identity as a pathological regression to some stage of infancy or childhood. We now consider such a view to be silly.

There is another view, advanced by John Bowlby, the creator of Attachment Theory. He posited a view that personality development isn't a single linear track. Instead, it is a multi-track phenomenon where we start out at a similar origin, but each point of interaction between the genetic inheritance, the emerging personality and the environment represents a possible branch of development. Bowlby states -

> *These two, alternative, models can be likened to two types of railroad system. The traditional model resembles a single main line on which are set a series of stations. At any one of them, we may imagine, a train can be halted, either temporarily or permanently; and the longer it halts the more prone it becomes to return to that station when it meets some difficulty further down the line.*

> *The alternative model represents a system that starts as a single main route that leaves a central metropolis in a certain direction but soon forks into a range of distinct routes. ... The further each route goes from the metropolis, however, the more branches it throws off and the greater degree of divergence of direction that can occur. Nevertheless, although many of these sub-branches do diverge further, and yet further, from the original direction, others may take a course convergent with the original ... In terms of this model the critical points are the junctions at which the lines fork ... [Separation: Anxiety and Anger. Attachment and Loss Volume 2]*

Bowlby's alternative model is one we would regard as being more consistent with a positive view of LGBTQ identities.

What if being an AB - that is the emergence of a baby/child persona in childhood - wasn't a regression per se, but a diverging branch of personality development?

In the same way that other minority, or LGBTQ identities are a diverging but healthy branch of personality development. It's only a speculation, but in the absence of empirical evidence either way, it is just as tenable as the single linear view. It certainly illustrates the pervasiveness of the latter view and how it prejudices our views of minority identities.

Numerically, ABs are a fairly small group. Rosalie Bent's guesstimate is that ABs are around 0.1% of the population, that is around one-in-a-thousand. Rosalie's guesstimate is likely to be as informed as any. That one-in-a-thousand number makes ABs a smaller population than transgender people, but of a similar magnitude. Transgender people, using a broad definition of that group, are estimated to be between 0.3% and 0.5% of the population (Wikipedia article 'Transgender').

ABs have probably existed for a long time. Prior to the internet and social media the vast majority would have lived their sense of self in secret, convinced that they were alone. That was my experience. My first experiences of having infantile needs and impulses began spontaneously, driven by my own psyche. It wasn't created by, or dependent upon, the internet or social media which didn't exist when I was an adolescent.

So, in essence, being an AB is no more threatening or confronting to the general public than a cross-dresser who identifies as having a persona of a different gender from their adult self. So why is public acceptance still lagging far behind that for crossdressers or LGBTQ people?

I believe that a key obstacle to public acceptance is that being AB is conflated with paedophilia – whether consciously, or unconsciously. AB related websites commonly carry prominent disclaimers distinguishing being AB from paedophilia and are vigilant in barring any content relating to biological minors, or the participation of biological minors on the website. ABs are genuinely concerned in their on-line posting or life stories to disavow any sexual interest in biological minors. Adult ABs are scrupulous in maintaining a rigid separation between the visible display of their baby/child personas and biological minors.

Yet I believe the conflation with paedophilia remains the 'elephant-in-the-room' when it comes to public acceptance. It was, and remains for me, my greatest fear in being known or 'outed' as AB. I suspect that is true for many other ABs. It doesn't help that being AB continues to be officially categorized as a paraphilia, a psychosexual disorder – a category which also includes paedophilia. It also doesn't help that males are far more visible as ABs than females. I understand from the work of Rosalie and Michael Bent that females are at least a significant minority of ABs. As women become more visible in the AB community, this will help lay the conflation with paedophilia to rest.

The fear of conflation with paedophilia does make it difficult for ABs like myself to disclose an innocent enjoyment of the wonder and innocence of happy, well-loved babies and young children. To see such tots and the way they light up at loving interactions with their parents is wonderful. It is a balm to my own childhood wounds and makes me feel hopeful for all of us. Being conscious of those wounds and the loss of trust and innocence they bring, I find any neglect or abuse of children abhorrent and utterly repugnant. I am sure any AB is the same. I fully support that our society has to be eternally vigilant to protect children against the scourge of paedophilia and sexual abuse. As ABs, we also need to remember that paedophiles will adopt any guise to further their evil purposes. As being AB becomes more readily accepted it will likely be more commonly used as a cover by paedophiles. From time to time, you see examples of paedophiles being outed and excluded from AB websites and social media.

The final word is that being AB is not paedophilia and conflating the two is a product of ignorance and prejudice. We need to remember being gay was once also conflated with paedophilia. It seems that any misunderstood identity becomes the target on which the fearful and ignorant can project their worst fears. Public understanding will eventually move beyond this.

It is a leap of the imagination for most non-ABs to understand what sharing your internal consciousness with a subjectively real baby or child is like. Yet that is the compelling, non-conforming sense of self which really defines being an AB and makes it a personal identity. On this basis, being AB has the same claim for recognition and respect as a healthy personal identity as any LGBTQ identity.

Rosalie and Michael Bent are the foremost public authorities on the Adult Baby identity. Rosalie is the wife of Michael, an Adult Baby. In 2012, Rosalie published the landmark book 'There's A Baby in My Bed' intended for the partners of adult babies. It was the first published work to seriously address adult babies as a personal identity, beyond a sexual fetish. It was updated in 2015 as 'There's Still A Baby in My Bed. Rosalie has also written a book for the parents of teenage adult babies. Michael has published a text 'Adult Babies: Psychology and Practices' and an anthology of insightful articles 'Being An Adult Baby'. Rosalie and Michael are the owners of the website abdiscovery.com.au which is dedicated to helping regressive adult babies understand themselves and fostering public understanding of the identity.

3 The Process of Identity Formation

We have established that being an AB is a personal identity. We can now apply an understanding of minority identity formation to ABs.

When I wrote an account of my life as an AB *('Living With Chrissie')* and it was published, I experienced a change in my sense of self that I can best describe as 'coming out'. I experienced this as a powerful and transformative process. The transition to full self-acceptance was relatively swift. However, it came after a prolonged period (decades) of internal conflict. 'Coming out' is evidently an internal process of struggle and acceptance – in my case a long and complex one.

'Coming out' is a term which originated with the transition that LGBTQ people make in perceiving themselves, and declaring to others, that they have a minority personal identity. My sexual orientation is heterosexual. Being AB is my sole experience of having a minority personal identity. After recognizing that, I was going through a process that was already understood by LGBTQ people, I looked around for writing that might help me better understand my own transition.

I found what I was looking for in the *Cass Theory of Lesbian and Gay Identity Formation* (referred to below as 'the Theory'). It is a theory of how people come to identify to themselves, and to others, as lesbian and gay. The Theory helps me to understand the process I was going through in fully accepting my identity as an AB.

In the sections below I outline the Cass Theory and, by way of example, apply it to my own life as an AB. I hope this may be helpful to other ABs, and to help non-ABs to better understand this identity.

The Cass Theory

The Theory was developed by Dr Vivienne Cass, an Australian clinical psychologist and lesbian. It was first set out in 1979 and subsequently developed in a 1985 PhD thesis and sequence of academic papers in the 1990s. It is applicable to the AB identity. Dr Cass states –

> *"In addition to its application to lesbian and gay identity, I also view my theory as being relevant to the formation of <u>any</u> minority identity that is given negative value by the wider community. On occasions, it has been adapted and applied to identities such as 'bisexual', 'woman' and 'transgender'."* [A Quick Guide to the Cass Theory of Lesbian and Gay Identity Formation]

The Theory is a compelling guide to the experience of 'coming out', reflecting its original purpose to help those struggling with the process. It is also nuanced and flexible, reflecting the author's background as a clinical psychologist, steeped in academic theory.

The essence of the Theory is that people who contemplate that they may have a minority personal identity go through a series of cognitive stages.

The Theory divides the formation of a minority identity into six sequential stages -

1. **Confusion**
2. **Comparison**
3. **Tolerance**
4. **Acceptance**
5. **Pride**
6. **Synthesis**

The identity formation process is powered by drives towards –

- self-consistency, where individuals seek to create and maintain a unified sense of self and avoid cognitive dissonance

- self-esteem, where individuals seek to develop positive feelings about themselves, and avoid negative ones

Stimuli, within the self and externally, can trigger these drives and prompt cognitive changes which propel the individual to move to another stage.

Each of the identity formation stages are discussed in a separate chapter below. I have paraphrased and interpreted Dr Cass' stage descriptions to make them generic to minority identities, rather than specifically refer to gay or lesbian people. This has also been done with an eye on how the stages apply to ABs. I have simplified Dr Cass' nuanced description of the multiple pathways through each stage to refer only to the outcomes of each of stage. I encourage those with an interest to refer to Dr Cass' original formulations (see the references section). (See also Ruth Fassinger's paper in the references for a summary of models of minority identity formation, and her own model of lesbian identity formation.)

Dr Cass cautions that *'the stages are simply markers in a process of identity formation'* and not to assume that *'people in each stage are identical in terms of behaviour or identity'*. Her writings suggest that there are likely to be significant differences between people's experiences and perspectives at the early, middle or later part of each stage.

The Theory takes account of the fact that a person may reject or accept the minority identity; that they may halt their identity formation and that they may traverse stages via different paths depending on their own perceptions and environmental factors.

Dr Cass uses the term 'foreclosure' to refer to the situation where a person halts their identity formation at an earlier stage, rather than progressing all the way to the final stage. Such a halt may be for an extended period of time or forever. It may represent that the person feels they have gone as far as they need to live with some kind of stability. With the objective and non-judgmental perspective of a counsellor, Dr Cass takes the view that no stage is better than another. I take a different view.

I foreclosed or halted my identity formation in an early stage for nearly three decades. In my case, it was a state of conflicted stasis because I was too fearful and unaware to move forward. I aspire, for myself, and for other ABs, to reach the final stage of identity formation. In my view, it is a better stage to reach than the others. It combines the benefits of self-acceptance, an integrated sense of self, and a broader inclusive view of the world and identity.

A key part of the Theory is the interaction between –

- the individual's perception of themselves

- their understanding of the minority identity in question, drawing on public information and understanding about that identity.

This means that the identity formation process will change as the availability and nature of public information on identity changes and grows. This is helpful in differentiating the experiences of older ABs who grew up prior to the internet/social media age, and those of the post-internet/social media generations.

In the LGBTQ community, an essential feature of 'coming out' and the culmination of identity formation is public disclosure of a person's minority identity. This is reflected in the Cass Theory of identity formation for lesbian and gay people. In this book, in the context of being AB, I am largely concerned with coming out **to self** and possibly, a life partner. Thus, 'coming out' means fully accepting the AB identity as real, permanent and healthy, and integrating that acceptance with the rest of the self. It does not preclude disclosure to a broader circle of people or to the public. However, my re-interpretation for ABs of the stages of identity formation of the Cass Theory does not require such broader disclosure.

Many LGBTQ people and some ABs consider that you haven't come out unless you have disclosed your identity in public. ABs with this perspective might consider that the approach of focusing on 'coming out **to self**' represents moral cowardice. I don't. I discuss this further in the final chapter on the way forward for the AB identity.

To illustrate the relevance and insights of the Theory to the AB identity, I apply the stages of identity formation to my life history. I am of the older pre-internet/social media generation. I was born at the beginning of the 1960s and first experienced thoughts and behaviours related to my AB identity when I was ten or eleven years old. I came out to myself and my wife, fully accepting my identity as real, permanent and healthy in my mid-fifties, in 2018. I have disclosed my identity only to my wife. My life as an AB can be found in the book 'Living with Chrissie'.

I also refer to five others whose life stories as ABs have been published in recent years. All are male. (I know there are female ABs but I don't know of any published life stories by female ABs). When their stories were published two were aged in their fifties, one in his forties, one in his thirties and one in his twenties. I don't cite these others by name (real or pseudonym) as it would be presumptuous and possibly offensive to offer comment on another identified AB's life history without their knowledge and consent. The life stories did not specifically refer to identity formation and stages. For each AB it is possible to identity the timing, duration and experiences of only a few out of the six possible stages. Never-the-less, it is still valuable to recognize the large variation in how the identity of ABs develops. There are key differences on three dimensions –

- older generations who grew up before the internet/social media age and younger generations

- those with accepting family and those not

- those who have disclosed to a broad circle of family and friends, and those who have not

4 First Stage - Identity Confusion - 'Could I be?'

The process of identity formation starts when a person experiences thoughts or behaviours which might indicate they may have a minority identity. This is typically at odds with their existing view of themselves. This leads to a questioning of self. This stage is associated with emotional states such as curiosity and bewilderment, or confusion, turmoil and panic.

The central experience of this stage is coping with the confusion about self.

There are three possible outcomes from this stage –

a. the prospect of the minority identity is viewed positively, and the person moves to stage 2 with a positive outlook

b. the prospect of the minority identity is viewed negatively, but the person is unable to successfully reject the thoughts or behaviours and moves to stage 2 with a negative outlook

c. the person successfully rejects the prospect of a minority identity, either confirming their prior view of self, or incorporating some of the thoughts or behaviours into their conforming self-image.

My Experience

For me, this stage commenced when I rediscovered nappies aged ten or eleven. I used to sneak flannelette sheets from the linen cupboard and safety pins from my mother's sewing cupboard and pin nappies on myself in the privacy of my bedroom. Stage 1 lasted until the end of my teens.

My experience conformed to category (b) above. I was unable to suppress my desire for nappies and babying fantasies and was deeply conflicted, ashamed and bewildered. My fantasies and behaviour was against everything I was supposed to be, and wanted to be – a responsible and mature grown-up boy, a credit to myself and my family. I was petrified by the fear that anyone would find out. I couldn't understand it and I'm not sure I tried (that came much later). I think I just locked it up inside me, something that could never be shared or known to anyone. I had no inkling of having a baby persona.

My key experiences of this stage included -

- The makeshift nappies felt wonderful - thick soft cloth swaddling my most sensitive parts - the soft bulk between my thighs – instant, reliable comfort and safety. I could only dream of proper towelling nappies and plastic pants, but how I longed for them.

- I can't remember if I masturbated in my nappies from the outset. I was certainly doing so by my early teens. It was always accompanied by fantasies of being babied by a loving strong mother figure (never my mother). The babying would always include being put in nappies. Sometimes I would just have these wonderful non-sexual daydreams of being babied by a warm-hearted loving woman, perhaps against my will.

- I got busted once, by my sister. It was in the latter years of high school. I had blocked the door to my bedroom with a chair, supposedly to reach some upper shelves. I was wearing a thick nappy made from a flannelette sheet. My sister pushed the door open and caught sight of me before I flung myself at the door and closed it. I think I made an implausible excuse about preparing for a fancy-dress party or a play at school. I felt like I wanted to die. The shame and embarrassment were biting and scourging. Strangely, nothing ever came of it. Looking back, I'm sure my sister dobbed me in to my parents and they adopted my family's customary coping strategy of 'ignore it and it will go away'.

Others' Experience

Of the other five ABs, all had covertly rediscovered nappies by no older than age ten or eleven. For some, this was much earlier, even as young as four or five years of age. For most, this involved purloining the nappies of younger siblings. Across the different generations there is a common experience at the onset of these behaviours – all were acting on strong impulses they didn't understand and acting covertly, conscious of breaking with parental expectations (this origin story also seems to be common to the four case studies cited by Rhonda Lipscomb in her insightful 2014 PhD dissertation, *'The Clinical Mental Health Experience of Persons with Paraphilic Infantilism and Autonepiophilia'*.) Most believed they were 'sprung' by their parents at one time or another and nothing came of it. At first, none were aware that others existed who shared the same need for, or satisfaction from, this covert behaviour. Only one was conscious of having a baby persona.

5 Second Stage - Identity Comparison - 'Maybe this is me'

In the second stage, the person contemplates that they may have a minority identity.

They also consider the implications of that identity, including negative implications such as estrangement from family and friends. They search for an explanation for themselves. There are feelings of isolation and estrangement. There may be a sense of loss of the certainties about self and the future life course. In the context of ABs, it needs to be recognized that for this stage to commence, the person needs to know that the identity exists, that there are others with whom they share these motivations and desires. The dearth of such information, particularly for ABs who grew to adulthood pre-internet/social media seems to be a significant factor in slowing the identity formation process compared to LGBTQ people.

The central experience of this stage are feelings of difference and alienation.

A person's experience of this stage can differ greatly. There are five possible outcomes –

a. the prospect of the minority identity is viewed positively, and the person moves to Stage 3 with a positive outlook

b. the person partially recognizes that they have a minority identity – they rationalize their thoughts/behaviour to make them more acceptable – typically rationalizing 'this is a temporary thing' (I'll grow out of it) or there were special circumstances

c. the prospect of the minority identity is viewed negatively, and the person seeks to minimize or lessen their personal responsibility for the non-conforming behaviour

d. the prospect of the minority identity is viewed negatively, but the person is unable to successfully reject the thoughts or behaviours and lives with strong internal conflict, possibly extending to 'extreme self-hatred that may lead to suicide or self-harm'

e. the person is successful in rejecting the minority identity

My Experience

For me this stage commenced at the end of my teens when I first became aware that there were other ABs. I discovered this through amateur fetish magazines bought in sex shops. In a reference library, I also tracked down an old academic book or article on 'infantilism' ('Patterns of Psychosexual Infantilism' by Wilhelm Steckel, dated

1952). Based on these slender and dismal sources I learned that I might be perverted or mad, but at least I wasn't alone.

Stage 2 lasted for nearly three decades until I was in my later forties! During that time I graduated from university, benefitted from a wonderful supportive marriage, and had a fulfilling career in the public sector. My experience was a mix of categories (b) and (d) above. Into my mid-twenties I hoped, somehow, that I would outgrow this weird obsession. I expected getting married would 'cure' me. I was wrong on both counts. I continued to be 'stuck', living with my baby 'thing', largely as a conflicted sexual fetish. It concealed from myself, and from my wife, the real understanding of my identity as an AB. It was a vicious cycle. The internal conflict drove a compulsive fetish. In turn, the fetish fed the internal conflict and self-loathing, which pushed genuine self-acceptance further away. Despite year after year of compulsive behaviour at odds with my adult self, I had no idea that I had a baby persona. I didn't know what a healthy, stable personal identity as an AB felt like, or how to get there.

Understandably, my wife reacted to my behaviour as to a harmful addiction or fetish that needed to be contained, rather than a healthy personal identity that could be safely embraced. Later, she told me that during these years she had no idea about most of my life as an AB. I was a lot more successful than I realized in keeping secret my motivations, behaviour and the contents of my collection of clothes. With hindsight, I see that I gave my wife no basis to know or understand that being an AB was an important part of my identity. For example she didn't know until much later that my baby collection included dresses, bibs, bonnets, dummies, and so on, which might have given a clue that it was something more than a nappy fetish.

There are cruel paradoxes in the conflicted stages of the AB identity. One of them is that the conflicted AB finds it less confronting to think of their 'thing' as sexual, rather than as a discrete persona. Yet the former identification is an obstacle to the understanding and acceptance of others of the AB's real nature. As a conflicted AB, I was not aware of the extent of my mis-channelled anger, secrecy, and mood swings. These can be very difficult for the AB's partner and family.

My deep internal conflict was clear in the repeated cycle of bingeing and purging. This is common to ABs. The term comes from the disease bulimia where the sufferer gorges on food and then, in deep self-disgust and loathing, makes themselves sick until they purge their stomachs empty. For ABs it means something different. The cycle starts with a 'binge' - buying a stash of nappies and baby clothes. This often comes after a period of suppressing our baby 'side'. The nappy fetish becomes stronger, accompanied by frequent masturbation. Pleasure is now fighting shame. The emotional 'let down' after each successive orgasm becomes more painful and demoralizing. Eventually, the growing internal conflict drives masturbation to a peak. The emotional 'let down' after the final peak orgasm is intensely painful. The disgust, remorse and self-loathing are scourging.

The only thing that will assuage the intense emotional pain is to 'purge'. We convince ourselves that we can now completely banish our baby 'thing'. This often means throwing away all our baby collection. Only then would the painful remorse occasioned by the binge be soothed. It would be replaced by a new transient kind of 'high' – a sense of being cleansed of our weakness and perversity and free to live a normal life. I would declare that I was giving up my 'nappy thing' forever. I meant it when I said it. I would pray for God to give me the strength to maintain my abstinence.

The aftermath of the purge would last a while. In my case my abstinence, at least in terms of physically wearing nappies, would last some months, sometimes nearly a year. I would masturbate without nappies for a time, but the comforting fantasies of being babied were always present. Eventually, the unmet needs of my baby persona would grow more and more insistent and I would 'binge' again. With each new binge I would fool myself that, this time, I could keep my baby 'side' under sufficient control so that things wouldn't get out of hand and I wouldn't be driven to purge again. Of course, that was a 'fool's hope'. The internal conflict hadn't gone away or being healed - it was just re-booted.

Another feature of my experience which is common to deeply conflicted ABs denying their identity is susceptibility to 'triggers' which could, at a moment's notice, prompt a compelling desire to wear a nappy. For years, I couldn't walk down the babies' aisle in a supermarket without 'triggering' the insistent need to get home and put on a nappy. This behaviour was in strong contrast to who I was otherwise – a person of strong emotional control, able to defer gratification.

Others' Experience

There is a big variation in the trajectory of the other five ABs. Two had supportive families and traversed this stage quickly, in their early teens. The supportive family environment was the key factor rather than their age or generation, with one being in his fifties and the other in his twenties. The other three did not have accepting family environments. They appear to have taken extended periods (likely a decade or two) well into adulthood to traverse this stage, likely living with a high level of internal conflict and turmoil in the interim.

6 Third Stage - Identity Tolerance – 'I can live with this'

In the third stage, the person acknowledges that they probably have a minority identity.

This acknowledgement is strongly coloured by recognition that the identity is viewed negatively by many. This is tolerance rather than full self-acceptance. Ambivalence, doubt and inner conflict are still present. The person is learning to manage incongruency between different aspects of self. The person is likely to reach out to others with the same identity, and perhaps to selectively disclose to others. The nature and quality, positive or negative, of those contacts is key to the person's trajectory and experience of this stage.

The central experience of this stage is the need to reach out to manage alienation.

There are three possible outcomes from this stage -

a.   the person's out-reach is positive, leading to a positive view of self as having the minority identity

b.   the person's out-reach has a negative outcome and they adopt a negative, conflicted view of themselves as having the minority identity

c.   the person's out-reach is negative and they are successful in rejecting the minority identity.

My Experience

For me, the third stage started in 2009 when I recognized reluctantly that my baby 'thing' would always be there. I stopped the binge and purge cycle and started a permanent collection of baby clothes. I was in my later forties. This shift came after a mid-life crisis several years before that had opened the door to a less driven and conflicted personality.

My experience conformed to category (a) above. What changed the previously negative trajectory of my AB life was buying the book *"There's A Baby In My Bed: Learning to Live Happily With the Adult Baby in Your Relationship"* by Rosalie Bent. It was a revelation and a Godsend! It was 2013 and I was aged in my early fifties.

For the first time, I could recognize myself in the book's honest and compassionate description of an Adult Baby! It was the first time I learned there was more to this identity than a sexual fetish. On two occasions over the next couple of years, I exchanged emails with Rosalie and her husband Michael. Their advice was compassionate and 'right on the money'. I was communicating with real, balanced, intelligent people who knew and lived this identity! After years of being stuck thinking of myself as an addict and my baby side as a fetish, my sense of self was starting to change for the better.

My key experiences of this stage included -

- I amassed a large collection of baby clothes of every style from onesies to bonnets to tights. I let myself buy baby dresses and even frilly nappy covers. But only in blue for a baby boy. Pink baby clothes and especially dresses had a guilty fascination for me, but I would never let myself buy any. Being an Adult Baby boy was as far as I could go at the time. Identifying as a baby girl was a step too far. It raised scary questions. Would it mean that I was a cross-dresser - that I really didn't want to be a male - that I wanted to be transgender?

- I was a bit more open to myself and my wife about my baby 'side'. Eventually, I took over the wardrobe in a spare bedroom for my growing collection of baby clothes. My wife didn't agree with me wearing my baby clothes in front of her, so unless she was out, I only dressed as a baby in the spare bedroom. Several nights each week I would sleep all or part of the night in the spare bedroom dressed in a nappy, plastic pants and baby clothes. It was a wonderful new freedom. My baby side was here to stay, but it was still, literally, in the closet

- Even though I had got Rosalie Bent's book, I still wasn't sure how to think about my baby 'side'. Despite my history of compulsive behaviours at odds with my adult-self, I wasn't ready to accept that my baby side was a distinct persona within my psyche. I didn't want to think I was crazy.

- Even though I had given up purging baby clothes I was still strongly conflicted. One form of this was that I now had mini-binges and purges of buying and then deleting digital copies of erotic Adult Baby fiction. I recognized the cycle for what it was, but still got caught up in it. I had a guilty fascination with stories of submission and 'sissification' where men and boys were forcibly dressed and treated as baby girls and came to love it. It fueled the same compulsive masturbation and shameful remorse as nappies had originally done.

- I felt ashamed about the masochistic fantasies. In retrospect, I realized they were a part of my internal conflict about my identity. They were psychologically unsafe, sacrificing emotional comfort and safety for sexual excitement. In hindsight, I know I was unconsciously punishing myself for having genuine emotional needs for nurturing in the first place. The coercion element of the fantasies was an indication that I hadn't fully accepted my baby persona and Adult Baby identity. At this stage, I needed the coercion element to pretend to myself that I had to be forced to comply with and enjoy the infantile need to be loved and protected by a parent figure.

Others' Experiences

Of the other ABs, two aged in their forties or older appear to have reached this stage in midlife after spending a lengthy conflicted period in the previous stage. The two older ABs do not seem to have disclosed their real identity beyond their partners. The two ABs aged in their twenties or thirties reached this stage much earlier, in their previous decade of life. The two younger AB's disclosed selectively, but to a wider group of people. Arguably, the longer period a person has lived with their formative AB identity in secret, the more difficult it is to disclose publicly and disrupt established adult relationships and life course. Traversing this stage no later than young adulthood more readily creates an option of disclosing and incorporating being AB into the forming adult identity, relationships and life course.

7 Fourth Stage - Identity Acceptance - 'I will be okay'

Arguably this is the pivotal stage in identity formation. The difference in perspective between this stage and the stages before is a watershed. At the beginning of Stage 4, the person has come to understand themselves as having a minority identity. The inner sense of the identity strengthens through this stage and the remaining stages of identity formation. There is likely to be more contact with others who share the identity and more disclosure of the identity to others. As a result of these processes, the person values their minority identity more highly, leading to a belief that it is just as good as a conforming identity. The sense of oppression or alienation from belonging to an out-group is reduced and tolerance changes to acceptance. There is a developing stable sense of self.

The central experience of this stage is coming to terms with the newly accepted identity.

There are two possible outcomes from this stage -

a. with continued positive interactions, both with those with the identity and others, there may be a sense of peace and fulfilment, and self-acceptance may be combined with a belief that the minority identity is a private matter

b. a negative reaction or the inadequate public understanding of the minority identity is felt strongly, heightening a sense of alienation and the person moves to Stage 5

My Experience

For me, this stage began when I went to a counsellor in 2015 and identified and accepted that I had a baby girl persona. It was a transformative experience. The stage culminated in 2018 when I wrote an account of my life as an Adult Baby at the invitation of Michael Bent. Writing it down made it 'real'. It was the first time I had been fully honest with myself about the ups and the downs of my life as an AB. The tipping point was writing about the future and contemplating a prospect, at the end of my life, of having to go into aged care as an Adult Baby – someone who needed to go to bed wearing a nappy and cuddling soft toys to sleep well. It was the deepest acceptance of a fundamental and permanent part of my identity. I could declare that I am an Adult Baby – an adult man with a baby girl persona.

My identity formation continued on its new positive trajectory. It largely conformed to category (a). I had a sense of freedom about my AB identity, and a sense of peace and fulfilment that I had never experienced before.

For the first time in my life as an AB, the tormenting internal conflict and struggle was gone! It felt like the outbreak of peace after a long war. I found I liked myself a lot more. I felt better about the world – it now seemed like a kinder place with more possibilities than risks.

For a few years, I was content to live with this new sense as an exclusively private matter. But with the freedom of retirement, the new compelling experience of self that I knew was not understood by the world-at-large propelled me to Stage 5.

For me, stage 4 was all about coming to know and love my baby persona. I named her Chrissie. To me she is a delightful, demanding, loving toddler. I wanted to make up for decades when my adult-self despised the as-yet-unnamed and unrecognized Chrissie and tried to bully and scourge her into silence and compliance. Sure, she could be a real 'little miss', at her worst a selfish brat. But she's also a shy, easily scared, innocent, loving, affectionate, warm-hearted, fun-loving little girl who melts my heart.

Contrary to what I feared, having a baby persona didn't feel crazy to me. It felt a bit strange at first, but quickly became the new normal. I now believe Chrissie has been there nearly all my life. She sprang from my distress at a temporary separation from my mother when I was aged three or four. Chrissie is still 'me'. But she's sufficiently distinct from my adult-self that it feels right for her to have her own name. She has different feelings and needs from my adult-self. Ultimately, Chrissie's infantile feelings and needs are also my feelings and needs – something my adult-self denied for a long time.

Chrissie is always with me, separately processing whatever is going on. Most of the time, when I'm my adult-self, she's in the background and I'm not consciously aware of her. Especially at work or other determinedly-adult spaces, I just 'get on with it'. Sometimes after especially stressful times I'll 'de-brief' with Chrissie to calm or comfort her. For example, dentists scare me. When I had to go for a particularly scary procedure, I imagined myself beforehand picking up Chrissie and comforting her. It worked. Both Chrissie and my adult-self were less fearful. Understanding when Chrissie is scared or needy, and being able to comfort her, has been a great help in managing my anxiety.

For the first time, Chrissie could be the proper baby-in-nappies she always wanted to be. Chrissie felt like an authentic baby with a wet nappy each morning, if she wanted. Best of all, this freedom to wear and wet a nappy doesn't feel sexual. Once I accepted Chrissie the dam broke when it came to pink baby girl clothes. Chrissie LOVES PINK! I think everything I've brought since is pink or mainly pink.

I brought Chrissie a soft clown doll and a large pink and white fluffy rabbit. She named them 'Dolly' and 'Bunny' and loves them dearly. She sleeps with them cuddled up either side each night, and even when she naps in the day. The wonderful comfort and security they provide has to be felt to be understood. Any little child would understand instantly. Likewise, the soothing comfort of a dummy.

With some caution, my wife agreed to let me wear my baby clothes around the house in front of her, under my dressing gown. It felt really great to be out of the closet. Later my wife accepted Chrissie wearing a nappy and baby clothes openly around the house. Despite Chrissie's big wardrobe of clothes, sometimes the nicest feeling is just to wander around in only a short baby pink T-shirt and a nappy and plastic pants – the freedom! The accepting gaze of my wife is more validating than the largest wardrobe. It feels like a deep acceptance of Chrissie as a real baby girl, a real part of me.

My wife feels safer, less afraid and irritated with my Adult Baby identity. Best of all, she gradually started to interact with Chrissie. She sometimes buys small toys for her. Even better, my wife will refer to Chrissie directly, asking 'how's Chrissie or 'what's Chrissie think of that?' Each and every time I feel a thrill. My wife has a great sense of humour. It spans a dry wit to laughing uproariously at physical comedy. For many years, understandably, my baby side wasn't a laughing matter for her (or me). One of the nicest and most healing things is that we now share a laugh *about* Chrissie, and my wife can share a laugh *with* Chrissie. And without the shame and the fear, there's a lot to laugh about.

My wife says she doesn't want to be Chrissie's mother. I know she is never going to change Chrissie's nappy or feed Chrissie a bottle. I've made my peace with that. It doesn't mean she doesn't love Chrissie or my adult-self deeply. She does. But some things would feel too wrong for her. She said it would be better if she was Chrissie's aunt. My wife had a wonderful relationship with her much-beloved aunt who taught her to have fun and enjoy being a girl, so it's a wonderful example.

My acceptance of Chrissie led to powerful cognitive and behavioural changes.

Astonishingly, my compulsive behaviour has disappeared. I no longer feel 'driven' by desires and impulses that I can't control. My compulsive masturbation has fallen away, and so has the heightened sexual excitement. After living with this demoralizing tyranny for so many years, it's wonderful to be free of it. Don't get me wrong - every so often is fine and good, but only so. It's proof, that for me, it's about identity, not fetish. The regularity of wearing a wet nappy has made it normal – a reliable source of security and comfort – it is no longer something edgy and exciting, just 'nice', just 'right'. My 'baby time' is now so 'every day' that I'm not thinking of a new dress, but instead, more nappies to rotate through the wash, and a nappy bucket, so I'm not washing every day.

Psychologically unsafe fantasies no longer hold any guilty fascination for me. I like fantasies or daydreams of being supervised and gently, but firmly disciplined by 'mummy', but I don't feel ashamed about that. For me, that's safe and fun. Masochistic fantasies just doesn't have any appeal anymore.

Accepting Chrissie has changed me in other, unexpected ways that have no direct relationship to being an Adult Baby.

- A lot, indeed most, of my anger disappeared. I experienced that difference on a daily basis. Only with hindsight can I see how much anger was generated by the conflict about my denied identity. I now understand that a great deal of mischannelled anger is one of the hallmarks of the conflicted stages of identity formation. I didn't see it in myself before.

- It influenced my faith for the better. Before I tended to over-think my faith. Chrissie has brought a more child-like character to it. I now find it easier to trust in the love of God.

- It unchained a great amount of creativity. For me that's writing (hence this book). It's like tapping into a formerly hidden, clear, fast-flowing stream within my psyche. It makes life fresh and hopeful.

- I identify more strongly with women and the movement for genuine equality for women and the freedom for all from sexual harassment and abuse. I identify more with LGBTQ people and their struggle for acceptance. Don't get me wrong – I'm not claiming that having a baby girl alter means I'm female or transgender or that I have walked in the shoes of women or transgender people. But accepting Chrissie has let me step aside from exclusively identifying with being a man and made it easier for me to be less defensive about the need for men to change.

I no longer seek or believe in 'a cure' that will see Chrissie disappear as a persona or sub-personality. That doesn't work for me. It's the equivalent of telling a gay man, 'it'll be okay, one day you'll meet the right girl'. A definition of psychological health that doesn't recognize my baby girl persona as having real feelings and needs, isn't me. It feels too close to the silent unremitting pressures of my upbringing to grow up quickly, be a mature responsible adult and leave childish things behind. I internalized that approach and it suppressed real feelings and needs to the detriment of my wellbeing.

Others' Experiences

Happily, all of the other ABs reached a point where they fully accepted their identity. All were concerned to seek some kind of peace with the experiences in childhood and adolescence that formed or expressed their identity. All seem now to openly share their identity with at least their accepting partners. Three had disclosed their identity to other family and received some level of acceptance in so doing. Of these three, only one AB was fully 'out' with their identity declared or known to a wider group.

Two, with supportive family environments, seem to have reached the stage of self-acceptance no later than their early twenties. The other three, who lacked such environments, attained full self-acceptance in middle life, ranging from their early thirties into their mid-forties. Three explicitly embraced having a baby persona, and of these two had baby girl personas.

8 Fifth Stage - Identity Pride - 'I've got to let people know who I am'

At Stage 5 the person is aware of the difference between their own complete acceptance of themselves and the rejection of this self by the society in which they live. They recognize that the desire to fully express their identity is made extremely difficult. The distinctive character of their minority identity is highly esteemed and contrasted adversely with those who are not empathetic or supportive of the identity (or are perceived not to be so). They may adopt an 'us and them' attitude. They become immersed in the identity sub-culture and experience a strong sense of group solidarity and pride. This leads them to confront issues such as perceived misunderstanding and discrimination.

The central experience of this stage is empowering pride and anger.

There are two possible outcomes from this stage -

a. those who receive consistently negative responses to their expressions of identity, and strengthen their immersion in the identity subculture

b. for those who receive significant or consistent positive responses to their expressions of identity, the division between 'us and them' cannot be easily upheld and the person moves to Stage 6.

My Experience

For me, this stage commenced in 2018 with the publication of my account of my life as an Adult Baby ('Living With Chrissie'). I was fortunate to subsequently have three more AB related books published by AB Discovery and Michael Bent that year. Writing these books and seeing them prepared for publication animated a powerful feeling of pride in my newly accepted identity. It also reflected an equally powerful need to let the world know who I am as an AB.

I feel proud of the courage and resilience it takes to come to terms with this identity. This pride is reflected in words from 'Living with Chrissie' -

> *Writing this account has been a powerful experience. It has let me see things with more clarity and less angst. I feel a bit naked having disclosed so much, counter to a lifetime's habit of secrecy. It is the first time I have fully 'come out' to myself and my wife and wholly accepted that I am a regressive Adult Baby. My baby girl persona Chrissie will always be a part of me. I like that.*

It will be nice to go forward without the dead weight of shame and secrecy, and to travel with a lighter spirit.

I am very conscious of the public ignorance and misunderstanding of the identity I now proudly acknowledge. Wanting to make some contribution to supporting ABs and to contribute to public education continues to motivate me to write.

I feel a strong sense of identification with ABs who are struggling with, or have acknowledged, the existence of a baby persona as a fundamental part of their psyche. They feel like 'my tribe'. I struggle to feel as empathetic towards other parts of the ABDL community, notably those for whom nappies are exclusively a sexual fetish. They feel a bit like a rival tribe. I'm not advocating this somewhat narrow or defensive 'tribal' identification – just citing it as conforming to the experience of being in this stage of identity formation. Hopefully, I will move to a broader identification in progressing to the next stage in the formation of my AB identity.

The powerful sense of wanting to be known for who I am as an AB, and my 'tribal' identification within the ABDL community, is also reflected in the final chapter of 'Living with Chrissie' -

I'm longing to be known and accepted for all of me, for the fellowship of intelligent and balanced people with alters like my Chrissie and those who love them. It's something I will look into. My initial look suggests that the on-line ABDL (Adult Baby / Diaper Lover) community is very broad and fractious. Those who approach nappies/diapers from a fetish perspective come from a different place from those with baby alters (Rosalie Bent calls the latter *regressive adult babies*). As you will know from reading my story, the fetish approach is not a comfortable or safe space for me. I don't begrudge people who come from the fetish side the same need for acceptance and fellowship but it's not my space. It seems that caution is a good idea.

At the time of writing this book, I feel myself to still be in this stage, yet to move to Stage 6.

Others' Experiences

As publication of one's life story as an AB is a fairly sure sign of the identity pride stage, I believe that all five ABs progressed from self-acceptance to this later stage of identity formation. In all their accounts, there is a sense of pride in having attained self-acceptance after navigating challenging life experiences, including isolation, self-doubt and inner turmoil. For all, there is a wish in communicating their experiences to help others with the journey to self-acceptance. All take issue in their own way with public ignorance and prejudice that makes this journey more difficult than it might otherwise be. This implies a positive identification with other ABs, consistent with this stage. One AB from a supportive family background reached this stage in his later twenties. For the others, this took until middle life, from the thirties, forties and fifties.

9 Sixth Stage - Identity Synthesis – 'I belong to the world'

When the person experiences their minority identity as being understood by at least some people with conforming identities the mutually exclusive alignment of esteemed and not esteemed between the two groups is rejected. Anger and alienation are reduced which strengthens self-esteem. The minority identity becomes integrated into the larger sense of self. The person is freed from the need to focus so much attention on managing their minority identity.

The central experience of this stage is a sense of belonging to the world at large.

There are two possible outcomes from this stage -

a.   the person maintains the integrated sense of self and its place in the world

b.   in response to adverse interactions or circumstances, the person again focuses on their minority identity and might adopt previous strategies such as non-disclosure of identity or limiting contact with some others.

Dr Cass herself seems to exemplify the broader post-tribal identification of this stage. Her writings suggest an over-arching commitment to the insight and benefits of her profession of psychology. She applies these insights objectively to the process of identity formation for both her own and other minority identities.

My Experiences

At the time of writing, I don't feel I have yet moved to this final stage of identity formation. I have only recently moved to stage 5 and the pride in my identity and 'tribal' identification of that stage is still a fresh and compelling experience. For the future, I aspire to the more integrated sense of self and the broader identification with anyone with an accepting heart associated with stage 6. The following words from a recently published article are an example of this aspiration -

> *In understanding ourselves as regressive adult babies, we are trying to understand what makes us different from others. It is important to remember that in fundamental ways we are the same as everyone else. All of us have a need for nurturing through our lives. We all suffer if those needs are not met, either as children or as adults. All children have comfort / transitional objects. These commonly continue in different forms into adulthood. For example, for smokers, cigarettes are commonly a transitional object. Many people other than adult babies have regressive*

impulses, and act on these, in both functional and dysfunctional ways. Everybody can be thought of as having an internal dialogue between their Inner Parent, Inner Child and Adult self. Many, many people have a conflict between these internal actors, and for some of these that conflict drives compulsive behaviours. We all have a true self and a false self. Many people struggle with self-acceptance. As regressive adult babies, we are so different from others, yet in other very important ways we are the same. Sometimes, it is not so different to be different.

Others' Experiences

It is difficult to establish if the other ABs have reached this final stage of identity formation. Most remarked on the importance of the other, non-AB parts of their personal identities. Arguably, for most, feeling unable to declare the identity beyond partners or immediate family, makes it more difficult to move beyond a compartmentalized sense of self to an integrated personal identity. More difficult, but hopefully not impossible.

10 The Intra-psychic Dimension of AB Identity Formation

The Cass Theory is couched exclusively in cognitive terms – that is the identity formation process is propelled by the interaction between changes in how people ***think*** about themselves and how they ***think*** about their minority identity. In turn, those cognitive changes are based on the drives to increase the self-esteem and congruency between the person's thinking about the self and their minority identity.

This description of the cognitive process does not differentiate between actors within a person's psyche. I believe it is essential to understand the process of identity formation in terms of the dialogue and conflict between the different parts of the psyche. This intra-psychic perspective is particularly important to understanding the conflicts in stage 2 and 3 of identity formation, and the resolution of those conflicts and self-acceptance in stage 4.

This intra-psychic dimension to self-acceptance and identity formation is discussed in my book *'Becoming Me'*. The book introduces this dimension as follows -

> *Internal conflict occurs when one part of our psyche is fighting with another part. It is a battle within, and against, ourselves.*

> *The idea of a conflict or dialogue within our psyche is a key feature of psychotherapy. For the purposes of understanding the internal conflicts of a regressive Adult Baby, this book uses the concept of a dialogue between our Inner Parent, Inner Adult and Inner Child. For those with an interest in psychology or psychotherapy this approach borrows the terms Parent, Adult and Child from Transactional Analysis but employs these to represent a dialogue within the psyche in the manner of the super-ego, ego and id of psychoanalysis. I find the concept of an Inner Parent, Adult and Child a simple and powerful way of understanding myself, and hope others will find it useful.*

Stage 2 – Identity Comparison – is the most challenging stage of identity formation because of the inner conflict. Dr Cass's description of the stage indicates that, for some, the experience of this stage can amount to 'extreme self-hatred that may lead to suicide or self-harm'.

Stage 2 represents the height of the conflict between the Inner Parent and the wounded Inner Child/baby persona. The Inner Parent denies the existence of the baby persona, trying to keep the latter locked 'in the closet'. The baby persona is fearful and desperate for recognition and nurturing. Faced with denial by the other parts of the psyche, the baby persona is angry, mistrusting and greedy. Episodically, they 'break out'. This typically manifests in compulsive masturbation wearing nappies to bondage-style fantasies. In response, the punitive Inner Parent brutally chastises and punishes the Inner Child so that the latter ends up cowering back in the closet. The raging Inner Parent also berates the adult self for the latter's weakness and lack of self-control in giving in to what the Inner Parent characterizes as an affliction, an addiction or a fetish (or all three). The adult self is weak and ineffective, unable to stop the brutal and damaging conflict between the Inner Parent and baby persona. In Stage 2 the height of this conflict manifests in 'binge and purge' cycles.

At Stage 2, this conflict largely plays out in the unconscious. The compulsive behaviours, shame and self-loathing of this stage are like the tips of icebergs, visible above the water, while the greater part of the conflict plays out, unseen beneath the surface.

The concept of 'polarisation' from Internal Family Systems (IFS) therapy is relevant and helpful to understanding the conflicted AB of Stage 2. IFS posits that everyone, including ABs, has multiple inner personas ('parts' in IFS terminology). Conflict or trauma produces a state of polarization within the psyche. In that state, parts take opposing or competing positions in the mistaken belief that this is necessary to protect the self. Each part reacts iteratively to the other, taking increasingly extreme positions. For ABs at Stage 2 of identity formation, the stronger the denial of the existence and needs of the baby persona, the more compulsive the behaviours driven by those needs. This accurately fits the extremes of the AB's binge and purge cycle (remembering that IFS was created by Richard Schwartz after working with bulimic clients).

At Stage 3, the strong and sometimes tormenting conflict of Stage 2 decreases. But this does not represent self-acceptance. It has the character of a 'ceasefire' or armistice between the opposed Inner Parent and baby persona, rather than genuine reconciliation and peace. In my case, this cease-fire was initially more the reluctant product of exhaustion. I was tired of beating myself up. I wanted a different way. That was my adult self (the self as leader of the parts in IFS) starting to grow stronger. Allowing a permanent collection of baby clothes was a signal to my baby persona that it was at least recognized, if not accepted. But from time to time, the cease-fire would still break down and my baby persona and Inner Parent would go back to opposing positions. But all of this was still playing out mostly in my unconscious. I did not recognize or understand my internal conflict.

For me, Stage 4 was about consciously accepting my baby persona as real, permanent and healthy. The conflict was resolved. My baby persona and my Inner Parent each found a recognized and accepted place in my psyche. That could only happen because my adult-self had strengthened to the point where it wasn't overwhelmed by the desperation of my baby persona and the fear of my Inner Parent. But it wasn't until Stage 5 that I consciously recognized and understood my inner conflict and dialogue. That recognition only happened with the benefit of self-acceptance and hindsight.

It would have been very helpful if, at Stage 2 or 3, I could have accessed information or counselling that allowed me to understand and resolve the conflict between the different actors of my psyche. Maybe it wouldn't have taken me thirty years to traverse the conflicts of Stage 2.

For readers seeking more information on the intra-psychic dimension of identity formation for ABs see: *'Becoming Me'*

11 Identity Not Paraphilia

Defining being AB as a personal identity overturns conventional psychological and psychiatric opinion which holds that being an AB is a paraphilia, a psychosexual disorder. This is how it is defined in the Diagnostic and Statistical Manual of Mental Disorders (the DSM), the standard diagnostic tool published by the American Psychiatric Association (APA).

At the level of popular understanding, things are improving, but on-the-whole, the public are more still likely to see being AB as a sexual fetish than a healthy personal identity. The growth in public knowledge about ABs at least means that the risk of it being conflated with paedophilia is reduced. However, greater knowledge is not synonymous with understanding or acceptance. It is noteworthy that Wikipedia still redirects a search for 'Adult Baby' to an article titled 'paraphilic infantilism'.

Even empathic health professionals like Rhonda Lipscomb and Thomas Speaker have an unwitting bias, in that they start from the unexamined assumption that being AB is primarily a form of sexual expression.

They are enlightened in seeking a non-pathological understanding of paraphilias, but they still essentially view being AB as a paraphilia. (In Rhonda Lipscomb's case this is not surprising, her insightful PhD dissertation was submitted to the American Academy of Clinical Sexologists.)

Defining being an AB as primarily a sexual behaviour or expression is wrong.

Defining being an AB as a psychosexual disorder is both wrong and offensive.

Here's why.

Not Primarily Sexual Behaviour or Expression

Dr Cass' first instruction to those counselling people with a minority identity is 'distinguish between sexual behaviour and identity'. It is the counsel of wisdom and experience. We need to heed it.

To date, it has been almost universally understood that being AB is fundamentally a sexual fetish. The public thinks so. Health professionals think so. Many ABs think so.

It's easy to understand why. Being AB invariably involves a nappy fetish. Compulsive masturbation using nappies is a universal experience at some point in AB's lives. Internal conflicts, emotional pain and psychological impairment are universally attached to this compulsive sexual fetish. These resulting states are also the starting point of the interest and perspective of health professionals.

However, we now understand that compulsive and conflicted behaviour, including sexual behaviour, is a feature of the conflicted early stages of the formation of minority identities. The vast majority of ABs have internalized at least some of the negative views about our identity. Arguably, at any one time most are in the conflicted stages of identity formation.

As a result, there has been little thought that the fetish is only the symptom of a deeper, and indeed positive phenomena, a personal identity. You don't look for what you can't imagine.

But once you remove the blinkers it's staring us in the face.

Many ABs recall that their first experiences with wearing nappies was before puberty and was linked to non-sexual emotional comfort. With puberty, nappies universally become sexual fetish objects. But even after puberty, ABs commonly indicate that they sometimes also derived non-sexual emotional comfort and security from their nappies and baby fantasies. This applies even to those in the conflicted early stages of identity formation. And as ABs progress to the less conflicted stages of their identity, the sexual fetish becomes less prominent. Conversely, the experience of non-sexual emotional comfort and security increases and comes to predominate. It is associated with a wider range of baby objects than those which are exclusively fetish objects.

Why does a non-sexual experience with nappies and baby things provide comfort and security? That isn't explained if being an AB is principally a matter of sexual behaviour.

Those experiences provide comfort and security because they touch an alternate sense of self. Specifically, a baby or child persona. But how does that work?

Nappies are a fetish object. But they were first, and more importantly remain, a transitional object (also called a comfort object). Transitional objects are a widely accepted concept in child psychology. The concept was developed in 1951 by the renowned psychotherapist and paediatrician Donald Winnicott. Transitional objects can be almost anything – but are typically a soft toy or security blanket – which are invested with special significance in the 'magical' thinking of a very young child. A transitional object 'stands in for' a very young child's nurturing figure. It becomes a psychological substitute for her when she isn't there. A baby creates transitional objects out of everyday things when they become aware of their separateness from the nurturing figure, and can experience a sense of loss when she isn't present. This generally occurs when the child is between 4 and 12 months of age.

I believe that the baby persona of ABs seeks comfort and security, nurturing, by using transitional / comfort objects. These transitional objects always include the AB's nappy, but may include many other forms – pacifiers, dolls etc. The baby/child persona seeks comfort and security through the same psychological mechanism, that a biological baby or young child uses. For me, this is further proof that the baby/child persona is subjectively real. In a most instinctual way they act like a biological baby/child.

So, yes, being an AB does involve a sexual fetish for nappies. But that doesn't explain the broader or deeper experience of being an AB. Because being AB is fundamentally about the non-conforming sense of self that comes from having a baby/child persona as part of the psyche. It is not surprising that such a compelling and pervasive sense of self will shape and colour sexual expression. But the identity is the fundamental feature and the sexual expression a derived or associated trait.

Not a Psychosexual Disorder

We can now move onto to consider why being an AB is not a pathological psychosexual disorder.

The Oxford Textbook of Psychotherapy (editors Glen Gabbard, Judith Beck & Jeremy Holmes) states -

> *Paraphilias are psychosexual disorders in which the individual experiences recurrent, intense sexual fantasies or urges to engage in unusual or unacceptable sexual behavior. To qualify as a psychiatric disorder according to the diagnostic criteria of DSM-IV-TR (Diagnostic and statistical manual of mental disorders, 4th edn), the behaviours, sexual urges, or fantasies must 'cause clinically significant distress or impairment in social, occupational, or other*

important areas of functioning' (American Psychiatric Association, 2000, p566). ... The most commonly diagnosed paraphilias listed in alphabetic order in DSM-IV-TR are : exhibitionism, fetishism, frotteurism, pedophilia, sexual masochism, sexual sadism, transvestic fetishism, and voyeurism.

The textbook was first published in 2005 and references the 2000 edition (DSM-IV-TR) of the DSM. This was superseded in 2013 by the DSM-5. However, the latter still defines being an AB as a paraphilia.

Adult babies – adults with a subjectively real child persona - are lumped together under the same broad category as flashers, gropers, paedophiles and peeping toms! Those perversions are coercive disorders in which the person forces themselves on non-consenting others. (I believe that, partly, it was Rosalie Bent's concern and outrage at adult babies being labelled as a psychosexual disorder, that caused her to write her landmark book 'There's A Baby In My Bed' in 2012.)

It is clear from the capricious changes across the successive editions of the DSM that the classification of being AB as a psychosexual disorder is based on ignorance and prejudice. Rhonda Lipscomb's description of the dismal history of the DSM on this matter makes it clear that the classification as a psychosexual disorder does not have a sound base in empirical evidence or a rigorous view of the human psyche. *(See her 2014 PhD dissertation in the references – the dissertation is available free, on-line.)*

It is instructive to know that being homosexual was also previously classed as a mental disorder. It was not removed from the DSM until 1974 (and not fully excised until 1980). Before that, being gay was also pathologised in inaccurate and offensive terms without any evidential basis. Aversive conditioning techniques were part of the treatment options for homosexuality. Being gay was removed from the DSM after a campaign by gay activists and medical professionals. That campaign is described by Dr Cass in a 2006 article -

'Political protests were also organized in the form of interruptions to conferences where proponents of the pathology model were speaking, and to strident demands that homosexuals be invited to participate in panel discussions on homosexuality. Leaflets railed against 'psychiatric propaganda'. Psychology and medical courses that used unfavourable reference material were picketed until they adopted gay-affirmative material. Therapists who advocated homosexuality as a sickness were boycotted.' [Sexual orientation and the place of psychology: side-lined, side-tracked or should that be side-swiped?' in the Gay and lesbian issues and psychology review Vol 2(1), 25-37]

I cite this to indicate that being gay wasn't removed from being classified as a disorder, and from the DSM, simply because the medical and psychology professions had a change of heart.

It is common for ABs experiencing a high level of internal conflict related to their denied identity to have compulsive sexual behaviours. This includes masturbating whilst wearing a nappy and having masochistic bondage-style fantasies about being coerced or humiliated by a parent like/substitute figure. It also includes compulsively seeking on-line erotic material related to these themes. On the surface, this would seem to fit the definition of a paraphilia. The distress and turmoil driven by the internal conflict about the denied identity might also seem to qualify being AB as a psychiatric disorder.

This is no more valid or accurate than identifying a person with a high level of internal conflict over being lesbian or gay as having a paraphilia (sexual) or psychiatric disorder. I liken the sexual fantasies and behaviour of conflicted ABs to the compulsive, furtive, emotionally empty sex in gay 'beats' that were linked to gay men in the days before there was broader social acceptance for being gay. When the world at large is ready to say you're perverted, some of that gets internalized as self-loathing. It seems to me that in both instances, compulsive sexual conduct is a product of internal conflict, specifically the denial of a fundamental part of your personal identity. It is a transitory release of the pressure of a deep internal conflict and shame.

As has been discussed, when the internal conflict is positively resolved and the identity accepted the compulsive behaviours, and the psychologically unsafe fantasies of the conflicted AB disappear. What remains is a stable, healthy personal identity. The adult self is fully functional and the child persona gives access to child-like wonder, security and contentment. Sexual expression continues to be defined by a nappy fetish but it is not associated with compulsive masturbation, nor does it cause distress. A sexual fetish for nappies is not the greater part of the healthy AB identity.

Being a non-conflicted AB is not inherently sexual in character. Nor does it drive compulsive behaviour, or cause distress or impairment. The definition of paraphilia is not valid.

12 Counselling Case Study - AB as a Paraphilia

Equipped with an understanding that being AB is a minority personal identity it is instructive (and confronting) to see what happens when, instead, it is treated as a psychosexual disorder.

This example is drawn from the 'Oxford Textbook of Psychotherapy' referred to previously. It is a mainstream text published by Oxford University Press. As at November 2018 on amazon.co.uk the publisher's 'blurb' states the following –

With the publication of this book psychotherapy finally arrives at the mainstream of mental health practice. This volume is an essential companion for every practising psychiatrist, clinical psychologist, psychotherapy counsellor, mental health nurse, psychotherapist, and mental health practitioner. … The first of its kind, this is a 'must-have' volume for all trainee and practising psychological therapists, whatever their background - psychiatry, psychology, social work, or nursing.

The textbook was first published in 2005 and from the above still appears to be current. Following the DSM, it categorises being an AB as a paraphilia. Helpfully, the chapter introduction includes the following caution for therapists –

Human sexuality is diverse and complicated. Practitioners must always remember that many individuals with unusual sexual fantasies, interests, or practices do not experience significant distress or impairment, and must be careful not to pathologize the diversity of human sexuality.

Unfortunately, the case study of a person we would recognize as an AB does demonstrate how this identity **is** pathologized. It also illustrates how the subsequent treatment based on this pathologized understanding is likely to have caused significant harm.

The case study is introduced as follows -

Case example: relapse prevention

Tom was a 32-year-old attorney whose marriage had recently been jeopardized by his wife, Joan, after finding several inexplicable changes to their credit cards totalling $480. She confronted him with the bills. At first, he said that there must be some mistake and that someone must be using his credit card number. But his wife persisted and eventually Tom admitted that he had been visiting the website 'babe-in-arms.com' and also a local massage parlour for the past 6 months and using them for sexual gratification. It did not help that during these 6 months Joan was caring for their newborn daughter, their first child. Tears flowed from both.

Upon his wife's insistence, but with agreement from him in order to save the marriage, Tom began both individual and group therapy. ... Tom admitted that he longed to be treated like a baby by his sexual partners and had in fact visited massage parlours that catered to this desire. He found it very arousing to imagine being cleaned and diapered by a woman. His experience in vivo was limited to being in diapers: being verbally scolded for soiling them, and engaging in noncoital cuddling. Apparently, the scene of his wife changing the diapers of his daughter brought back sexual fantasies that had long lay dormant. The admission of this paraphilic arousal pattern was very embarrassing to Tom, but he also admitted relief that his secret was now shared with others who he had found on the internet. The group responded with support, and to the best of their abilities, understanding.

My first response, as I am sure is the reader's, is deep compassion for Tom, his wife and his baby daughter. This is an awful situation for all three. The birth and care of a child is not a good time to deal with the deep and confronting personal and marital issues associated with being 'outed' as an AB. This is particularly so with a partner who evidently had no prior knowledge of this deep-seated and long-standing identity.

It is almost certain that Tom is an Adult Baby – in the deeply conflicted stage 2 of identity formation as per the Cass Theory. He is living a double life. On the one hand, he is establishing his career in a private law firm – a notoriously competitive environment. He is likely to be concerned to be the employee and person that he is expected to be. Yet, inside he is driven by a deep need to experience being cared for and nurtured as a baby; a need he clearly doesn't understand and is deeply ashamed of. When he presents for therapy that need is a compulsion. It is so great he is willing to put his marriage and likely his career at risk.

The case study refers to his fantasies as long dormant. What we know, and the textbook doesn't, is that these fantasies and the needs which drive them are likely to have been present since childhood and persistent through his life ever since. Dormant? I suspect, in a climate of judgement and effectively 'shaming', Tom may not have volunteered the persistent and ongoing presence of his fantasies. I further suspect, given the risk of his visits to the massage parlour being discovered from his credit card statement, that Tom was at the peak of a binge and purge cycle which is a feature of stage 2, specifically the binge part. He would have been caught in gut-wrenching internal conflict with a maelstrom of self-loathing, shame and remorse. Very likely that conflict would include a self-sabotaging impulse to be punished for his need for nurturing, and having acted on it, as well as a positive cry for help and recognition of that need.

Tom's behaviour and distress seemingly meet the diagnostic criteria of the DSM for a paraphilia in that 'the behaviours, sexual urges, or fantasies must cause clinically significant distress or impairment in social, occupational, or other important areas of functioning'. The unwitting therapist would have been satisfied that Tom's case was a fetishistic paraphilia.

Based on the subsequent treatment plan the therapist evidently identified three grounds for therapy –

1) Tom's compulsive behaviours – he does not have control over his impulses and actions and at the peak of his compulsion is behaving like an addict seeking 'a fix'

2) Tom's infidelity to his wife in visiting massage parlours, and the issues for his marriage related to his behaviours and his need for nurturing

3) the obstacles that Tom's distress poses for him being the father his baby daughter needs, and that he wants to be for her.

Each of these are grounds that validly merit therapy.

So let us see how therapy progressed. The case study continued -

The methods used in both Tom's individual and group therapies were cognitive-behavioural. Especially helpful was his recognition of the envy he felt at the attention his wife gave to their newborn. He replaced thoughts of sibling envy with the correct thought that this was his daughter and she was entirely dependent upon him. Behaviourally, he countered this envy by helping his wife care for their daughter. What Tom was surprised to learn was that the more he cared for his daughter, including changing her diapers, the more he felt love for his daughter and a grateful love from his wife for sharing the child-care.

With treatment and the threat of divorce, the behaviours of utilizing the website and going to the massage parlours ceased immediately. After 9 months of treatment, even the infantilism fantasies had decreased in frequency and intensity. For 6 months he had not masturbated to the thought of his being cared for like a baby. Tom considered his problem a sexual addiction, and in addition to therapy, attended group meetings of Sex and Love Addicts Anonymous (SLAA). He felt when therapy was concluded, he could continue to attend the 12 step group for the support and program it gave to his 'sobriety'.

Based on an understanding that Tom is a conflicted AB we can see that the therapy included a mix of good and negative elements – unfortunately mostly the latter.

The positive and appropriate components of the therapy include –

a) Tom disclosing his envy of his daughter and becoming more engaged, alongside his wife, in the care and nurturing of his daughter

b) him ceasing visit to massage parlours (which would have fueled his internal conflict about being an Adult Baby).

By contrast, the harmful features of the therapy are fundamental. They include –

i. identifying Tom's issues exclusively as a sexual addiction, an exclusively negative trait – thus precluding a therapeutic exploration of its source or the possibility of disclosing a positive personal identity beneath the internal conflict and compulsive behaviours;

ii. failure to address Tom's deep need for nurturing and any healing of the wounded inner child desperate for that nurturing

iii. failure to address the savage and harmful internal conflict associated with a conflicted stage of identity formation

iv. failing to heed that Tom had made positive contact on-line, likely with people in the ABDL community – and this may have provided a resource for the therapist and Tom to navigate a positive path of identity formation

v. basing a long-term solution solely on maintaining abstinence in a manner akin to a drug addict - essentially the solution is based on, and relies on a denial of, any ongoing needs for nurturing or a positive personal identity as an Adult Baby.

The failure to recognize Tom's need for nurturing is incomprehensible and reprehensible. He is desperately acting in the most obvious fashion on a deep-seated need to be nurtured and this forms no part of the therapeutic diagnosis or treatment! Tom was diagnosed as having a sexual fetish, ignoring the glaring fact that the culmination of this 'sexual fetish' is described as 'non-coital cuddling' with a mother-substitute!

The case study illustrates the need for care regarding a malign alliance between an unwitting therapist and the conflicted AB's punitive Inner Parent. The latter is seeking to punish and exile the AB's wounded Inner Child – locked away 'out of sight and out of mind'. An AB in crisis or distress will be desperate for help, likely deeply shamed and remorseful, with their punitive Inner Parent in the ascendant.

The treatment program largely reflects the worst errors and gaps in the therapeutic approach. The case study continues -

Tom recognized that it was important for him to establish a relapse prevention program (RPP) to employ for the post-therapy future. ... This is the RPP that Tom and his therapist developed:

1. Identify risk states before sexually acting out: negative emotions, like being ignored by my wife; being criticized by partners or clients at work; feeling ineffective or lonely; being bored. Feeling that I deserve a reward and to be cared for.

(a) What I can do instead: use the ... Daily Mood Log and Cognitive Distortions Checklist. Do something positive and fun for myself – rent a DVD, buy a CD, take my wife out to dinner; get more involved in caring for and playing with my daughter. Don't be a PIG (problem of immediate gratification)!

2. Recognise Seemingly Unimportant Decisions (SUDS) that place in high-risk situations: carrying extra cash beyond what I would need; driving by areas where there are massage parlours; leaving work early for 'unaccounted for' time; being in a private area at home with the computer.

(a) What I can do instead: never carry more than 15 dollars. Do not carry an ATM card; carry only one credit card, which wife pays the bill for each month. Post picture of wife and child in prominent place on car dashboard. Work out map alternative routes so that never have to drive by high-risk areas. Call wife before leaving to establish time record if feeling tempted to drive by risky areas. Look at relapse prevention card (carry in wallet). Move the computer to a room into which privacy is not given and face the screen toward the entrance door of the room.

3. Avoid lapse in thoughts or behaviour: thinking about past experiences with massage parlour women or images and chats on the internet. Masturbating. Driving near areas where massage parlours are located. Reading the ads for sexual services in the newspaper.

(a) What can I do instead: talk to SLAA sponsor, attend extra meetings. Call therapist to discuss. Substitute a positive activity such as a regular exercise program.

4. Relapse: surf on the internet for sexual sites. Go to massage parlour.

(a) What I can do: remember that this is not the end of the world. I can be sober. Don't give up hope!! Go to SLAA meetings and therapy sessions.

This treatment approach contains significant harmful elements, including -

i. It is based on the denial of the underlying needs for nurturing (renting a DVD or buying a CD is not a substitute for nurturing).

ii. The behavioural management techniques – in terms of cash, credit cards and citing of the computer - deepen Tom's mistrust of himself (exacerbating a negative feature of his conflicted and denied identity). By giving Tom's wife oversight of his behaviour it also creates a co-dependency which will have a corrosive longer-term effect on the marital relationship.

iii. An apparent proscription on masturbation which is unsustainable (to be fair, this may not be the intention of the abbreviated reference in the treatment plan).

Given the deficits of the therapy, Tom is likely still very much a conflicted AB. This is because the therapy has done nothing to address the savage internal conflict of a denied personal identity. In light of this, there are significant doubts regarding the prognosis. The case study concludes –

Two years following treatment, Tom continues to employ the RPP that he developed. He and his wife were in marital therapy for six months, which helped to clarify the expectations each had of the other in areas such as domestic chores, sex and affection, and leisure activities together. He had one 'relapse' within the first 3 months of ending therapy in which he went into a massage parlour. He immediately felt guilty and remorseful and left without having sexual contact. Tom called his SLAA sponsor and reported the incident. They agreed he would increase the frequency of meetings to three times a week. Tom also had a consultation with his therapist. The therapist helped Tom to recognize how he had allowed risk states and SUDS to creep back into his life. They agreed that he would return every six months for a 'check-up' consultation.

Tom relapsed relatively quickly and is principally 'protected' from further relapsing by shame and remorse. Many ABs will recognize that Tom is still caught up in the binge and purge cycle and its' savage internal conflict. These cycles can have long intervals, especially after the deep shaming and fear of detriment which occasioned Tom's entry to treatment. It is very unlikely that Tom would have been able to sustain the unreasonable objective of abstinence which cruelly set him and his family, up to fail.

In the textbook, it is noteworthy that the section immediately after the case study is titled 'Behavioural modification' and includes treatment options for paraphilias generally, including aversive therapy with electric shocks or nauseating ammonia odour. This is followed by a section titled 'Biological treatment' including drugs to reduce the sex drive and psychotropic medications. This highlights mainstream psychology's pathological view of being AB.

Thanks to the historic struggles and victories of the gay and lesbian community we now understand personal identity. We know that it can't be 'cured' away by psychology, therapy or religious faith. It can be denied – at great cost to a person's wellbeing – but it can't be wished away. If a person presents to a therapist in crisis or distress related to their LGBTQ personal identity we now understand that the therapeutic issue is the crisis or distress and how to positively resolve it – not to deny or change the underlying personal identity.

Once we accept that being an AB is a personal identity then Tom's treatment program can be seen as very similar to 'gay conversion therapy'. That is, it is based on denying the minority personal identity, not because it is intrinsically harmful or unhealthy, but because it is seen as unacceptable to society at large. We now understand that gay conversion therapy is professionally unethical, causes great harm and doesn't work.

Therapy for a conflicted AB needs to be based on the fact that it is a personal identity – a healthy identity if the internal conflict is resolved – and not a fetishistic paraphilia. This applies even if the client presents in crisis or distress.

We need to revisit the case study to consider how Tom's therapy might have proceeded if the therapist had recognized that Tom had a personal identity as an AB. Key features of a positive approach include –

1. being open to the prospect that Tom's distress relates, not to an intrinsic deficit in his psyche, but to the internal conflict about his denied identity, the behaviours it drives and the prospect of rejection by others

2. identifying and addressing Tom's internal conflict and its' internal actors, starting with his shame and remorse and obvious need for nurturing

3. being open to finding and addressing the wounded Inner Child behind the obvious need for nurturing

4. exploring with Tom a model for a healthy, sustainable personal identity as an AB – recognizing that he will, initially, have no notion of what this might look or feel like; and

5. addressing the issues for Tom's parenting of his daughter and his marriage, of self-acceptance of a healthy, sustainable identity as an AB.

To enable effective therapy there needs to be an alliance between the therapist and the AB's adult self (the self of IFS), the custodian of the self-acceptance of the AB's personal identity and broader personal and social responsibilities including as a father and a husband.

There is a fundamental difference in the effectiveness of counselling based on the two views of being an AB. The actual counselling, based on the view that it is a psychosexual disorder, left Tom believing his psyche was pathological. He would have to live with his pathology and attempt to control it for the rest of his life. In essence it left him believing himself irrevocably perverse and broken. He is not able to fully trust himself, and must depend on his wife to monitor and control his behavior. That sets up a co-dependency which will damage his marriage over the longer term. His real need for nurturing which prompted his compulsive 'binge' behavior was not acknowledged, bottling that pain up inside him and closing the door on the prospect of healing. He must spend the rest of his life denying a real and important of himself. The outcome is very similar to using 'gay conversion therapy' to try and convince a person with an LGBTQ identity that they cannot ever be themselves.

By contrast, counselling based on a view that being an AB is a personal identity would have identified the internal conflict that tormented Tom and drove his compulsive behaviours. It would have recognized that his obvious need for nurturing was real and lead to an identification of the wounded inner child. That would open the door to the healing of the buried emotions linked to that wounded child. All of this would have opened the door to Tom accepting that he had a minority personal identity, which is capable of being psychologically healthy and sustainable – that he is not irrevocably broken and perverse.

Even positive counselling is not a panacea. The prognosis for Tom's marriage would still have been uncertain at best. The shock for Tom's wife of discovering her husband's deep-seated and longstanding identity at a time when she is caring for their newly arrived, firstborn child would be very difficult to overcome. Even with the best counselling, Tom's wife would be faced with accepting that her partner, and the father of her child, had a minority heterosexual personal identity. She couldn't be blamed if she couldn't accept that. But if she could, it would open the door to healing the wounds to her marriage caused by Tom's internal conflict and compulsive behaviours.

13 Benefits of the Theory – Individuals

Understanding the process of minority identity formation helps our understanding of ABs at both the level of the individual and the AB community. The following chapter outlines the benefits at the individual level.

The troubling thoughts, feelings and conflicts ABs' experience in relation to their non-conforming sense of self can be understood as belonging to the process of their identity formation. That process follows stages and pathways which are very similar to those for LGBTQ people.

I believe that this offers important reassurance and strength to ABs. Those same troubling thoughts, feelings and conflicts are way-stations to a healthy, stable personal identity if we have the courage to face them. There are times we may be conflicted but we are not perverted or crazy. The healthy identity that is our destination is as deserving of recognition and respect as the other minority identities – both our own respect and that of others.

More concretely, a knowledge that we are engaged in a process of forming our identity can help ABs navigate that process with less doubt, pain and delay. Accepting that you have a minority identity is often going to be challenging, but having an idea of what is involved at each stage is certainly an advantage. Honest self-reflection, and perhaps the compassionate and honest feedback of a partner, friend or counsellor, will assist in using a knowledge of the stages of the identity formation process to help navigate the process.

Counselling

In contrast to the uninformed and harmful example of the previous case study, the Cass Theory of Identity Formation supports an empathic and genuinely therapeutic approach to counselling ABs, and particularly conflicted ABs.

Dr Cass intended her Theory would assist counsellors to -

- customize counselling by better identifying where the individual is located in the process of identity formation

- recognize people who have foreclosed their identity formation at a particular stage and may be having difficulty with that resolution.

Dr Cass developed eleven guidelines for counselling using the Theory. I cite the seven that seem most relevant to ABs, below -

a. *Distinguish between sexual behaviour and identity*
In the context of the AB identity this injunction is especially important given that for the first three stages of identity formation it is common for compulsive fetish behaviour to mask the real nature of the AB identity, the existence of a subjectively real baby or child persona. Seeking what lies behind sexual behavior, especially compulsive sexual behavior, is key to a genuinely therapeutic approach to counselling ABs.

b. *Focus on the specific issues of the stage in which individuals present.*
It is sound in any counselling context not to get ahead of the client. For a conflicted AB in stage 2 or 3 it may be helpful to introduce the notion of dialogue and conflict between actors within the psyche (Inner Child, Inner Parent). However, as has been discussed, the idea of sharing consciousness with a subjectively real baby/child persona may be very confronting. Exploring this prospect too soon, such as early in Stage 2, is likely to be traumatic for the client and counter-productive. It may be that a client might only be able to countenance such a concept if they have already reached Stage 3.

Richard Schwartz states a similar caution regarding the introduction of such concepts in Internal Family Systems (IFS) Therapy. He states –

> *"It is not a good idea for a therapist to open the door to the inner world [of subjectively real personas] with a highly polarized [conflicted] client, especially for the purpose of releasing exiles [the IFS term for personas such as the AB's baby/child persona], if the therapist cannot stay with the client at least long enough to help him or her integrate those exiles. I have the same reluctance to expose exiles when a client's external environment is dangerous or intractable, or when a client is in a position in his or her family or job that allows little room for vulnerability."*

c. *Do not assume people in each stage are identical in terms of behaviour and identity.*

d. *Remember the stages are simply markers in a process of identity formation and clients' experiences may represent the early, middle or later part of the process occurring at any stage.*

e. *Recognize that identity formation occurs within the context of other processes and issues taking place in an individual's life, and that any of these may interact with the development of identity.*
Points (c) to (e) are a reminder that in a counselling context the Theory is a therapeutic aid, not a road map. The counsellor's use of the theory should not constrain or obscure the exploration of the client's experiences, and unique experience of self.

f. *Recognize the importance of appropriately timed and positive contacts with others, of the same identity, and those with other minority identities or conforming identities.*
It is particularly important that ABs in the earlier stages of identity formation have access to information about what a non-conflicted, healthy identity looks and most importantly, feels, like. Direct contact with ABs in this space is very important. Counsellors need to be able to refer those ABs at an appropriate stage of identity formation and the counselling process to such contacts.

g. *Do not judge any stage as better than other stages, or any individual as better than any other based on their stage of identity formation.*
In a counselling context, such an empathic and non-judgmental approach is sound and ethical.

h. *Accept clients as being in the stage they describe themselves to be, not where it is thought they should be.*
Dr Cass is concerned not to infringe upon, or harm, a client's sense of self. In her writing she also argues to

accept at face value a client's view that their minority identity is biologically determined. This is notwithstanding that her own view as a clinical psychologist is more nuanced and contemplates that identity is a product of the interaction between biology, self and public notions of identity. This is a complex ethical matter. I can see the therapeutic wisdom in working from where the client 'is at'.

The bottom line is that anyone counselling an AB, especially a conflicted AB in the early stages of identity formation, needs to understand that they are relating to someone who has, or may have, a minority personal identity. At a minimum, the counsellor needs to observe the honoured injunction for medical professionals – 'do no harm'.

There are hopeful signs that some health professionals see the need for a constructive understanding of ABs. In her well informed PhD dissertation Rhonda Lipscomb states -

Just as the attitudes about treatment approaches for gay, lesbian and bisexual individuals have changed dramatically in the past 40 years with the changing cultural attitudes, it is time for the mental health profession to catch up with AB/DL community attitudes.

14 Benefits of the Theory – Understanding the AB Community

Understanding the process of minority identity formation can also help the understanding of ABs as a group and a community.

Online Forums

In the process of coming out to myself, I started to look at online forums for ABs. I had mixed impressions. In the positive, there were genuine, much needed public meeting spaces where people sought and shared information. Some participants responded with kindness and the benefit of their experience to the requests of others. In the negative, there seemed to be a preoccupation with the surface dimension of being an AB to the exclusion of a deeper understanding of the identity, sometimes with acrimonious and defensive posts. To me, the on-line AB community looks like a mixed bag.

Understanding the different needs and perspectives of people at the six different stages of identity formation helps understand some of the dynamics and pitfalls of the on-line AB community. ABs from the different stages of identity formation are interacting simultaneously in the same forums. Some of the different needs and perspectives in play are outlined below –

- people at Stage 1 – they are very likely just observing forums without interacting.

- people at Stage 2 and 3 – some will be actively seeking information in the process of determining whether they identify as an AB. Others will be conflicted ABs, some struggling with the tormenting binge and purge cycle, some with mis-channelled anger. Many will be strongly invested in the fetish dimension.

- people at Stage 4 – they may be more likely to observe or interact less frequently. When they interact, their contributions are more likely to be constructive and honest.

- people at Stage 5 – they are in a position to be well informed about being AB, but are also driven to publicly claim their identity and hold strong opinions. Some will be 'keepers of the faith', seeking an exclusive sense of community with those that share their own specific sense of self. From this source comes 'identity politics, with its negative elements of 'us and them' and prickly defensiveness.

- people at Stage 6 – perhaps like those at Stage 4, being less driven, they are more likely to observe, and to interact selectively. When they do interact, these are likely to be the 'elder statespersons' and mentors of the community with empathy for the perspectives and experiences of those in the preceding stages.

A significant level of miscommunication is likely in any forums where people from different stages of identity formation are interacting simultaneously. The stages of identity formation represent a cognitive sequence, each stage building on the experiences and perspectives of the one before. Empathy and awareness of another's perspective will tend to flow in one direction – from those at the later stages of identity formation towards those in the previous stages. It won't work so well in the other direction.

You have to experience a stage to fully comprehend the perspective it brings.

In particular, there is a great difference in perspective between fully accepting yourself in mid to late-stage 4, compared to the perspectives of the previous stage. For example, if you're in Stage 3 and heavily invested in the fetish side, you may not have much interest in a deeper understanding of the identity.

It is likely that active participants in on-line forums will be disproportionately those from Stage 3 and Stage 5. They are particularly driven to reach out to others and participate. This may be associated with some of the negative features of on-line AB forums – a focus on the surface dimension and fetish side of being AB (Stage 3), hostility (conflicted Stage 3 and prideful Stage 5), and the defensive 'gatekeeping' of a diffusely understood identity (Stage 5).

It seems to me that the key unmet need in on-line AB forums is for those at stages 1 to 3 to find information on what a healthy stable AB identity looks and feels like, and how to move from a conflicted stage to full self-acceptance. Hopefully, in the future, this is a need that people in the latter stages of identity formation, especially those in Stage 6, will be able to meet.

Other Contexts

A knowledge of the different stages of identity formation is also useful in better understanding and interpreting case studies and surveys of ABs. The perspectives, behaviours and experiences of people with a minority identity will be differentiated, in significant part, by their stage of identity formation. Knowing, or being able to surmise, the stage of a person in a case study helps to interpret the lessons and conclusions of the study. This was demonstrated in the case study of Tom the lawyer, husband, father and conflicted AB in the previous chapter. It is likely that many ABs identified in clinical case studies are people in the conflicted Stage 2 and 3 of identity formation. Those people are not representative of the healthy self-accepting AB identity.

Similarly, an uncritical use of surveys will not produce an accurate understanding of the AB identity. Survey populations will be disparate – they are likely to include those who are validly categorized as fetishists, as well as ABs from most stages of identity formation, including those from the conflicted stages. This would be equivalent to seeking to understand the gay personal identity from an uncritical use of surveys which included bisexual people, gay people who are 'out', gay people 'in the closet', and those who engage in sex with same-gender partners but who reject identifying as gay. As with most surveys of complex matters, surveys of ABDLs need to be analysed using explanatory models which segment the population across the key differentiating variables. These variables should include the stage of identity formation, or proxies for those stages.

15 The Way Forward for the AB Identity

Coming out to myself as AB was both a positive and confronting experience.

It was confronting because I felt bound, both willingly and unwillingly, to a diverse group of people who share that identity.

As with anyone, my sense of self is my own.

But as the Cass Theory of Identity Formation indicates, a minority identity is also a collective property. For better or worse, defining myself as AB gives me a personal stake in that collective identity.

I am both proud and dismayed by the state of the collective identity of being an AB.

The best example of this was a recent (2018) lengthy thread about the AB identity on an AB forum. It was constructive in tone, with little of the grandstanding that sometimes mars on-line forums. It had posts from about two dozen ABs, of both younger and older generations, and both conflicted and self-accepting ABs.

Reading the thread made me proud of the courage and resilience of my fellow ABs. It takes a great deal of both to hold to your true sense of self in the face of pervasive isolation and public misunderstanding. There was much-shared experience of living with self-doubt, and the sometimes oppressive sense of having a hidden minority identity. I was especially moved and proud of the ABs in middle age and older, my contemporaries. They were unbowed after a lifetime of struggle, and had often reached an accepting place within themselves.

I was dismayed at the lack of a clear and shared view of the fundamental nature of our identity. Usually, our identity was thought of only in superficial terms (nappies). Despite their resilience, many had internalized some of the negative public views and were conflicted about our identity.

I am dismayed because we, as an identity, and as a society, are a long way from where I want us to be.

In my lifetime I aspire for myself and other ABs to be able to openly avow a personal identity that at least a significant minority of the public understand as healthy and deserving of recognition and respect.

I would like to disclose that, as an adult male, I have a subjectively real baby girl persona.

Let's be clear, that doesn't mean I want to *share* that persona in public, or with anyone except those I love and trust. My nappies, baby clothes, soft toys etcetera belong to a very young, vulnerable persona – they are not public property.

Why disclose at all? Why isn't it exclusively a private matter?

Because my baby persona is an essential part of who I am. It's not all I am - but you don't really know me unless you know I have a baby persona as a healthy part of my psyche. Self-acceptance has already made a big and positive difference in my life, after decades of self-doubt and isolation. I would like that positive journey to continue.

Disclosing our AB identity will always be a personal choice. Likely, there will always be risks and detriments. No one should ever feel pressured to disclose. But I would like to have an option to disclose based on a better environment than presently exists.

For those who say – impossible! – I say, nothing changes until we can start to imagine and articulate the change we seek. What's the alternative? Staying completely in the closet is a recipe for isolation and neurosis. As an older AB, I want something better for the next generations of ABs. I am sure we all do.

How is change going to happen?

How is the collective AB identity going to move forward?

We need a positive shared direction. I believe that collectively ABs need to -

1. reach a shared view of the fundamental nature of our identity

2. reject pathologising views of our identity
3. clarify the public permissions we seek for our identity
4. better support other ABs in the formation of their identity

These are things that ABs, and those that love them, need to do for themselves.

Shared View of Identity

Being an AB is about having a subjectively real baby or child persona as a fundamental, permanent and healthy part of the psyche.

That's the positive understanding that we want the world to have about us.

Of course, the baby or child persona is expressed in concrete behaviours. Almost universally, that includes nappies. But after that the range of behaviours is diverse and individually unique. Nappies are universal and important because they express, and in part, meet a deep need within us. The need is to recognize and accept our baby or child persona as *real*.

But focusing on nappies as the defining feature of our identity is wrong, and counter-productive.

Gay and lesbian people won recognition and respect for their identity because the public came to understand that it was about universal positive values. Not just sex. Love. Being true to yourself. The public eventually got it. It was unconscionable to shame and discriminate against people for heeding a universal and positive motivation. In the end, society understood our common honour for love was more important than the differences in who we choose to love. As a society, we all benefitted from the successful struggle of gay and lesbian people – it affirmed fundamental positive values for all of us.

For ABs there is a bridge to public understanding. Everyone has an inner child (except the emotionally dead). The healthy inner child is a well spring of psychological well-being and creativity. It is a concept with wide currency. Many, besides AB's, struggle with owning their healthy inner child.

The AB identity deserves respect because it is about honoring positive universal motivations – accepting and nurturing our inner child – being true to our self. That is to the benefit of all.

Reject Pathologising Models

One of the first things LGBTQ people campaigned for and won was to discard false, offensive, pathological models of their identity. Arguably it was a pre-requisite for any other positive acceptance. As long your identity is officially regarded as a psychiatric disorder, it's going to be pretty hard to make much progress with public acceptance.

In the DSM, being AB is grouped in the same category as flashers, gropers, paedophiles and peeping toms! Those are all disorders which are defined by their sexual character and coercive in that they are forced on non-consenting others. Being AB is neither defined by its sexual character nor is it coercive.

This pathological view of being AB is highly offensive and empirically invalid. It is an ongoing source of harm when health professionals act on this invalid understanding to counsel ABs.

Being in any way conflated with paedophilia is one of the biggest obstacles to public acceptance of the AB identity.

As a start, ABs need to avoid health professionals that use a pathological model of our identity.

Seeking professional counselling when you need it is a sign of maturity and psychological health. However, it is important to find the right kind of counselling and to recognize that the wrong therapy can be harmful.

If a person is seeking counselling and that counselling may touch on their identity, or possible identity, as an AB, I recommend the following. Check that the counsellor can conceive of being a non-conflicted AB as a healthy personal identity. If they can't they will likely be working with a pathological model of being AB (whether they tell you that or not). That may cause harm when you are at your most vulnerable. Look elsewhere until you find a counsellor who can consider being AB as an identity. This is likely to be an LGBTQ friendly counsellor or perhaps one who has some experience of working with DID. The empathy and therapeutic skill of the counsellor is the central requirement. But all-things-being-equal in that respect, a counsellor with experience in Internal Family Systems (IFS) therapy would be a good prospect. A counsellor working with a Rogerian framework (based on the work of psychologist Carl Rogers) should be non-judgemental and positive about the client's capacities but may not offer the guidance about the experience of identity formation.

Public Permissions

I contend that we need to seek public permissions for our identity which are consistent with what fundamentally defines that identity.

Being an Adult Baby is about having a persona that has infantile or child-like feelings and needs. That identity is vulnerable, and like any very young child needs to be protected from unsafe environments. Therefore, an identity as an Adult Baby is going to have a significantly private character.

I aspire to live in a society where I might disclose that I have a baby girl persona. But I don't need or want to share that persona in public, or with anyone but those who love me. It would be nice for no one to be fazed when I discretely wear nappies under adult clothes for my baby persona to experience being out in the world, feeling the sunshine on her face and the wind on her skin. But I don't aspire to show my nappy, wear baby clothes, suck a dummy or play with dolls in public.

In my view, the distinction between these two permissions is akin to the difference between public acceptance of shows of affection between LGBTQ people (positive/affirming), and having gay sex in public (not positive). Making an exhibition or public show of my vulnerable child persona seems to be me to reflect a conflicted stage of identity formation rather than full self-acceptance.

That doesn't mean that all public images of ABs in nappies, baby clothes, hugging soft toys etc are bad. They have a positive and necessary role – principally *within* the AB community. They can provide positive modelling for ABs seeking to discover and accept their AB identity. Many ABs are alone with their identity – with none or few to share it with. Seeing other ABs can be a bit like looking in the mirror. It helps to see and think to yourself – 'that's me'. In my journey of self-acceptance, I benefited from the you-tube videos of articulate, camera-friendly ABs. Also, being able to share positive images – selfies - on social media with other ABs is one of the few ways of validating our experience of ourselves (often with the safety of 'clipped' images and an on-line identity protecting us from being 'outed').

The key point is these images have positive value within and for the AB community. While there is no firewall between them and the wider public, you have to go looking for them to find them. That's different from the public permissions we seek for our identity. It doesn't mean we all want to walk down the street, or through the mall, like we're going to daycare.

Better Support Healthy AB Identity Formation

It is very important that ABs create a more supportive environment for the formation of their identity. In every new generation, there will be young people with emerging AB identities. There are also many adult ABs who are struggling with their internal conflicts, and with external disapproval and detriments, in relation to their identity.

There are three dimensions to a more supportive environment -

a. permission and encouragement for the exploration of identity
b. access to information regarding the non-conflicted AB identity
c. access to supportive contacts that affirm a healthy, stable minority identity.

It is particularly important to positively influence the views of parents. Remember the first consciousness of the AB identity commonly occurs around ten years old. From the discussion of the early stages of identity formation, we know the fundamental importance of a supportive family environment. In the absence of such an environment, the all-too-common pattern is for the beginning of the identity to be solitary and covert, with a consciousness of parental disapproval and the absence of reassurance or guidance. This can start a life course of secrecy, shame and estrangement from others. Rosalie Bent's book *'So Your Teenager is Wearing Diapers: understanding why some teenagers want to wear diapers'* is the first example of a resource targeted at this key need.

There is a dearth of information on the healthy, non-conflicted AB identity. The internet is awash with AB fetish content and inane posts about the best diaper. That is no help when you're in the tormenting throes of the binge and purge cycle. In fact, it's completely counter-productive. Conflicted ABs need information and resources to help them understand and resolve their inner struggles and conflict. They need to know there is a self-accepting, healthy, happy space on the other side of their struggles – not just an endless re-boot of binge and purge. The AB Discovery website is an important source of information about the non-fetish AB identity. More power to it. We need more like it.

Thirdly, we need on-line meeting spaces that better affirm the healthy AB identity. Online and social media interaction meets a fundamental need for ABs. Everyone - people with conforming personal identities as well as minority identities - have a human need to be understood and accepted for who they are. With being AB being a largely private identity, on-line/social media platforms will be the most accessible means to interact positively with others.

For all the above needs it is for ABs who have reached non-conflicted stages of identity formation to contribute to the positive picture of the identity.

The Way Forward

Writing about a way forward for a collective personal identity is pretty presumptuous. There will be some who think so and question my credentials to do it. Hang it! It needs to be done – if for no other reason than to challenge other views and move things forward. If you're an AB and disagree with what I have to say – great, write your own book or blog, and put your views out there.

In this spirit, until someone comes up with something better, I propose the following credo –

We are functional adults with a child persona as a real and healthy part of our psyche. It is a core part of our sense of self. We have held true to that sense of self in the face of lifelong public misunderstanding. We are adult babies, ABs. We deserve and claim respect for our personal identity. ⏾

References – annotated list

Bent, Michael		Adult Babies: Principles and Practices (2015) (Amazon & Abdiscovery.com.au)
		The first text taking an analytical approach to the AB identity, written by an AB.
		Being an Adult Baby: Articles and Essays on Being an Adult Baby. (2016) (Amazon & Abdiscovery.com.au)
		A collection of insightful and thought provoking articles on the AB identity. Notably – 'My Story', 'Identity Confusion in the Adult Baby', 'Finding Balance Between the Baby and the Adult', 'Binge and Purge', 'My Story as an Adult Baby'
Bent, Rosalie		There's Still A Baby in My Bed: Learning To Live Happily With the Adult Baby in Your Relationship. (2015) (Amazon & Abdiscovery.com.au)
		A revised version of the 2012 book that first articulated that being an AB was a personal identity, not just a fetish. Written by the wife of an AB. Evergreen.
		So, Your Teenager is Wearing Diapers! Understanding why some teenagers want to wear diapers (2015) (Amazon & Abdiscovery.com.au)
		The first published resource to help younger ABs and their families.
Bowlby, John.		Separation: Anxiety and Anger. Attachment and Loss Volume 2 (1973) (Basic Books & Amazon).
		Second, and most useful, of the three volumes setting out Attachment Theory.
Burch, Brian M.F.		The Adult Baby's Guide: the Life Struggles of the Perpetually Diapered (2014) (Amazon)
		A courageous book by an AB who survived a very difficult 'coming out' as a young adult. I don't agree with all the author's views but he's one of the few outside AB Discovery.com.au who's published a book that sees being AB as more than a fetish.
Cass, Vivienne		Homosexual identity formation: A theoretical model. Journal of Homosexuality, 1979, 4(3), 219 – 234
		The original 1979 paper setting out the Cass Theory.
		Dr Cass academic papers, including the three cited here, are available free from the following website -

	http://www.brightfire.com.au/publications/	
	Sexual orientation identity formation: A Western phenomenon, In R. Cabaj & T. Stein (Eds), Textbook of Homosexuality and Mental Health American Psychiatric Press, Washington, 1996 I prefer this to the original 1979 paper for the exposition of the Cass Theory.	
	Sexual orientation and the place of psychology: side-lined, side-tracked or should that be side-swiped? Gay and lesbian issues and psychology review. 2006, Vol 2(1), 25-37 Includes a history of how gay and lesbian activism changed the official classification of homosexuality as a psychiatric disorder.	
	A Quick Guide to the Cass Theory of Lesbian and Gay Identity Formation (2015) (Amazon) Worthwhile purchasing for the author's compelling retrospective on her own theory.	
Fassinger, Ruth E. & McCarn, Susan R.	Revisioning Sexual Minority Identity Formation: A New Model of Lesbian Identity and its Implications for Counseling and Research. The Counseling Psychologist 1996. A model of identity formation for lesbians. Separates the development of the sense of self, from group identification, with a 4 phase model for each. This insightful model is more lesbian specific than the Cass Theory. I preferred the Cass Theory for ABs. The bipartite Fassinger model involved additional complexity without additional benefit. The guidance for counsellors in the application of the Cass Theory was also key. This article has a useful summary of other models of identity formation. Available, free on-line at - https://studysites.uk.sagepub.com/thomas2e/study/articles/section6/Article107.pdf	
Ingram, Ben	Fear and Joy: A Life In and Out of Nappies (2018) (Amazon & abdiscovery.com.au) Inspirational story of someone who grew up loving nappies and later became a soldier who served his country three times overseas.	
Lewis, Dylan	Living With Chrissie: My Life As An Adult Baby (2018) (Amazon & Abdiscovery.com.au) My account of my life as a very late bloomer as an AB ('better late than never').	
	Becoming Me – the Journey of Self-acceptance: a Guidebook for Adult Babies Traversing Life (2018) (Amazon & Abdiscovery.com.au) Focuses on self-acceptance, the intrapsychic dimension of identity formation, and the childhood origin of the identity	
Lipscomb, Rhoda J.	The Clinical Mental Health Experience of Persons with Paraphilic Infantilism and Autonepiophilia. A phenomenological research study. PhD dissertation (2014). An excellent study of being AB by an informed and sympathetic health professional. Good up-to-date review of literature and research, including an informative history of the official classification of being AB as a mental disorder. Available free, on-line at - http://www.esextherapy.com/dissertations/Rhoda%20J.%20Lipscomb%20The%20Cli nical%20Mental%20Health%20Experience%20of%20Persons%20withParaphilic%20I nfantilism%20and%20Autonepiophilia.pdf	

Lyra, Henry.		The Epitome Of Love: An ABDL Novella (2018) (Amazon)
		Life affirming fictional story about a teenage AB coming out to his supportive family, inspired by the author's true life experience (the latter included as an appendix).
Marshall, John.		Australian Baby – A Life of Nappies, Bottles and Struggles. (2018) (Amazon & Abdiscovery.com.au)
		A landmark. The only account I know of an AB who cites identifying from an early age as having a baby (girl) persona.
		Oxford Textbook of Psychotherapy (editors Glen Gabbard, Judith Beck & Jeremy Holmes) (2005) (Oxford University Press)
		Claims to be an authoritative text on psychotherapy for all mental health professionals – cites an appallingly pathological view of the AB identity.
Rowan, John		Subpersonalities: The People Inside Us (1990) (Routledge [paperback] & amazon)
		Demonstrates that multiplicity models of mind and consciousness have a long and respectable pedigree.
Schwartz, Richard C.		Internal Family Systems Therapy (1995) (Guildford Press [paperback] & amazon)
		Original exposition of IFS, the school of psychology which may be best suited to counselling ABs.
Speaker, Thomas John		Sexual Infantilism in Adults: Causes and Treatment. Masters thesis (1980)
		Psychosexual infantilism in Adults: The eroticization of regression. Doctoral thesis. (1986)
		Opens the door to a non-pathological understanding of ABs. Proceeds from an unexamined assumption that being AB is principally a sexual expression. Includes large number of brief case studies, some of which have references to the non-sexual dimension of being AB.
		Available free, on-line at –
		http://understanding.infantilism.org/surveys/
W, A.T.		Got Parts? An Insider's Guide to Managing Life Successfully with Dissociative Identity Disorder. (2005) (Amazon)
		A compelling short description of the nature of DID and the road to psychological health by someone with the identity.
Wikipedia		See articles on –
		'Comfort Objects'
		'Coming Out',
		'Cass identity model' – caution, note Wikipedia did not heed Dr Cass as the authority on her own theory, preferably see also the Cass references above, including free on-line articles
		'Dissociation (psychology)'
		'Fassinger's model of gay and lesbian identity development'

		'Transgender'

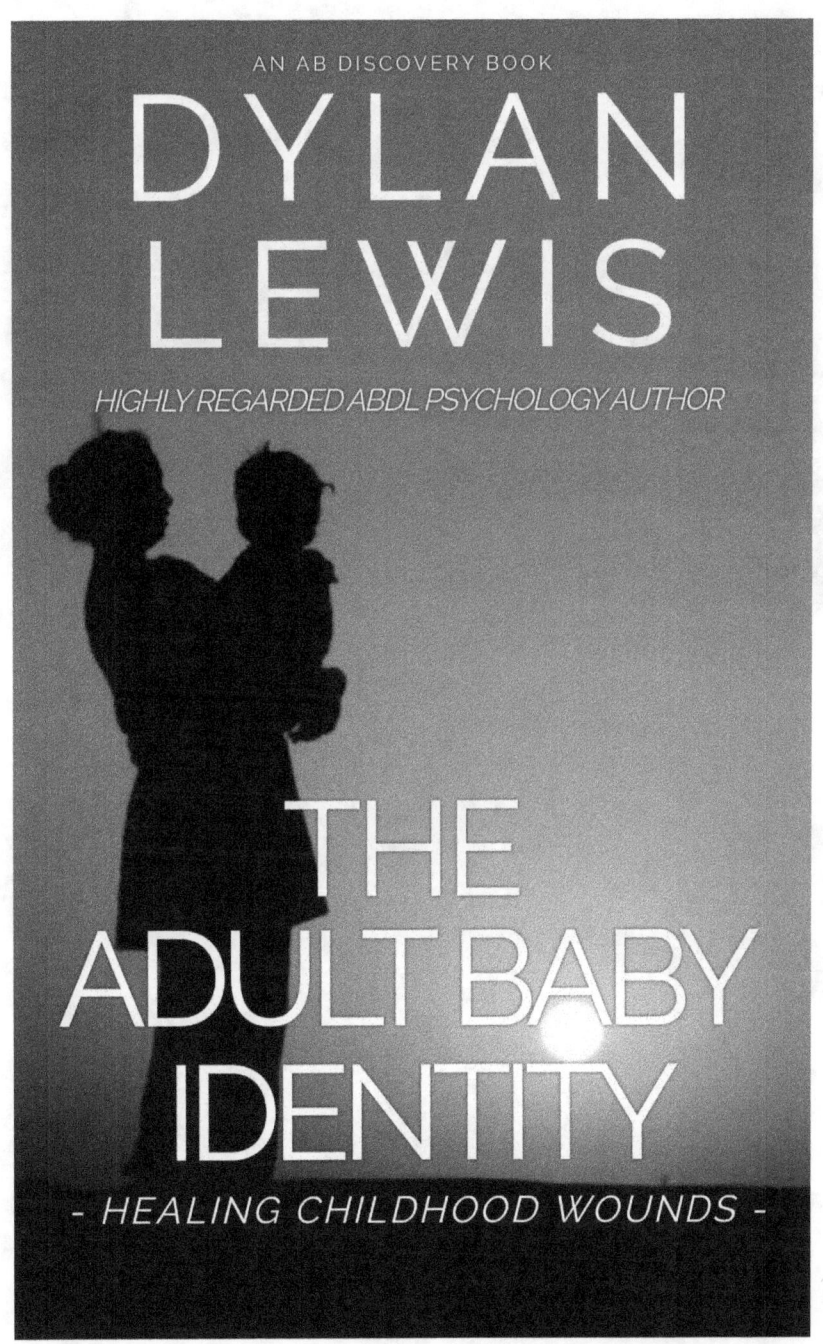

The Adult Baby Identity –
Healing Childhood Wounds

by
Dylan Lewis

First Published 2019

Copyright © Dylan Lewis

All rights reserved.

Dedication:

To my wife for her constant love and wisdom.

To Rosalie Bent and Michael Bent who let the world know adult babies aren't mad, bad or alone.

To Donald Woods Winnicott for his profound humanity.

Foreword

It is said that *'no one gets out of child-hood unharmed'*.

This is one of those truisms that understands that we all carry some scars and drag around some burden that developed in childhood. Despite the best efforts of parents, family, teachers and those around us, there are always things we pick up along the way that cause us a measure of trouble or difficulty later on. Parents are not perfect and Mary Poppins is not real. Life is full of mistakes, failings and weakness, even in the best of people. Fortunately for most of us, these childhood-grown issues are relatively small and well within our capacity to manage and live with.

But not everyone is so lucky.

For some people, *'just get over it'* or *'just say no'* is a grossly inadequate – and ignorant – response to the problems they face. For Adult Babies, this is very much the case.

We have known for some time that the drive to wear diapers, to act like a baby or to desire to re-experience infancy, is more than some mere affectation that we can choose to do or to discard by our own choice. It is, however, not an addiction that can be cured, nor a fetish that can be explained away. It is something much more complex and intertwined with our being. It also had its seeds in very early childhood, ironically, often as actual babies and toddlers.

But what is it that sets one-child-in-a-thousand on a path of life-long desires for diapers and the elements of infancy? Most of us come from what we would call 'good homes' and yet, we still wear diapers or wet the bed and crave the intimacy and experience of babyhood.

Dylan Lewis' book goes down that particular rabbit hole and seeks to understand why we are who we are, despite those good homes and good parents.

We are all to some degree… A Wounded Child. But for some of us, those wounds affect us very deeply in a bizarre and powerful fashion – diapers.

May understanding flourish and healing flow through it.

Michael Bent

1. Introduction

Being an adult baby is a minority personal identity.

It is based on a non-conforming sense of self – adult babies have a subjectively real child persona as an essential and permanent part of their psyche. That persona, often long denied, drives the AB's characteristic behaviours – a love for nappies, soft toys, pacifiers, baby clothes etcetera.

The AB identity keeps these symbols of infancy or childhood very much in view. It's like a bright neon sign pointing to the origins and essence of the identity.

Yet paradoxically, many ABs don't want to look too deeply inside themselves, or back into their childhood. I am an adult baby. For me, looking within was a painful and fearful prospect.

Why? Because if I looked too deeply, I was afraid I would confirm my worst fears – that I was broken – irrevocably broken beyond hope of healing. Specifically, I would confirm that being AB was the source of that brokenness. I suspect it is the same for many ABs. Better to live in the present, sometimes comforted, often distracted by nappies, than to delve too deeply inside.

Anyhow, how could I look back into the unknowable past, into early childhood or infancy? It is beyond recall.

But what if it is possible to look into the childhood origins of our adult baby identity?

What if looking within didn't confirm the worst?

What if looking inside was the road to understanding and healing?

That is what this book is about.

We can look deep inside the AB identity. We have two means to do so. The first is with the help of two eminent and renown psychotherapists, John Bowlby and Donald Winnicott, who understood personality development in very young children. In particular, Winnicott was a paediatrician and gifted psychotherapist who had decades of direct experience with mothers and babies. He documented a profound and compelling understanding of the psyche of infants and young children.

The second means is through reflection on the character of our child persona. I believe that for many ABs, their child persona originated in childhood trauma. The full experience of that trauma and the child persona is commonly denied in what is called dissociation. So, the childhood mould from which that persona was formed was unique and is long gone. But our child persona is a cast from that mould. We can tell much about the mould from the cast which is still with us.

When we look into the infancy and childhood of an AB, there *is* pain and brokenness.

It is the bond between mother and child which was broken.

It is the child's trauma and dissociation which was broken.

Our Inner Child is wounded.

But our AB identity, our child persona, is *not* broken.

Our child persona is a positive, redeeming response to what *was* broken. It has kept a vital, spontaneous and creative part of us – our True Self - alive and safe when we feared we would lose ourselves to despair.

Our AB identity embodies courage and hope – love for our wounded Inner Child. We have kept faith with our Inner Child and our True Self, even when we didn't understand ourselves. It is a redemptive part of our psyche – of which we can be proud.

The key audience for the book are ABs and those who love them. ABs need to have the understanding, and the language, to explain why being AB is a healthy personal identity so that we are not defenceless in the face of the ignorance or prejudice of others. That is why I have drawn on the work of eminent psychotherapists and contemporary experts.

This book is my best attempt to understand our shared identity. It reflects my personal experience as an AB. I have a layman's lifelong interest in psychology. I have no formal qualifications in psychology. Every adult baby is different and some will disagree with my views. I do not intend to disparage any who's views are different from mine. Take what is useful or helpful from the book and leave the rest behind.

The other audience is health professionals. Those who counsel AB's need a deep understanding of the psyche of infants and young children. Not only what can go wrong, but how it feels from the inside when it does. They need to know John Bowlby and Attachment Theory, Donald Winnicott, childhood trauma and dissociation, multiplicity in consciousness and parts. Only then can they genuinely understand the AB identity. I believe that equipped with that understanding, they will sooner see that the AB identity is ultimately healthy and redeeming.

This book is based on the pioneering work of Rosalie Bent and Michael Bent in identifying and understanding adult babies as a personal identity. I recommend their books and website www.abdiscovery.com.au . I refer to their insights and understanding throughout the book.

By 'adult baby' I exclude role players and diaper lovers for whom diapers, baby clothes or baby activities are an optional extra they can freely live without, and fetishists for whom these things are confined exclusively to sexual expression.

This book is the third in a trilogy. The first, 'Becoming Me', deals principally with self-acceptance. It has one chapter on the childhood origins of being AB. That was insufficient to do the topic justice and hence this book. The second book, 'The Adult Baby Identity – Coming Out as an Adult Baby', makes the case that being AB is a minority personal identity and deals with the stages by which that identity is formed.

This book is about the healing that comes from understanding the childhood origins of our identity. If you are an AB, that is likely to raise troubling issues and feelings. Those hurts can be healed. The journey of healing and self-acceptance is not an easy one to undertake alone. You need a confidant who you can trust, and who will be an ally in your healing.

If there is no one in your life with whom you can safely share your feelings about your life as an adult baby, seek professional support – preferably from an LGBTQ-friendly counsellor who understands issues of personal identity. If you are in crisis or deep distress about being an adult baby seek professional counselling.

2. The Lost World of Infancy - Attachment Theory

The pioneers in understanding the adult baby identity, Rosalie and Michael Bent locate its origin in early childhood.

We need to start off once again by stating the sometimes-controversial fact that the beginnings of AIR (Adult Infantile Regression) is in the first three years of life. Although some may only become aware of it in later years, detailed discussions always point back to feelings and experiences that occurred in the pre-school age range. A majority will also point to an age of around 3-4 years of age when they first became aware of 'something different'. No toddler of that age is going to have much of an idea of what it is – only that something is there. What we can infer is that since age three is the point at which memories remain, it is not only possible but probable, that the causes of AIR are in the sub-three-year-old level.

Rosalie subsequently refined this to locate the origin of the identity, very early, in infancy.

As most of us can't remember anything specific about the first several years of our lives, this might seem to place the origin of our AB identity in our unknowable past.

But the life's work of two renown psychotherapists, John Bowlby and Donald Winnicott, allows us to understand the lost world of our infancy. Armed with that understanding, we can fill in key missing pieces which are beyond our conscious memory.

We begin by understanding the development of the child's personality when all goes well.

Attachment Theory explains the most important influence on child development. It was created by John Bowlby (b.1907 d.1990), an English psychiatrist and psychotherapist. Bowlby was a theorist, but he also ran a mother's group in a child clinic for twenty years. He sought to show the importance of environmental factors, like parenting, on the formation of the child's personality, and to base this on empirical evidence.

Attachment Theory is applicable to all stages of life but has enormous relevance to young children. It tells us that the first human need is for affectionate attachment to another. (Note Attachment Theory is not the same as Attachment Parenting or Attachment Therapy.)

Bowlby states –

> *...For not only young children, but human beings of all ages are found to be at their happiest and able to deploy their talents to best advantage when they are confident that, standing behind them, there are one or more trusted persons who will come to their aid should difficulties arise. The person trusted provides the secure base from which his (or her) companion can operate.*

The Theory holds that the attachment between mother and baby, and particularly the continuity of that attachment, is fundamental to the development of the child's personality. We now take this understanding for granted. Before Bowlby developed his Theory in the 1950s and 1960s, it wasn't so. Children were treated as mini-adults, expected to 'tough it out' in difficult circumstances without any long-term adverse effects. Very young children were routinely separated from their mothers, or any consistent mother substitute, in all manner of settings – such as hospitals, residential nurseries, children's homes, and boarding schools – because there was no formal learning that recognized the importance of the bond between mother and child.

Patterns of attachment are formed in childhood. Bowlby states –

> *"... the period during which attachment behavior is most readily activated, namely about six months to five years, is also the most sensitive in regard to the development of expectations of the availability of attachment figures; but that nevertheless sensitivity in this regard persists during the decade after the fifth birthday, albeit in steadily diminishing degree as the years of childhood pass."*

The relationship with the mother forms a key part of the child's personality because the child develops an 'internal working model' of relationships, based on what it has learnt. Essentially, the child internalizes the pattern of interaction with their mother, to provide the predictability necessary to function successfully.

Attachment Theory and its importance for young children is best demonstrated through the 'Strange Situation' studies. Attachment Theory holds that a child with a secure attachment to their mother will feel better able to explore their environment. The *Strange Situation* is a procedure designed to test the effect of one-year-olds' attachment to their mothers, on the babies' exploration and play in an unfamiliar setting. The procedure was developed in the late 1960s by Mary Ainsworth (b. 1913 d. 1999) an American psychologist and colleague of Bowlby.

The procedure involves short, timed episodes of interaction, separation and reunion between the mother and child. A stranger is present for some episodes, both with the mother and baby, and with the baby alone in the absence of the mother. The procedure is filmed and the child's reactions to these episodes categorized. As at 1993 the procedure had been used in over thirty academic studies and is regarded as a reliable and valid instrument. (See Ainsworth's article *'Attachment, Exploration, and Separation: Illustrated by the Behaviour of One-Year-Olds in a Strange Situation'* cited in the references and available free, on-line.)

The Study strongly confirms Attachment Theory. The babies' exploratory activities are strongest when the mother is present and decline significantly in her absence. The absence of the mother causes the babies to seek to recover the physical proximity of their mother (crying, searching etc). The babies react very differently to the stranger than to their mother indicating that their attachment is specific to the latter.

The 'Strange Situation' studies also revealed another major finding – one central to our interest. The studies revealed significant differences in how babies responded to the return of their mothers after separation. The optimal relationship between mother and child is called a secure attachment. Babies with secure attachments were upset, but not unreasonably distressed when their mother left. When their mother returned, these children sought comfort and soon returned happily to their explorations and play. A secure attachment points a child towards a trusting relationship with themselves and with others – a kind of *'I'm okay, you're okay'* space.

Therapist Jasmin Lee Cori states -

> *'Secure attachment creates a deep sense of belonging, because it anchors you, giving you a place in the web of life. That place is bigger than any one relationship, but mother as our first relationship sets the stage. Later, we may find belonging by knowing that we are part of a team, a tribe, a neighborhood, a club, a community, a nation, or a social movement – or by having our own child and partner. When we have a sense of belonging, we feel embedded, part of something.*

*Feeling valued and known are also part of this belonging.' ['The Emotionally Absent Mother:
How to Recognize and Heal the Invisible Effects of Childhood Emotional Neglect']*

Jasmin Lee Cori indicates a child with a secure attachment takes in the following messages from their mother –

"I'm glad you're here; I see you; You are special to me; I respect you; I love you; Your needs are important to me. You can turn to me for help; I am here for you. I'll make time for you; I'll keep you safe; You can rest in me; I delight in you."

The Strange Situation studies suggest that in advanced western countries, about two-thirds of the child population have a secure attachment. Subsequent research identified that children's attachment styles persist into adulthood (some people change their attachment style as adults, but most don't).

Feminists have criticized Bowlby for placing sole responsibility for the raising of children on mothers, and not considering whether society adequately supports mothers, or recognizing that women have lives and aspirations beyond motherhood. This is valid. In this respect, Bowlby was a product of his time. Fathers now take a much greater role in raising their children and men may be the primary carer. When Bowlby or Winnicott say 'mother' we now would say 'primary caregiver'. I have continued to refer to mothers because that was true when they wrote.

Bowlby's focus on meeting the attachment needs of babies and children remains entirely valid, but we now accept that these needs can and should be met by more than the child's mother alone.

Rosalie and Michael Bent are the foremost public authorities on the adult baby identity. Rosalie is the wife of Michael, an adult baby. In 2012 Rosalie published the landmark book 'There's A Baby in My Bed' intended for the partners of adult babies. It was the first published work to seriously address adult babies as a personal identity, beyond a sexual fetish. It was updated in 2015 as 'There's Still A Baby in My Bed. Rosalie has also written a book for the parents of teenage adult babies. Michael has published a text 'Adult Babies: Psychology and Practices' and an anthology of insightful articles 'Being An Adult Baby'. Rosalie and Michael are the owners of the website www.abdiscovery.com.au which is dedicated to helping regressive adult babies understand themselves, and fostering public understanding of the identity.

3. The Lost World of Infancy - The Child's Psyche

Attachment Theory tells us that the development of a child's personality is founded in their attachment to their mother. This is based on empirical observation of mothers and babies – notably the external behavioural effects of long and short term separations of mother and baby.

The work of Donald Winnicott allows us to understand how attachment works *within* the psyche of mother and baby. Later in the book, we will see that Winnicott's key formulations are central to understanding ABs.

Donald Woods Winnicott (b.1896 d.1971) was a paediatrician and a gifted psychotherapist. He has been described by the contemporary philosopher Alain de Botton as the greatest British psychoanalyst who ever lived. From decades of interaction with thousands of mothers and babies, Winnicott gives us an extraordinary insight into the psyche of infants and young children. A colleague, speaking at Winnicott's funeral said -

> *"I first got to know Donald Winnicott twenty-two years ago when I became a physician at the Paddington Green Children's Hospital. I went there with a poor opinion of the general usefulness of child psychiatry, but I soon found that, however difficult and damaging a child's past and present circumstances, the situation always changed for the better once Dr Winnicott became involved. ... Donald Winnicott had the most astonishing powers with children. To say that he understood children would to me sound false and vaguely patronizing; it was rather that children understood him and that he was at one with them. ... within a few minutes of a child entering his consulting room both the child and Dr Winnicott were oblivious to the presence of anyone else." [Boundary and Space: An Introduction to the Work of D.W. Winnicott]*

Winnicott has a warmly positive view of the human condition and its origins in the child psyche. A colleague said of him -

> *Perhaps the most important temperamental influence on Donald Winnicott's work was simply his belief that life is worth living. There was nothing romantic or sentimental in this: he was fully aware that 'life is difficult, inherently difficult for every human being, for every one of us from the very beginning', and he could identify with the people who came to consult him because he knew about anxiety and doubt. ... His faith in human nature embraced the whole person ... He could not believe that human beings are born with the seeds of their own destruction in themselves. He was unable, for instance, to accept Freud's explanation of aggressiveness in terms of a death instinct." [Boundary and Space: An Introduction to the Work of D.W. Winnicott]*

Winnicott saw the first year of life as a vital and enormously creative period in the development of the human psyche. From the outset, he does not see the infant psyche in isolation. He famously said, "*there is no such thing as a baby - there is a mother and a baby*". The mother's care is the basis of the healthy development of the baby's psyche. Winnicott coined the term the 'good enough mother' to mean that mothers didn't need to be perfect, but rather sufficiently attuned to the needs and feelings of her baby.

Winnicott recognized that the loving way a 'good enough' mother held her baby was very important. It epitomized the bond between mother and baby. He used the term 'holding' to describe how the mother created a physical, and especially a psychological, space that protected and nurtured her baby. It applies particularly to young infants, but it also extends to older children when they are frightened, or sick, and return to their mother for reassurance and comfort. Winnicott saw a mother's nurturing touch as very important to a baby and child's healthy psychological development. That touch was the beginning of how the baby discovered and felt alive in his or her own body.

In the first weeks and months, the baby's psyche is fragile. The mother's close care protects her baby's psyche from intrusions that would overwhelm the latter. At this stage, the baby experiences the mother and her care as part of the baby's undivided psyche. There is no 'me', no 'other'.

But even at this stage of total dependency, Winnicott sees the baby's psyche not as passive, but vital and creative. The baby ruthlessly 'attacks' the mother's resources and the mother has a hunger to be so attacked, in a relationship of mutual reciprocity. The baby's psyche 'imagines' the mother's breast or bottle as it appears. The mother's reliability in presenting the breast or bottle instils a sense of 'magical' omnipotence that is the baby's first sense of safety – when the breast or bottle is needed, it appears, created by the baby.

From the earliest stage, the baby is forming its psyche from the relationship with their mother. The mother attuned to her baby accurately mirrors in her face her baby's state of being. The baby sees itself in that mirror. Winnicott saw this as vitally important. It is a foundation of the True Self, and beyond that, the baby's healthy psychological development. He summed it up with the phrase –

"When I look, I am seen, so I exist. I can now afford to look and see."

The baby has a True Self, which is embodied in the spontaneous gestures as the baby discovers itself and meets the challenges of development that will continue throughout life. The True Self is what makes the baby feel 'real'. It is the seat of what makes the baby, and later child and adult, feel authentically and distinctively 'themselves'. For someone writing in the secular discipline of psychotherapy, Winnicott's conception of the True Self approaches the notion of a spirit or soul. The real nature of the True Self is beyond being communicated with others. It can only be experienced.

Throughout the life of a baby and young child, Winnicott believed that the continuity of the mother's care and attunement to her baby's feelings and needs was the key to the child's healthy psychological development. This continuity allowed the baby to keep 'going on being' and focus on its own enormous developmental challenges and tasks.

In the next stage, the small lags between the baby's need for feeding or care and the mother's response gradually develops the baby's sense of being separate from the mother. This is a milestone for the baby's psyche and appears in the second six months of life. Now there is a 'me' and an 'other'. The mother's attunement to her baby is still fundamentally important. The lag between the baby's need and the mother's response is not so long or unreliable as to overwhelm the baby's psyche, but enough to erode the 'illusion' of omnipotence, that the breast or bottle is created by the baby.

The creation of a 'me' with a boundary containing within it the experiences and memories of the baby, is the beginning of the personality. But the recognition that the mother is external, creates anxiety for the baby at the prospect of separation from her. The baby learns gradually to be alone for short periods, initially learning to be alone in the reliable presence of her or his mother. The baby can hold in his or her mind the image of the mother for a short period of time and tolerate separation for that short interval. If the mother is attuned to her baby and reliably meets the baby's needs, the baby's ability to hold the image of the mother gradually lengthens, and with it the ability to tolerate longer separation.

It is in this stage that the great majority of babies acquire comfort objects like a security blanket or soft toy. In the 'magical' thinking of the baby, the object comes to stand in for the mother. It becomes a psychological substitute for her when she isn't there, typically helping the baby to tolerate the mother's absence and sleep securely. Winnicott called these 'transitional objects'.

He recognized them as belonging to a very important development in the baby's psyche. The baby has created a comfort object by investing it with special significance. It is neither wholly subjective, an 'illusion' solely within the psyche – nor is it wholly external like the mother. It is transitional between the subjective inside world of 'me' and the external world of 'other'. Yet the meaning the baby has endowed the security blanket or teddy is tangible enough to be understood by others – 'want your teddy?'

The discovery by the baby that it is distinct from others is a milestone that ushers in major developments in the baby's psyche. This includes relating to others, aggression, fantasy and guilt. The baby now learns that to get his or her needs met, it must relate to others, initially the mother, but a progressively wider group. The healthy capacity to 'use' others is a key developmental milestone. It is still founded on the reliable attunement of the mother to the baby's needs that allows the baby to learn in psychological safety without being overwhelmed by interruptions and intrusions that it cannot make sense of.

Lesser, tolerable, delays in meeting the baby's needs, prompt the baby's aggression. With the distinction between self and others, this is now genuine aggression towards another, not simply the discomfort of an earlier stage. In fantasy, within the baby's psyche, its powerful anger 'destroys' the mother. But the 'good enough mother' neither rejects the angry baby nor retaliates. The baby learns that the mother destroyed in the baby's fantasy is not destroyed in reality. Through this, the baby learns safety with others, and with its own powerful anger.

Winnicott considered that the capacity to play was the epitome of a baby or child's psychological health.

> *"Winnicott believes that the ability to play is the benchmark for the entrance into a life*
> *of health and vitality. All that goes right in child development leads to play, and play, in turn,*
> *allows every subsequent task and obstacle of the humanizing process to be accomplished."*
> *[Steven Tuber. Attachment, Play and Authenticity: A Winnicott Primer]*

He had a unique and compelling understanding of play. When a child at play make-believes that a spoon is an aircraft, that is a creation, an illusion, of the child's mind. Yet in play, the child can share that illusion with another and in turn, the other person can share their own illusions. Play is neither wholly subjective (contained within the self) nor wholly objective (the spoon is not an aircraft) – it is transitional between the two. Winnicott was the first to understand this unique category – transitional phenomena. Play is the prime example of this phenomena, along with transitional objects like security blankets and soft toys. Winnicott understood that all culture belongs to the same category of transitional phenomena as play. When we share sports, political beliefs or religion with others, they are neither wholly subjective nor wholly objective – we agree with others to invest shared activities with common meanings which are not inherent in objective forms.

At first, the baby learns play from her or his mother.

> *"Play is good because the baby delights in the magical control, the omnipotent feelings,*
> *the incredible confidence he derives from his 'magical' to-and-fro with his mother. Critically, the*
> *good enough mother 'gets it', she goes along with the baby's illusory omnipotence, that he's*
> *pulling the strings."*

In play, the child experiences an empowering sense of omnipotence and learns gradually to surrender that omnipotence and accept external reality. Later, the baby learns to play by themselves, and still later to play with other playmates. Winnicott viewed play as the epitome of health because it embodied creativity, the healthy capacity to 'use' others (playmates) to satisfy needs, the capacity to be alone, and the spontaneous authentic character of the True Self.

Summary

So, with the help of Bowlby and Winnicott, we understand healthy personality development in the first years of life. The baby's psyche is vital and active. From the outset, the 'good enough mother', attuned to her baby's feelings and need, is building a secure attachment. Her care allows the baby to feel omnipotent and safe. She gradually lets external reality intrude so that her baby learns to deal with it without feeling overwhelmed. The mother takes her baby's rages and fears in her stride. As a result, baby learns to trust others and their own feelings. They have a True Self based on their spontaneous delight in their discovery of themselves and the world, and in being alive and grounded in their bodies. They learn slowly to tolerate mother's absence, initially for short periods, because they can hold a trusted image of her in their minds. The mother teaches her baby to play and the baby experiences empowering omnipotence, and creativity. That omnipotence is again gradually surrendered so that the baby learns to deal with external reality without being frightened and overwhelmed. Through play their creativity can be shared with others.

4. When It Goes Wrong

Unlike adult babies, the vast majority of adults do not need or enjoy reliving infancy with nappies, soft toys and pacifiers. Once was evidently enough. It is clear that for ABs something went wrong in infancy or childhood. Bowlby and Winnicott can guide us to identify what that was.

The 'Strange Situation' studies identified that two-thirds of children have secure attachments. What about the rest? Not so good. They have insecure attachments. In the studies for children with insecure attachments, the short separations from their mother were much more problematic. The babies' healthy explorations were more curtailed in the absence of their mothers, either by outright distress or concerned preoccupation. But the greatest differences were when their mothers returned. Instead of being readily comforted and then returning to their healthy explorations, babies with insecure attachments showed very different reactions.

Based on these behaviours Mary Ainsworth and other researchers divided the children with insecure attachments into three groups –

1. avoidant,
2. ambivalent
3. disorganized.

Each of these insecure attachment styles are described below.

Babies with an **avoidant attachment** reacted in an unexpected way. They did not seek reunion with their mothers, either ignoring her or hovering at middle distance, but keeping an eye on her. If picked up, they protested to be set down again. These children are associated with mothers who were dismissive of the needs of the child. Therapist Jasmin Lee Cori describes children with avoidant insecure attachments.

> *"The largest of the insecure categories is a style that has been called by several names – compulsively self-sufficient (Bowlby), avoidant (Ainsworth), and dismissive (Main, referring to this style in adults).*

When the mother is consistently rejecting or non-responsive and emotionally unavailable, the child gives up, learns it is futile or dangerous in relationships to need, and consequently turns off his or her needs and attachment feelings. This, in essence, is what this style is all about.

More specifically, mothers of avoidant children have been found to:

- reject the infant's need for attachment and the behaviours the infant uses to try to get attachment
- be uncomfortable or hostile to signs of dependency
- dislike affectionate, face-to-face contact

- be more aversive to cuddly contact and physical contact
- show less emotion

When mothers don't show enjoyment holding their babies, babies eventually seem to turn off their more natural desire to be cuddled. When held, they seem to go limp, like a sack of potatoes.

These children have 'turned off wanting'. Of course, you can't fully turn off wanting; you just disconnect from your awareness of it. Your wanting gets relegated to the unconscious, where it remains in a very primitive form and has a sense of great urgency attached to it.

By contrast, babies with an **ambivalent attachment** became 'clingy', insisting on being picked up or holding on to their mothers. These children are associated with mothers who were inconsistent in meeting the needs of the child – perhaps sometimes being smothering or over-intrusive. This does not meet the need for genuine nurturing. Jasmin Lee Cori describes this style -

> *This second style has been called anxious attachment (Bowlby), compulsive care-seeking, ambivalent (Ainsworth), dependent, and preoccupied. All of these names reflect some important quality in the pattern. The dependence and care-seeking are obvious; the ambivalence, slightly more complex. Children with this style show a heightened need for closeness and an angry, rejecting quality. In the Strange Situation, a much-used research design, one-year-old children are extremely distressed at being left by mother but have a difficult time in accepting her ministrations when she tries to patch things up. They go back and forth between being very demanding and clingy and being hostile. I've chosen the term preoccupied because through both sets of behaviours, these children (and later adults) are so anxiously tied up with how available others are, that it dominates their lives.*

This style of attachment has been correlated with mothers who are less consistently rejecting than the self-sufficient children had, but not consistently responsive enough to create secure attachment. Sometimes they're there; sometimes they're not. Sometimes they are experienced as loving; other times as inexplicably rejecting. The preoccupied child (and later adult) doesn't know what to expect.

The third group, babies with a **disorganized attachment**, seemed to be most affected, and fluctuated between being 'clingy' and avoiding or distancing behaviours. This attachment type is much less common than the other two. Jasmin Lee Cori states -

> *Some children fit a pattern that is called disorganized or disorientated attachment. Here, there isn't a consistent pattern. These children show behaviours characteristic of one or more other attachment styles alternating between moments of fear and confusion. This is the pattern found in the majority of children who are abused.*

> *Of course, abusive parents aren't only abusive; sometimes they provided needed care. So, they are both a source of fear and a source of reassurance, and this is understandably confusing.*

> *The behavior of the child is likewise inconsistent. Such a child may appear confused or apprehensive in the presence of that parent or even dazed at times. How can you know if it's safe to go to Mommy if sometimes she comforts you and sometimes, she seems to spiral out of control and hits you?*

Research shows that attachment types persist into later childhood and adulthood. Insecure attachments have an ongoing adverse effect.

Children with avoidant attachments are likely to create psychological defences such as denying their own needs. They are likely to become reserved and aloof and parent themselves to a significant degree. Jasmin Lee Cori indicates that these children often experienced their parents valuing them 'not for being a child, but for growing out of it'. She states -

Children in this situation perceive that their parents don't want to deal with their needs and feelings and learn to conceal their emotions. The same child who goes limp like a sack of potatoes as an infant is the school-aged child with one-word responses when mother asks about his day or who keeps mother at arm's length. This child will not go to mother for help. Even if she wanted to connect with him later on, the child is now on guard, hidden behind a wall. ...

People who predominantly have this attachment style, have turned off their attachment needs, and, as one researcher suggests, become deaf to attachment-related signals. Better to be self-sufficient as possible. A person with this style is more armoured in relationships and tends to allow not much closeness. Letting others close enough to develop real feelings of attachment - even much later in life - feels scary. It is too close to the unbearable pain of feeling rejected as an infant when one was so utterly dependent.

In the second group, children and adults with *ambivalent attachments* are more likely to develop a dependent personality and have difficulty in trusting in themselves. Jasmin Lee Cori states -

Unfortunately, the strategies used to secure the desired attachment often drive people away. By the time we reach adulthood, these include –

- *heightened needs for closeness;*

- *hypervigilance about attachment signals;*

- *always questioning and testing the other's commitment;*

- *emphasizing need and helplessness in order to get others to stay;*

- *punishing others for not providing what is desired;*

- *anger when attachment needs are not met.*

Being alone, especially in times of distress, is upsetting for those with anxious attachment, and they don't do well when their attachment figures are away. In later relationships, they are likely to feel insecure when their romantic partner goes away, and are more likely to be jealous. Those with an anxious attachment style are always looking for love.

Children with this style appear too caught up in attachment concerns to explore their world, and there is some evidence that adults with this style are so preoccupied with relationships that they turn into under-achievers.

A disorganized attachment is the most problematic for the child's healthy psychological development. (Note that the disorganized attachment category is not the same as the clinical Attachment Disorder which affects a much smaller proportion of the population.) Jasmin Lee Cori states -

These children are often found to take on caretaking roles with their parents, in essence abandoning the child role altogether. It's a pretty smart response if you think about it. Children in these situations often see that adults can't really be trusted or aren't competent, so taking a provider role is probably safer.

- *Some of the effects associated with disorganized attachment include –*

- *marked impairments in emotional, social and cognitive functioning;*

- *not being able to soothe yourself;*

- *feeling that you are to blame for what was done to you and that you have no value;*

- *feeling alienated from the world around you;*

- *being vigilant, distrustful and avoiding intimacy ...*

The three insecure attachment patterns – avoidant, ambivalent, disorganized – are not completely distinct. Individuals may combine different elements of the three patterns. Personally, when I'm feeling insecure, I mostly display the behaviours of an avoidant attachment, but I do also have some ambivalent attachment behaviours.

Children and adults with insecure attachments are prone to anxiety which is an isolating, insidious and sometimes debilitating trait. They are over-represented in terms of developing neuroses or dysfunctional behaviours. Not all, or even most, individuals with insecure attachments develop such outcomes, but they are more likely to do so. Speaking as a person who grew up with an insecure attachment, I can say that there is a less visible but everyday price, in finding it difficult to trust in relationships. The second-guessing of yourself and others created by an insecure attachment can be a cruel self-fulfilling prophecy.

Jasmin Lee Cori indicates that children with insecure attachments 'heard' their mother telling them one or more of the following –

> *"I don't have it to give; You ask/take too much. Your needs are too much; I don't really care about you."*

Perhaps the deepest wound of an insecure attachment is missing out on the sense of belonging. Those with insecure attachments often go through life mostly feeling like the 'outsider', the one who doesn't fit.

So, what went wrong?

This can span the gamut from abuse and neglect at one end of the spectrum to more usually, at the other end of the spectrum, simply a mismatch between the mother's care or sensitivity and the feelings and needs of the child.

If the mother is not sufficiently attuned to her baby, she is too late meeting the baby's needs, or she meets the wrong need. Every mother misreads her baby sometimes, but the non-attuned mother is unable to repair those miscues. When the baby becomes enraged at her or his needs not being met, the mother retaliates with her own frustration, or distances herself, rejecting the baby's feelings and needs. Likewise, she is unable to fully comfort the baby's fears and distress. When the baby looks into her face, instead of seeing the baby's feelings and state accurately reflected in that mirror, the baby sees instead the mother's preoccupations and concerns. The baby's delight in her or his spontaneous discovery of itself and the world – the baby's True Self - goes unrecognized and unaffirmed.

In essence, the mothering is not 'good enough'.

How did that affect the baby or young child's psyche? For that we to turn again to Donald Winnicott.

Instead of feeling empowered and safe, the baby is sometimes afraid and overwhelmed. Children with an insecure attachment learn to doubt that they can completely rely on their mothers for comfort and safety. This can adversely affect the development of their confidence to explore their environment, be alone without anxiety, trust in others and to play freely.

The baby's healthy 'going on being' is interrupted. The baby must turn aside from discovering itself and working through its developmental challenges to instead focus on the mother and her mood. The child must try to repair the mother's mood so that she becomes available to the child again. The child learns to comply with the mother's mood and expectations. This precocious compliance creates a False Self. That brings a loss of creativity and the feeling of being 'real'. The child has to be something other than its True Self to get its needs met. The child learns that it's rage or fear cause his or her mother to not be available to them. The child learns not to trust their own feelings.

One of the deepest and most insidious wounds of an insecure attachment comes from the absence of nurturing touch, or from insensitive, callous or abusive touch. Nurturing touch helps a baby and child 'live' in their bodies. That is a core part of Winnicott's conception of what creates the True Self. The absence of nurturing touch separates us from us from our bodies.

Jasmin Lee Cori says –

> *"Appropriate touch also helps us locate ourselves in our bodies. The untouched child may be alienated from his or her body and experience feelings of unreality. The sense of reality comes from being grounded in the body, and touch is part of what accomplishes this. A lack of touch or abusive touch may also encourage dissociation, a psychic separation from the body. ... a child who has not been sufficiently touched becomes locked inside his or her own skin and then experiences normal touch as threatening. This is called tactile defensiveness. Such defensiveness can manifest as insensitivity or hypersensitivity to being touched or in being touch avoidant. Children who do not receive enough positive touch will often (unconsciously) feel untouchable, as if there must be something terribly wrong with them."*

I believe people with avoidant insecure attachments will be particularly susceptible to this tactile defensiveness. It is certainly true for me.

A secure attachment can also be fragile. A child can have a secure attachment in infancy and lose it later in childhood, through separation from their mother or other traumatic events. Bowlby's writings indicate that often the mother's extended absence for the birth of a subsequent child may have been distressing or traumatic for a young child.

Anyone who grew up with an insecure attachment as a baby or child has a wounded Inner Child. They have grown up experiencing a deficit in nurturing. Needs for nurturing that go unmet for a long time can deaden the spirit and the heart. It constricts the emotions, inhibiting our ability to love, and to experience the love of others. It can make us more susceptible to anxiety and depression. At its' worst it feels like living in a lifeless desert.

Without nurturing, psychological comfort and safety, the True Self wilts and retreats, and with it the feeling of being 'real' and distinctively yourself. The False Self grows.

The False Self

Winnicott recognized that we all need a False Self to some degree. The False Self has a dual role. Firstly, it serves to comply with the demands that the world makes on us. It allows us to fit into society, to conform enough with social customs and expectations to 'get by' without wearing 'our heart on our sleeve' and being either too vulnerable or abrasive.

Secondly, it hides and therefore protects the True Self. In this second role, its relationship with the True Self, Winnicott indicated that there are levels of health or pathology.

At the most negative, the False Self is completely dominant. The person may see themselves entirely in terms of their False Self, the Self that exists to meet the expectations of others.

At the second level, the True Self is 'acknowledged as a potential and allowed a secret life'. It may underlie a clinical illness which is serving a positive purpose, to preserve the individual in adverse circumstances.

At the next levels, the purpose of the False Self is to 'search for conditions which will make it possible for the True Self to come into 'its own'.

In health, the person lives their True Self, with the False Self only serving the minimum necessity of avoiding unnecessary social friction.

We shall see later that this understanding of the True Self and False Self is central to understanding ABs.

Summary

We have seen how a mother's lack of attunement to the feelings and needs of her baby or child creates an insecure attachment. The child learns that they cannot fully trust either others or themselves. They will become dependent and clingy, or reserved and aloof. That insecure attachment generally persists into adulthood. It makes a person prone to anxiety, and to other neuroses or mental illnesses.

A person with an insecure attachment has a wounded Inner Child and a deficit in nurturing. That deficit causes the True Self to retreat, diminishing the person's experience of themselves as being 'real' and engaging with life and others in a vital and spontaneous way. The False Self grows to unhealthy levels.

If you're reading this and recognize that you had an insecure attachment as a child, don't be dismayed. Recognizing the pain of that insecure attachment can be troubling. But you have already survived it, and that pain can be healed. Therapist's Jasmin Lee Cori's book *'The Emotionally Absent Mother: How to Recognize and Heal the Invisible Effects of Childhood Emotional Neglect'* is a good self-help resource for healing.

5. The Origins of the AB Identity – Insecure Attachment

I believe that ABs had insecure attachments with their mothers as babies and young children.

I can offer no proof of this. However, consider that empirical observations, replicated in different countries, indicate that around one-third of children have an insecure attachment. The AB identity uniquely keeps the symbols of infancy and its unmet needs, nappies, stuffed toys, pacifiers etcetera, very much in view. It is reasonable to consider that ABs are a subset of the much larger population who had an insecure attachment as a child.

I don't mean to offend the ABs who remember a good childhood relationship with their mother. Having an insecure attachment as a child does not require that a mother was abusive or neglectful. It is simply that the mother was not attuned to the needs of their child. This can occur for many, common reasons.

For example, I believe that as a child I had an avoidant (insecure) attachment. My mother was not a 'bad' mother. Initially, I was a sickly baby and she was anxious. In my first years, she lived far from the support of family and friends with a husband who, as per the time, took no role in caring for children. She brought up her first-born child (me) according 'to the book'. At the time, that meant there was a set way to bring up a child. For example, a mother wasn't supposed to pick up a crying child when they'd been put down to sleep in case they grew up dependent and 'clingy'. With the best of intentions, my mother wasn't attuned to my needs but to what 'the book' said.

Jasmin Lee Cori states –

> *"Holding mother responsible for our insecure attachment is not saying she is somehow bad or even uncaring. There are many things that may be going on. For one, she may love her baby but be frightened or repulsed by being needed. Unfortunately, this often leads to a vicious cycle, because the more she withdraws or withholds her care, the more the baby signals his need, and it is this signaling of need and urgency behind that may frighten the mother. Other contributors include being unskilled at reading a baby's signals; being preoccupied, overwhelmed or depressed; being insecure and overly sensitive to rejection; or having been under-mothered herself. If her mother was not able to graciously give to her or attune to her needs, if her mother was too busy or too cold, then this is the pattern that is branded into her, which she unwittingly repeats."*

Locating the source of the adult baby identity in an insecure attachment between mother and baby is consistent with Rosalie Bent's research on ABs. The 'Strange Situation' studies which identified children's attachment types were undertaken with children who were between 9 and 18 months old. This is consistent with

Rosalie's view that the formation of the adult baby identity is located very early, in infancy. It is also consistent with a key need for ABs. Rosalie identified the most important thing to ABs is to have their baby persona recognized as real, and the second most important requirement is to be in a parent/child relationship to some degree. This reflects the importance of the insecure childhood attachment and the unmet need for nurturing.

Knowing that AB's had an insecure attachment helps cast light on a key part of the AB identity. AB's very obviously have issues with their toilet training. A child with an insecure attachment is already experiencing a deficit in nurturing. Might a child in these circumstances be reluctant to surrender the intimate contact of nappy changing, which holds at least the possibility of nurturing?

In my case, I believe that toilet training was a milestone by which my mother judged her success as a parent. I've read the childcare manuals that were around in my infancy. Toilet training was supposed to be completed at an early age, again whether the child was ready or not. My mother wasn't toilet training me, she was toilet training the model child from the childcare manuals.

I suspect that toilet training was experienced by ABs as a demand for compliance and a diminution of nurturing that was already too scarce. Perhaps the child believed their compliance was a condition for their mother's continuing approval and affection. Remember also that precocious or forced compliance drives the False Self – the self that meets the needs of others. It seems likely that ABs experienced toilet training as a further distancing from their True Self, from feeling 'real'.

Differences Between ABs

I suspect that the different types of insecure attachments may align with important differences between ABs. These differences are likely reflected –

1. in their life history as ABs; and

2. in their relationships.

ABs with avoidant insecure attachments as children tend to unhealthily deny their feelings and needs. It seems more likely that they will –

- as children and adolescents, seek to be as independent of their parents as possible, and thus be less likely to show 'childish' needs through bedwetting or incontinence

- keep their AB side secret from everyone until later in life, concealing much of their AB needs and life from their partner for a long time, and be later in life in accepting themselves as AB or 'coming out' to others

- not seek or accept a partner being a mother to their child persona, and perhaps more likely to substitute AB fetish/fantasy material/pornography; and

- as an AB, not sustain sexual intimacy with a partner

I belong to this category of ABs. As an AB I was a 'slow learner/late developer', only fully accepting myself in my fifties. I had internalized my parents' silent demand to leave any display of the needs of early childhood behind.

ABs with an ambivalent or disorganized attachment as children are more likely to display their needs to engage the attention and care of others, although also possibly sabotaging that care. It seems more likely that they will -

1. as children and adolescents, unconsciously display their need for attachment through bedwetting and incontinence;

2. disclose their AB side to their families or close friends and accept understanding and support from these sources;

3. seek and accept a partner who will be a mother to their child persona, although also more likely have a troubled history in primary relationships through partners feeling overwhelmed by their AB needs; and

4. as an AB, sustain sexual intimacy with a partner.

Several published life stories by ABs seem to be consistent with this pattern for an ambivalent attachment.

I know what an avoidant attachment and behaviours feel like from firsthand experience. I am conscious that is not true for an ambivalent attachment. If you think I'm not reading the latter accurately, go with your own experience.

The above differences are important to understanding the dynamics, and sometimes conflicts, within the AB community. Although all ABs with an insecure attachment have deficits in nurturing and a wounded Inner Child, they will have different ways of responding to those deficits and wounds.

6. The Origins of the AB Identity – Trauma and Dissociation

For some ABs, it is possible that an insecure attachment to their mother, and an unmet need for nurturing, was enough to give rise to their child persona, and hence their AB identity.

But for many ABs, I think there was more to it.

I believe that for many ABs their child persona emerged within the psyche during a time of trauma. For some ABs that relates to abuse or neglect. For most, the trauma relates to the 'ordinary catastrophes' of childhood.

In my case, my baby persona originated in a traumatic temporary separation from my mother when I was aged three or four. My book *'Living With Chrissie – My Life as an Adult Baby'* describes the event.

> *"My mother went to a sporting club, presumably for some much-needed respite from caring alone for two small children. While she was playing, I was left with my [two year younger] sister in the care of other adults. My sister became inconsolably distressed at the separation. I felt responsible, either for caring for her, or at least for showing a good example. But in the face of her distress, I couldn't contain my own and ended up bursting into tears and wetting my pants. I couldn't see my mother and she seemed to have gone beyond hope of return. I felt terrified, overwhelmed and abandoned. I had failed to be the 'big boy' I was expected to be. My sister was picked up and comforted by the other adults, but I don't remember being so comforted. My mother recalled the event as sufficiently traumatic that visits to the sporting club were not soon repeated. The event necessarily passed from my mind but when it was recounted by my mother in later childhood, I could recall it vividly. Many, many years later I would understand this was where Baby Chrissie sprang from."*

My mother's subsequent account indicated that she recognized that the event was distressing but evidently was not aware that I was traumatized. This is not surprising for the mother of a child with an avoidant attachment.

I suspect an experience like mine is common amongst ABs. Remember that for a young child, separations from their mother can be deeply traumatic. What may seem to a casual observer as simply distress, may, in fact, be trauma. There is a greater propensity for children with insecure attachments to be traumatized – both in terms of their own greater vulnerability, and because their parents are unaware of their child's real needs and feelings.

Winnicott indicates that separation from the mother goes beyond distress to trauma when it exceeds the time the child can hold the image of their mother in their minds. The length of time the child can hold that image is affected by whether the child has a secure or insecure attachment. Trauma leaves a lasting effect. The child experiences it as '*a break in life's continuity so that primitive defences now become organized to defend against a repetition of 'unthinkable anxiety' or a return of the acute confusional state ...*"

In essence, it becomes a wound.

The origin of a persona within the psyche in such traumatic circumstances is referred to as 'splitting'. The traumatized persona is split off from the self and quarantined within the psyche.

We commonly associate this phenomenon and the existence of sub-personalities or personas with Dissociative Identity Disorder (DID), formerly known as Multiple Personality Disorder (MPD). A person with DID has multiple personas or 'parts'. In an unhealthy state, the parts act independently of the self.   However, with therapy and self-management, the parts work cooperatively and there is a healthy sense of self. In the absence of dysfunction, the person has a minority identity, not a disorder. There are many high functioning people with dissociative conditions. Dr Steinberg states that they:

> "*... run the gamut from PhDs to prostitutes and are generally highly intelligent, creative, brave, articulate and likeable. Many are accomplished professionals, married, raising children, holding down responsible jobs.*"

Friends, colleagues and acquaintances are often not aware the person has a dissociative condition. I have a relative in my extended family who has DID. He is a teacher who has taught special needs children at schools around the world. It was our experience with our relative that prompted my wife and myself to consider that I may have a child persona, and to seek a counsellor experienced in such matters.

A parallel between DID and being AB is that the latter's child persona can be a different gender from the adult self. Rosalie Bent indicates –

> '*... around half of physically male Adult Babies and Little Ones identity as female infant/toddler, indeterminate or sissy. ... 'Sissy' and 'girl' are quite similar and when determining your Little One's gender, keep in mind the sissy option. It is a subset of the female gender, but for simplicity, I have used it as a separate one.*'

In most cases, the male adult self and the baby/little girl persona happily coexist, each in their own space, there is no sexual dysphoria as for a transgender person.

I believe that ABs and people with DID are on the same continuum. Both have discrete personas or sub-personalities. For both, psychological health lies in accepting the existence of those personas, meeting their valid needs and having a cooperative relationship with the self.

Dissociation

Dissociation is significant for both DID and being AB. Dissociation is where the painful memory of the trauma, and resulting persona, has been deeply repressed to enable the self to function. Dr Marlene Steinberg is the psychiatrist who developed the standard diagnostic questionnaire for identifying dissociative conditions. She states -

> "*To help us survive, certain perceptions, feelings, sensations, thoughts, and memories related to the trauma are split off from full awareness and encoded in some peripheral level of awareness. Miraculously, dissociation alters reality but allows the person to stay in contact with it in order to help himself.*" [The Stranger in the Mirror: Dissociation The Hidden Epidemic]

For both ABs and people with DID, the existence of personas within the psyche is commonly denied for a long time for fear of being thought crazy. It often takes a long time for an AB to accept that they have a baby/child persona, notwithstanding a lifetime of compulsive child-like behaviour completely at odds with their adult self.

Let's look further.

Dr Steinberg distinguishes five elements of dissociation –

1. Amnesia – gaps in memory or 'lost time';

2. De-personalisation – a feeling of detachment from yourself or looking at yourself as an outsider would;

3. De-realization – a feeling of detachment from your environment, or people that were previously familiar to you;

4. Identity confusion – a feeling of uncertainty, puzzlement or conflict about who you are - perhaps a continuing struggle going on inside you to define yourself;

5. Identity alteration – a shift in role or identity, accompanied by such changes in your behaviour that are observable to others – you may experience the shift as a personality switch or loss of control over yourself to someone else inside you.

Dissociation is evident in two behaviours common to conflicted ABs (those denying the existence and needs of their child persona) –

1. 'triggering', and

2. the 'binge and purge' cycle.

Triggering

'Triggering' is a common indication of dissociation. For conflicted ABs, it commonly arises when a sight, smell or touch creates a compelling need to act out their baby 'side'. This is typically the need to put on a nappy but may extend to other baby paraphernalia or activities. The need may be so strong as to be an irresistible compulsion.

Rosalie Bent describes these triggers -

> *"... some attribute about an object that can trigger a regressive episode. It is almost never a generic object, but rather something very specific that triggers a memory or emotion which in turn, triggers the regression. For example, it may be a soft toy, but not just any soft toy. It may be a Care Bear toy, but not just anyone, but rather a pink one, of a specific size and style that clearly has a deep-rooted memory attached to it."*

My experience with triggers is described in *'Living With Chrissie – My Life as an Adult Baby'* -

A compelling desire for a nappy could be set off at a moment's notice from any number of visual 'triggers'. It could be seeing a magazine advertisement with a baby in a nappy; anything to do with breastfeeding – especially pictures of women wearing maternity bras; a line of cloth nappies drying on a clothesline would do it every time. For years, I couldn't walk down the babies' aisle in a supermarket without 'triggering' the insistent need to get home and put on a nappy. This behaviour was in strong contrast to who I was otherwise – a person of strong emotional control, able to defer gratification.

Triggering involves the dissociative components of 'identity alteration', 'identity confusion' and past amnesia. The sudden compulsion to don a nappy is clearly outside usual adolescent or adult behaviour. Depending on the level of compulsion, it can represent either identity confusion or identity alteration. In the latter case, it is the AB's child persona 'breaking through' and demanding that its' needs be met. Amnesia is involved because the source of this compulsion is initially unexpected and mysterious – it arises from a persona whose existence and origin has been veiled by past amnesia.

Binge and Purge

The 'binge and purge' cycle is an even more stark example of dissociation. The following description is from my book *'Becoming Me – the Journey of Self-Acceptance'* -

The term [binge and purge] comes from the disease bulimia where the sufferer gorges on food and then, in deep self-disgust and loathing, makes themselves sick until they purge their stomachs empty. For adult babies, it means something different. The cycle starts with a 'binge' - buying a stash of nappies, baby clothes and baby paraphernalia. It's like a drug addict going on a 'bender'. Our nappy fetish becomes stronger and accompanied by frequent masturbation. The internal conflict grows stronger. Pleasure is now fighting shame and remorse. The emotional 'let down' after each successive orgasm becomes more painful and demoralizing. But we are on a runaway train we can't stop, even if we wanted to – and we don't want to. Eventually, the growing internal conflict drives masturbation to a peak. The emotional 'let down' after the final peak orgasm is intensely painful. The disgust, remorse and self-loathing are scourging and gut-wrenching.

The only thing that will assuage the intense emotional pain is to 'purge'. We convince ourselves that we can now completely banish our need for baby things. At its worst, this often means collecting every last item of our baby collection and throwing it away. In my case, I would throw everything into neighbourhood clothing recycling bins, as a way of making the purge irrevocable. Only then would the painful remorse occasioned by the binge be soothed. It would be replaced by a new transient kind of 'high' – a sense of being cleansed of our weakness and perversity and free to live a normal healthy life of which we can be proud. In my case, I would declare to my wife that I was giving up my 'nappy thing' forever. I meant it when I said it. I would pray for God to give me the strength to maintain my abstinence.

The aftermath of the purge would last a while. In my case my abstinence, at least in terms of physically wearing nappies, would last some months, sometimes nearly a year. I would masturbate without nappies for a time, but the comforting fantasies of being babied were always present. Eventually, the unmet needs of my baby side would grow more and more insistent and I would 'binge' again. With each new binge, I would fool myself that, this time, I could keep my baby side under sufficient control so that things wouldn't get out of hand and I wouldn't be driven to purge again. Of course, that was a 'fool's hope'. The internal conflict hadn't gone away or being healed - it was just re-booted.

In my experience, the binge and purge cycle has a powerfully negative effect on the personality and moods of adult babies. We are tense, anxious, irritable, distracted, and have difficulty concentrating on anything other than nappies. At the crescendo of the cycle, just before the final crash and purge it's like a complete personality change, for the worse. I really hated and despised myself at those times. It must be awful for our partners to live with.

The binge and purge cycle is a truly 'Jekyll and Hyde' experience. At its peak, it overpowers the adult self. Like triggering, it involves the dissociative components of 'identity alteration', 'identity confusion' and past amnesia. However, binge and purge involves two internal personas – the child and the AB's punitive parent. Identity confusion and identity alternation are evident in the seesaw as these two personas successively 'breakthrough' and drive the AB's compulsive behaviour. The inner source of this disturbing cycle is mysterious and incomprehensible to the conflicted AB – arising from personas whose existence and origin has been veiled by past amnesia.

In my firsthand experience, at its peak, the binge and purge cycle represents a level of behavioural and emotional disturbance which approaches that of someone with moderate DID. Dr Steinberg states -

"In the most basic terms dissociative identity disorder, or DID, formerly called multiple personality disorder, is what happens when your 'inner child' or some other hidden part of yourself operates independently, seizes control, and makes you act inappropriately or impairs your ability to function."

That is an accurate depiction of the ABs' binge and purge cycle.

The Character of Dissociation for ABs

I had long remembered-in-outline the traumatic event when I was a child. But it was only with an experienced counsellor that I fully recalled the terror it engendered and understood that my sense of trauma was so overpowering that it split off a distinct persona. It was a kind of psychic 'death'. To this day, occasionally in a strange and emotionally challenging physical environment, I will find myself catastrophizing and preparing to deal with dying in a fashion which has no connection to the present reality. I now realize that I was re-experiencing that original childhood trauma and fear of dying.

The delay in recall and the emotional 'flashbacks' are consistent with what Dr Steinberg explains about dissociation and the memory of traumatic events. Those memories are divided and compartmentalized within the mind – the memory of each sense is stored in a different 'compartment' – sight is separated from sound, from touch, from smell, from feeling. That was why I had a visual memory of the incident, but didn't understand the trauma until the memory of my feelings was reclaimed and joined with my visual memory. It also explains that it is the memory of my feelings as a traumatized three or four-year-old that floods back when I catastrophize in strange and confronting physical surroundings.

Dr Steinberg indicates that *'the younger a child is when the trauma occurs, the more likely it is that the event will be dissociated'*. She indicates that dissociative symptoms are common, although often masked by, and misdiagnosed for, other conditions such as anxiety, depression or bipolar. She cites a recent study which estimates that dissociative symptoms affect fourteen per cent of the US population. She also suggests that DID is not as rare as once thought and affects an estimated one per cent of the US population. Given the likely link between dissociation and the AB identity, it is possible that for some ABs, symptoms of anxiety or depression or other conditions may also be related to undiagnosed dissociated trauma in childhood.

Using the questionnaires in Dr Steinberg's book *'The Stranger in the Mirror: Dissociation, The Hidden Epidemic'* I assessed the extent to which I displayed the five elements of dissociation – amnesia, de-personalisation, de-realisation, identity confusion and identity alteration. I got scores showing no or mild symptoms for the first three elements. However, I got scores for moderate levels of identity confusion and identity alteration. This is consistent with my experience of being a functional adult with a subjectively real child persona.

However, this doesn't seem to fit neatly with expected patterns of dissociation. Dr Steinberg seems to expect that those with a distinct persona or sub-personality, as indicated by moderate or higher levels of identity alteration, would have moderate or higher levels for the other four elements of dissociation. They would be diagnosed with Dissociative Identity Disorder (DID) or Dissociative Disorder Not Otherwise Specified (DDNOS). Dr Steinberg states -

" ... research has found that identity alteration, as with all the dissociative symptoms, occurs along a spectrum of intensity: mild levels in the general population; mild to moderate levels in people with non-dissociative psychiatric disorders, but also with people with dissociative disorder not otherwise specified (DDNOS); severe levels of identity alteration in people with dissociative identity disorder (DID).

A person with moderate levels of identity alteration may act as if he or she is like two (or more) different people, but it's not clear whether these identity alterations assume complete control of a person's behaviour or represent separate personalities. A normally shy person who gets drunk at a party, for example, may turn into a lampshade-on-the-head scene maker or an X-rated sexual provocateur but maybe disinhibited from constraints on his or her usual self rather than under the control of a distinct identity fragment.

Severe identity alteration, the sina qua non of DID, involves a person's shifting between distinct personality states that take control of his or her behaviour and thought. These alter personalities are more clearly defined and distinctive than the personality fragments that characterize moderate levels of identity alteration. Each alter has its' own name, memories, traits and behaviour patterns.

Identity alteration differs from identity confusion in that identity confusion represents the internal dimension of identity disturbance, whereas identity alteration represents the external dimension. A person with identity confusion, in other words, has thoughts and feelings of uncertainty and conflict related to his or her identity; a person with identity alteration manifests the uncertainty and conflict behaviourally."

Compared to Dr Steinberg's research, ABs appear to follow a different pattern. They have a distinct child persona which manifests behaviourally, but without some of the other elements of dissociation. I didn't experience the mental confusion – the chatter of many internal voices – that is experienced by those with out-of-control DID. Nor did I suffer from present-day amnesia. People with uncontrolled DID can sometimes become aware of gaps in their recent memory – such as finding things they don't remember buying or waking up in locations they didn't remember going to. That doesn't seem to be the case with ABs. Even in my worst 'binge and purge' times, I was always aware of what was happening – my adult self just felt powerless to stop it.

I suspect that for many ABs, dissociation is a chronic background factor. Dr Steinberg states –

"One of the trickier aspects of dissociation is that the more chronic some symptoms are, the less stress they may cause because you've adapted to them and they have become as normal to you as breathing."

That is so true for me. In researching and writing this book, the pervasive influence of dissociation on my personality and experience of life, has been a revelation. No wonder I didn't see it before. It's always been there from childhood – by what standard would I know that it isn't usual? And to the extent that I did have to recognize that my behaviours were atypical, denial came into play. I simply refused to explore or accept the implications of just how differently my psyche as an AB was hard-wired. It doesn't scare me. I've already been living it. But it has explained a lot. I now realise that, as a conflicted AB, my experience of dissociation included a background level of internal conflict – guilt and self-loathing; compulsive fetishistic masturbation at least every few days; and widely spaced episodes of turmoil, manifested in the binge and purge cycle.

I suspect that being AB has a similar relationship to dissociation, as do crossdressers or transvestites, who have a subjectively real persona of another gender within their psyche.

Two Factors – Insecure Attachment + Dissociated Trauma

I believe that being AB originates with an insecure childhood attachment, *together* with the emergence of a child persona from a dissociated traumatic event in childhood. Health professionals working in the field of dissociation have linked the two phenomena. (See 'Recognizing Dissociation in Preschool Children' by Fran Waters, The International Society for the Study of Dissociation Volume 23 Number 4 July/August 2005 which includes an extensive list of references. See the annotated list of references.)

The combination of these two phenomena is consistent with the comparative rarity of ABs. Empirical studies found that up to one-third of the population had an insecure childhood attachment. By contrast ABs are much less common. Rosalie Bent estimates that ABs represent 0.1% of the population – or one-in-a-thousand people. This suggests that dissociation is a key factor in distinguishing ABs from the larger population with an insecure childhood attachment. ABs appear to be a small subset of those with stronger dissociative symptoms – the latter constituting up to one per cent of the population (one in a hundred).

If you're an AB and you've experienced, or are still experiencing, triggering or the 'binge and purge' cycle, then you may have dissociated trauma in your past. Don't be afraid - that trauma can be healed. Dissociated childhood trauma is a serious issue. I urge you to seek counselling with a professional counsellor experienced in identifying and treating trauma and dissociation. This may be a counsellor who has some experience of working with DID, or an LGBTQ friendly counsellor used to working with minority identities. The empathy and therapeutic skill of the counsellor is the central requirement. But all-things-being-equal in that respect a counsellor with experience in Internal Family Systems (IFS) therapy would be a good prospect.

If you want to read further about dissociation see Dr Marlene Steinberg's book *'The Stranger in the Mirror: Dissociation The Hidden Epidemic'*.

7. Beginnings, Denial, Repression and Internal Conflict

The sequence of things is important.

For ABs, I believe it is most likely that the insecure attachment came first. The dissociative childhood trauma and the splitting off of a child persona came next. Remember, attachment patterns are established very early in life. They are well developed by the time a child is 12 months old. The insecure attachment made us more vulnerable to being traumatized by the 'ordinary catastrophes' of childhood, such as temporary separations from mother. Alternatively, for some, it is possible that they initially had a secure attachment in infancy, and a traumatic event in childhood led to an insecure attachment. Whatever the relationship between insecure attachment and trauma, the AB behaviours and identities only came much later.

In my case, I believe that I developed an avoidant insecure attachment with my mother in my first year of life. When I was around three or four, I was traumatized by a temporary separation from my mother. I believe that was when I split off my baby girl persona. I didn't become aware of a fascination with, and need for, nappies until about age ten. The fascination with nappies was accompanied by fantasies of being babied by a warm, caring mother-substitute. The age of ten is before puberty. In those initial years, I believe that my need for, and experience of, wearing nappies was about obtaining non-sexual emotional comfort. Of course, I didn't understand at the time, but this was my child persona 'breaking through'.

I believe my life history is representative of many ABs. From published life stories and studies by health professionals, the onset of the AB identity is typically around age ten. (See my book *'The Adult Baby Identity – Coming Out as an Adult Baby'* for a discussion of these initial stages of the AB identity). This usually takes the form of rediscovering nappies. Like me, this is not a casual interest, but rather a compelling, irresistible need. That suggests dissociated trauma. It is consistent with a traumatized baby or very young child persona seeking comfort at a deeply instinctive and infantile level.

The key point is that the first manifestation of the AB identity came well after the insecure attachment was established, and well after the first traumatizing event.

We were living with pain and despair long before we become AB.

Our Inner Child was wounded long before we became AB.

We felt we didn't belong, long before we became AB.

Being AB is a response to a broken childhood – not the cause.

It is clearly an attempt at self-comfort. Presumably, that was because as children with insecure attachments, we didn't trust that we could get the comfort we needed from our parents. From the life histories and clinical studies of ABs it is clear that from the outset, around age ten, the fascination with nappies is covert. While we didn't understand our identity or its origins, we *did* understand that it would not be approved of, or accepted, by our parents. We were on our own.

Puberty complicates matters. Our awakening sexuality is grafted onto a non-sexual AB identity which is already present. Of course, from the outset, that existing identity shapes and informs our sexuality. Nappies go from being a comfort/transitional object to a fetish object. Winnicott explicitly recognizes the possibility of such a progression. And, as for any teenager, our sexuality becomes an outlet, and a release, for the powerful drives within the psyche. And ABs bring a lot to that table!

Denial and Repression

Being an AB is a big deal.

It's a mind-fucking, one-in-a-thousand identity, that stays with you for life - whether you want it or not!

It's all too much to digest quickly or easily. And like everyone else the world over, ABs don't digest the big stuff quickly or easily. We refuse to accept just how big a deal being AB is. Our psyche is hard-wired very differently from everyone else we know. WTF! We fear if we accepted just how different and life-changing being AB is – it would all be bad, or we couldn't handle it. A big part of the mind-fuck is *why?* - where did the identity come from? We didn't just have a bad day and become ABs. We suspect, and fear, something deep or big must have happened.

As we have seen, I believe that for many of us, being AB comes from the combination of an insecure childhood attachment with our mothers/parent *and* childhood trauma. Both are difficult to deal with.

The insecure childhood attachment is painful to acknowledge. It means accepting that as children, we often felt lonely, fearful and unloved. So, we deny it. Denial is a conscious or active refusal to acknowledge the full significance of something we, deep down, know is true. Denial commonly involves minimizing or distorting unpleasant experiences – "it wasn't so bad" or "there were good times." We twist our minds to avoid (re)experiencing what will cause us pain. If you had an insecure childhood attachment, you know it. You lived it. But we just don't want to touch that hotplate again. A person in denial can push back pretty hard against someone, or a situation, that touches on the unwanted truth.

Jasmin Lee Cori talks about the difficulty in accepting unpleasant truths about our childhoods -

> *"Often it will take quite a bit of time in therapy for someone with significant mother wounds to really begin to tell the truth about their childhood. There's a considerable difference between the story one tells at first and the lived experience, and it is the lived experienced, stored in the unconscious, that takes time to get to. As this is unearthed, the story that was constructed to protect the wound slowly crumbles.*
>
> *Even for those who are quite aware that their relationships with their mothers somehow fall short, opening to the full depth of what was missing is likely to be resisted and happens only slowly over time. Because the wound is so painful, we naturally shy away from it. We become less sensitized only as some of the pain is carefully drained away and we have grown stronger."*

Although the under-mothered often have some sense that there was something they missed and that this 'something' affects them yet today, we seldom see the correlations in a direct way."

The childhood trauma is different, and even more difficult. It was too much for us to handle when it happened. So, we dissociated. Our psyche split-off a child persona. We split-off the overwhelming fear and hurt. Our psyche buried both deep. It's called repression. It's not the conscious mind at work – it is the unconscious safely quarantining things that are too difficult for us to handle, so we can continue to function. If a persona and memories are repressed, we genuinely don't know they are there. It is amnesia.

But it doesn't stay that way forever. Present-day experiences can trigger the return of fragments of those repressed memories. As we saw in an earlier section, the repressed persona will sometimes 'breakthrough' and influence or control our behaviour. After that has been happening for a while, repression can start to shade into denial. Our conscious mind has become aware that there is something *'behind the curtain'*, but we consciously refuse to accept the significance of what we are experiencing. And for ABs, the repression starts to break down very early. That is the hidden gift of being AB, as we shall see in the discussion of the False Self below. We know at times our adult selves don't have full control over our behaviour, but we refuse to consider what this implies.

Dr Steinberg states –

" ... people suffering from a dissociative disorder often have a huge amount of denial. ... Their worst fear is that if they talk about their symptoms to a therapist, they'll immediately be labelled as a freak or a crazy person.

Very often people who have separate parts of themselves keep them hidden, because they don't think of them as well-defined personalities, but more as 'aspects' of their own personalities or different internal voices or puzzling 'sides' of themselves with which they are not in touch with all the time."

That was me!

I denied the existence of my child persona for around fifty years! Despite decades of compulsive behaviours at odds with my adult-self, I would not accept that I had a distinct child persona within my psyche. I was three or four years of age when I was traumatized and the persona I now recognize as Chrissie, emerged within my psyche. I was in my early fifties when I went to a counsellor experienced in dissociation, who helped me identify and accept my child persona. In the interim, Chrissie was unrecognized and unnamed, but she created merry-hell with my life. She was a source of seemingly bizarre, confronting and disruptive behaviours that were completely out of character with my reserved, responsible adult self.

My denial took the form of preferring to think I had a bizarre sexual fetish. That fitted with the compulsive behaviours. But it didn't explain why I sometimes got non-sexual emotional comfort from wearing nappies or fantasies of being babied by mother-substitutes. Paradoxically, despite my inhibited personality, I found it easier to fear I was a pervert than to accept that I shared my consciousness with an innocent child persona. I suspect this is true for many conflicted ABs.

Further, I suspect a good number of diaper lovers (DLs) are actually adult babies in denial – *"it's just a thing for nappies/diapers"*. Many DL's may be genuine fetishists, for whom a diaper/nappy is exclusively associated with sexual expression. Many 'littles' / 'kinksters' / age players may not consider they have a subjectively real child persona. But if someone gains any non-sexual comfort from a nappy/diaper, if they have experienced any triggering or 'binge and purge' cycles, then there are probably deeper processes at work within the psyche – whether this is acknowledged or not. Suggesting to people in denial, that they are in denial, doesn't work too well. Things just have to take their course.

Internal Conflict

Denial and repression leave ABs with an internal conflict deep in our psyche. For the purposes of understanding the inner life of an adult baby, I use the concept of a dialogue between our Inner Parent, Adult and Inner Child. The idea of dialogue within our psyche is a key feature of psychotherapy and is applicable to everyone (not just ABs).

With conflicted ABs, the three internal actors are at war with each other.

- The Inner Parent is brutally critical and punishing toward the Inner Child.

- The Inner Child is wounded - hurt, angry, greedy, selfish and rebellious.

- The Adult Self is weak, like an ineffective umpire in a very rough sporting match. It is unable to stop the critical Inner Parent abusing the wounded Inner Child or to stop the latter from rebelling and throwing tantrums.

The punitive Inner Parent doesn't accept the baby persona as real or healthy. This is the kernel of the internal conflict. It is a denial by one part of the psyche of another part – in effect a denial of the AB's own identity. The punitive Inner Parent denies any need for nurturing. They say *'Pull yourself together! You're a grown up!'* As a result, the wounded Inner Child re-experiences the original wound created in the insecure attachment. Their genuine needs are not met and they again feel hurt, alone and abandoned.

With the need for nurturing brutally denied, the conflicted AB feels their heart and spirit deadened. To recapture a sense of being alive they are driven to compulsive masturbation. Their adult baby identity is largely expressed as a sexual fetish. Though they put on a nappy to masturbate and perhaps have other baby clothes or paraphernalia, these are not much more than sexual 'props'. They resort to the 'high' of psychologically unsafe masochistic fantasies or behaviours, or risk unsafe exposure. The masochistic fantasies can best be understood as attempts to revisit the original insecure childhood attachment with mother, in the desperate, unconscious hope of a different outcome. Such fantasies involve being dominated by a parent-substitute figure. The masochistic component includes coercion, intentional humiliation and shaming. These elements intensify the identification with being a helpless, dependant baby who wants and needs love and protection. This is our wounded Inner Child screaming for nurturing.

But because the psychologically unsafe fantasies are a product of deep internal conflict, the AB's need for nurturing is not met. They are still guilty and ashamed about the existence and needs of their child persona. For me, at this point, I needed the coercion element to pretend to myself that I had to be forced to comply with, and enjoy, the infantile need to be loved and protected by a parent figure. You can't give comfort to a part of yourself you are at the same time denying and berating.

Masturbation temporarily relieves the tension of the savage internal conflict. Episodically, the compulsive behaviour takes control of, and tyrannises the lives of conflicted adult babies. In turn, we feel remorse for our lack of self-control, which intensifies the internal conflict. Eventually, this builds to a peak of the 'binge and purge' cycle.

But ultimately denial and repression don't work. They start breaking down. It's a bit like trying to force an angry, unwilling cat back into a box. It commonly gets harder to maintain dissociation the older you get.

False Self

When we are trying to deny the baby persona in our psyche, this is our False Self at work. It is trying to keep the façade in place that will be acceptable to others.

But remember that the other role of the False Self is to protect the True Self. The False Self does that in several ways. It hides the True Self, so that it is 'acknowledged as a potential and allowed a secret life'. So even when we are hiding our identity as a secret sexual fetish, our False Self is keeping our identity, our True Self alive.

Because as awful as a conflicted dissociated life can sometimes be, it is better than losing all hope of recovering our True Self.

With hindsight, I can see that my False Self served a useful purpose in keeping my deepest wounds and needs away from further trauma at the hands of my unaccepting, emotionally austere family. I would have been too fragile to protect myself from their disapproval of my secret identity.

But the False Self also searches 'for conditions which will make it possible for the True Self to come into its' own'. In my experience, the savage internal conflict of denying my baby persona eventually becomes too debilitating and exhausting to maintain. It takes too much psychic energy to keep the dissociation holding the feelings of an insecure childhood attachment and childhood trauma at bay. Eventually, whether through exhaustion, or a crisis that represents a cry for help, we are brought to the road to acceptance.

That is the hidden logic of the False Self discerned by Donald Winnicott! Even as we are consumed finding the energy to deny our identity, this is laying the groundwork by which our True Self will win out.

There is a parallel understanding in Internal Family Systems (IFS) Therapy developed by Richard Schwartz. In IFS there are internal personas, called 'parts' led by a unifying Self. There are several categories of parts – 'exiles' and 'protectors'. An AB's child persona would be an exile and their Inner Parent would be a protector. Richard Schwartz indicates that 'protectors' will only let the 'exiles' out into the light of day, and acceptance, when the protectors feel it is safe to do so. IFS therapy involves working with a counsellor to facilitate that process.

In my case, I didn't fully come out to myself as an AB until I had retired from my job, and with it, my family's livelihood and financial security didn't need to be protected from me being 'outed'. This is example of the hidden logic of the False Self or the IFS 'protectors' at work.

When I accepted my baby persona, the internal conflict stopped and the compulsive behaviours stopped. What remained was a healthy adult baby identity that is a source of innocent comfort, security, happiness and wonder. For me, this is compelling proof of the existence of a subjectively real child persona within my psyche. I still have a nappy fetish, but it's not a compulsion.

Summary

The AB identity is a response to a broken childhood. It is not the cause of that brokenness. The insecure attachment with our mother, and the first traumatic event, came well before the first manifestations of the AB identity. The latter generally occurs around age ten, before puberty. It commonly consists of a fascination and deep irresistible need for nappies. That mysterious compulsion is consistent with dissociated trauma. It is an attempt to self-comfort. It represents a traumatized baby or young child persona seeking non-sexual nurturing at a deep instinctual and infantile level. But as children with insecure attachments, we know deep down we are on our own, that our need for nurturing comfort won't be accepted or met.

Puberty grafts our new sexuality onto an existing AB identity. Nappies go from being a source of comfort to a fetish object. AB's deny and repress their child persona, and its origins. Typically, we live for many years with a savage internal conflict about our identity. Our fetish becomes a way of distracting ourselves from a recognition and acceptance of who we are. In one sense, that is our False Self keeping a publicly acceptable façade in place. But in another, deeper sense, our False Self is protecting our identity, our True Self, by keeping it hidden until we are ready to accept ourselves.

8. Winnicott and the Child Persona

The most important quality of the AB's child persona is that it is subjectively real. Accepting this is what resolves the internal conflict for Adult Babies.

For non-conflicted ABs, one of our greatest fears is that others will not understand or accept our child persona is subjectively real. We fear others will instead, think we are neurotic, indulgent or just plain crazy. Many health professionals work with models of psychology which cannot accept a healthy identity based on a multiplicity of consciousness.

Donald Winnicott understood child personas and their origins. In his book '*Playing and Reality*', published just before he died in 1971, he cites working with an adult client with a subjectively real child persona. The client is not AB, but his child persona seems to share many of the characteristics of AB's child personas.

Winnicott was counselling a middle-aged, married, successful professional man. After listening to his client Winnicott said –

> *"I am listening to a girl. I know perfectly well that you are a man, but I am listening to a girl, and I am talking to a girl. I am telling this girl: You are talking about penis envy."*

Winnicott, an experienced and expert psychotherapist, identified that his client was speaking from the standpoint of child persona of another gender. That persona was sufficiently real within the client's psyche to replicate the subconscious of a biological female child or adolescent. (The concept of penis envy is understandably problematic from a feminist perspective. Feminists might take some comfort from the fact that, in this instance, it is being attributed to a biological male! The concept might be okay, provided that vagina/womb envy is also recognized.)

In subsequent exchanges –

> *The client stated – "If I were to tell someone else about this girl, I would be called mad."*

> *Winnicott stated – "The girl that I was talking to … What she wants is full acknowledgement of herself and of her own rights over your body. … she has always hoped that the analysis would in fact find out that this man, yourself, is and always has been a girl …"*

> *Winnicott reflected – " … I had never before fully accepted the complete dissociation between the man (or woman) and the aspect of the personality that has the opposite sex. In the case of this man the dissociation was nearly complete."*

"Now the new position had been reached the patient felt a sense of relationship with me, and this was extremely vivid. It had to do with identity. The pure female split-off element found a primary unity with me as an analyst, and this gave the man a feeling of having started to live."

Winnicott sees the child persona as a matter of identity!

He understands its origin in dissociation. He doesn't describe his client's identity as pathological or in terms of mental illness. The client's acceptance of his child persona is welcomed in terms - 'a feeling of having started to live' – which indicate that Winnicott saw the acceptance as bringing the client closer to the client's True Self. Remember this is 1971, nearly fifty years ago! This is exactly what ABs are struggling to get others to recognize and accept now - in 2019.

In the short description of the case, there is no reference to any behavioural manifestations of the client's formerly dissociated persona ie. crossdressing. But given the brevity of the discussion, it is possible that this may have been present.

Further, Winnicott evidently had sufficient experience working with such clients as to make some very insightful generic observations. He evidently encountered child personas of the opposite gender, in both male and female clients.

It is rewarding to review one's current clinical material keeping in mind this one example of dissociation, the split-off girl element in a male patient. The subject can quickly become vast and complex, so that few observations must be chosen for special mention.

(a) One may, to one's surprise, find that one is dealing with and attempting to analyse the split-off part, while the main functioning person appears only in projected form. This is like treating a child only to find that one is treating one or other parent by proxy. Every possible variation on this theme may come one's way.

(b) The other-sex part may be completely split off so that, for instance, a man may not be able to make any link at all with the split-off part. This applies especially when the personality is otherwise sane and integrated. Where the functioning personality is already organized into multiple splits there is less accent on 'I am sane', and therefore less resistance against the idea 'I am a girl' (in the case of a man) or 'I am a boy' (in the case of a girl).

(c) There may be found clinically a near-complete other-sex dissociation, organized in relation to external factors at a very early date, mixed in with later dissociations as a defence ... The reality of this later organized defence may militate against the patient's revival of the earlier reactive split.

(d) The split-off other-sex part of the personality tends to remain of one age, or to grow but slowly. ...

(e) ... It is interesting that the existence of this split-off female element actually prevents homosexual practice. In the case of my patient he always fled from homosexual advances at the critical moment because (as he came to see and tell me) putting homosexuality into practice would establish his maleness which (from the split-off female element self) he never wanted to know for certain.

Winnicott identifies that the child persona likely originated in dissociation at a 'very early' point in life; may have been completely denied by the client; nevertheless is an important and influential feature of the psyche; may be permanent, and evidently need not be pathological. Again, all this in 1971!

Winnicott also finds that the character of the child persona can be influenced not just by the psyche of a client, but by their parent's disposition. In this case, he and the client identified that the client's mother would have preferred the client was a girl. For me, an adult male with a baby girl persona, this was a confronting perspective – as Winnicott suggested it would be. I want to think that my baby girl persona is entirely a product of my own psyche. But on reflection, I can see there is truth in Winnicott's perspective. My mother is more comfortable with women than men. She is uncomfortable with overt masculinity or men in positions of authority. I can see that this had an influence on the gender of my child persona.

Winnicott, a deeply intuitive and humane person, was ahead of his time. Fortunately, the idea of personas or sub-personalities is becoming more accepted. Since the 1980s a school of psychology has emerged which views having multiple personas as normal – applicable to all. Internal Family Systems Therapy (IFS) was developed by Richard Schwartz based on his work with bulimic clients (see the book of the same name, published in 1995). It posits that we all have multiple personas (termed 'parts') lead by a unifying self. Conflict or trauma produces a state of polarization within the psyche. In that state, parts take opposing or competing positions in the mistaken belief that this is necessary to protect the self. Each part reacts iteratively to the other, taking increasingly extreme positions. This is certainly consistent with the situation for conflicted ABs.

The therapist Jasmin Lee Cori - who I often cited in relation to insecure childhood attachments - also works with client's sub-personalities in healing those insecure attachments. She does not refer specifically to Richard Schwartz' Internal Family Systems (IFS) theory but evidently works in a very similar manner. She refers to this as 'parts work'.

Summary

There are intuitive therapists and schools of psychology that accept personas or subpersonalities within the psyche, as both subjectively real AND psychologically healthy.

9. Saving Grace

S o being an AB originated as a response to an unhealthy insecure attachment between mother and child, and dissociated childhood trauma. That trauma split off a child persona. That is commonly denied for a long time and results in savage internal conflict for the AB. Surely being AB must be unhealthy, pathological?

Isn't it all broken, as we feared?

No!

Attachment Theory allows that an insecure attachment in childhood can be healed. That can happen through mechanisms such as self-nurturing, accepting our real identity, a good marriage, a redeeming personal faith, or therapy. That healing changes the internal working model that shapes a person's present and future relationships, and in adulthood, they can move from an insecure to a secure attachment. A person who had an insecure attachment as a child, cannot 'wipe that slate clean,' but they heal (or at least make peace with) the wounds that damaged themselves and their lives. Dissociated trauma, too, can be healed.

The adult baby identity is a source of this healing.

It is a saving grace!

Our baby persona, our Inner Child, is an aspect of our True Self. When we accept our baby persona/Inner Child, we have an invigorating feeling of being 'real', we feel vital, and capable of responding to life with spontaneous, innocent happiness and wonder. It opens the door to healing and health.

For ABs (or anyone), self-acceptance is not a simple straight-forward process. It has hidden depths and complexities. But it is worth the journey. By self-acceptance, I don't mean a 'cure' that would see our child persona disappear, rather accepting that persona as a real, permanent, fundamental and healthy part of our psyche. See my book *'Becoming Me – the Journey of Self-Acceptance'* for a guide map for self-acceptance that AB's can customize for themselves.

Self-acceptance removes the internal conflict that comes from denying the subjective reality of the child persona. In turn, the removal of the conflict, drains the compulsive energy from the fetish/False Self dimension of the AB identity. The end of the compulsive fetish changes the character of the AB identity. It shifts from masking the pain and despair, to healing it. Self-acceptance is the pre-requisite to healing.

To understand how and why accepting our child persona opens the door to healing we need to turn again to the work of Donald Winnicott. Remember that for Winnicott, the True Self is as close to a conception of the human spirit or soul, as it is possible to render in secular writing. Keeping faith with your True Self is powerfully healing and healthy.

There are five ways in which our AB identity can heal our wounded Inner Child and lead us to health and wholeness. They are -

1. self-nurturing using transitional objects;

2. reconnecting with the true self;

3. inhabiting our bodies;

4. innocent healthy play; and

5. if needed, by liberating and completing the self by accessing the identity of another gender.

Each of the five healing mechanisms is discussed below.

Self-Nurturing and Transitional Objects

Accepting our baby persona allows ABs to nurture themselves (and to genuinely receive nurturing from others). In turn, that self-nurturing strengthens self-acceptance in a virtuous cycle.

The nurturing is what our wounded Inner Child needed and didn't receive when we were a baby or a child. These are needs for comfort and safety felt at a deep, child-like level. These are not needs that can be satisfied in an adult way with a nice warm beverage and a biscuit in a comfy armchair. The comfort sought has a strongly tactile dimension. The safety is psychological safety – to feel protected and 'held', to return to a time when the worries and dangers of the world were held at bay beyond the cot or nursery.

A non-conflicted AB meets their need for nurturing when they have 'baby time'. But how? Why is a soft or wet nappy so comforting? Why is a favourite soft toy so calming? Or favourite baby clothes? Or a dummy? Or a bottle? After all, a wet nappy or any of these are not intrinsically comforting for most adults – most would find them annoying, if not downright discomforting. They ARE, however, deeply comforting and calming for adult babies.

I believe ABs gain nurturing by using comfort or transitional objects to unconsciously recreate the presence of a loving mother. We are recreating the circumstances of the original insecure attachment with our mother with the unconscious purpose of changing that to a positive outcome. In the unconscious mind, this time, we will be loved and mothered as we needed to be. And we will be - because in a healthy AB it is our nurturing Inner Parent who meets our baby persona when we have 'baby time'. (Or if you have faith in a personal God or Saviour, it is a loving God as our mother or father).

In a healthy, non-conflicted AB, all the three parts of our identity (Parent, Child and Adult) are 'pointing' in the same direction to see our child persona's need for nurturing is met.

The Inner Child, our child persona, is confident they are loved, and their needs will be met. As a result, they are mostly happy, and playful or calm – and readily comforted.

The Inner Parent is a nurturing, protecting parent – attentive to the needs of our child persona.

Our adult-self safeguards our adult baby identity, ensuring that there is space for our Inner Parent to nurture our child persona.

For the non-conflicted AB, 'baby time' is a happy, soothing, nurturing experience. When we return to being our adult selves, we are calmed, refreshed – grounded in our true selves – better adults as well as better babies or children.

Remember in the psyche of biological babies, transitional objects stand in for the mother's presence. That is why they help babies go to sleep or help the baby to tolerate their mother's temporary absence.

For Adult Babies, our nappies were a transitional object long before they were a fetish object. One of the reasons ABs wet their nappies is that a wet nappy is more powerful as a transitional object – better at making us feel comforted and safe. It unconsciously harkens back to the time when the wet nappy might soon mean the presence and attention of mother.

Of course, the AB's transitional objects commonly extend to soft toys, pacifiers, bottles, soft baby clothes and blankets etc.

Remember too, that the creation of comfort/transitional objects runs very powerfully and deep in the psyche. Biological babies create transitional objects when they are aged between 4 and 12 months. This is before they have much, if any, language before they can use abstract symbols. The child persona of ABs uses comfort / transitional objects to gain comfort and safety in exactly the same way that a biological baby or child does. For me, this is further proof that the child persona is subjectively real. In a most instinctual way, they act like a biological baby/child. You can't fake the deep child-like comfort that an AB gets from their nappy and other comfort/transitional objects.

Non-conflicted ABs, and those who love them will instinctively create a 'holding' environment as Donald Winnicott meant, an environment that is experienced by our child persona as nurturing. I can give an example from my own life.

My wife has decorated my bedroom as though it were a guest bedroom for the grandkids. There are piles of fluffy toys in several corners, a white wooden bed in a style that wouldn't look out of place as a baby's cot, and bed linen in soft pastel colours, again not out of place in a nursery. My baby persona is nurtured to wake up and go to sleep in a space that recognizes and accepts her as real, as having real needs. Every time I take a quiet moment, that passive nurturing is there. I know that other ABs do the same. How many times on YouTube or Twitter have you seen a nursery style backdrop to an adult baby's selfie?

Self-nurturing is a deeply healthy and healing capacity. Being an adult baby is a declaration and a challenge to ourselves about our need for nurturing. ABs show great courage in not turning away from the need for nurturing, despite the unconventional way that need presents itself.

As we grow up, we learn to be embarrassed or ashamed about a need for nurturing – it's being childish, or indulgent. *'Grow up and get over it'*. *'Suck it up, princess'*. These are the admonishing voices we hear in our minds. These messages are WRONG! No one should never be ashamed or embarrassed about needing nurturing. We all need it, not just adult babies. We all have an Inner child. Nurturing is a human need and many ills of the world would be solved if those needs were met. At its heart, it is an innocent need.

Learning to recognize, accept and meet our own need for nurturing is key to a healthy sustainable identity as an adult baby. Don't get me wrong, it's lovely to experience the nurturing care of a loving partner, but if we are to be psychologically healthy, that can only be a complement to our own capacity to meet the nurturing needs of our baby persona.

Reconnecting with the True Self

Accepting and embracing our AB identity also lets us reconnect with our True Self. As children with insecure attachments AB's experienced much of their parent's love as conditional. We felt we needed to please our parents to keep their love. That strong need to comply with what others wanted from us became a life time habit. It strengthened our False Self and distanced ourselves from our True Self - who we really are.

Unsurprisingly nappies or bed wetting are central to this. Nappies are central to the AB identity. Michael Bent sums it up –

> *Nappies so clearly represent the age of infancy, the dependency of infancy and the security and comfort of infancy.*

We have seen that nappies are the most important of the AB's comfort/transitional objects that allows self-nurturing. But there is another dimension. For ABs, nappies put us in touch with our True Self.

For me, it is a powerful experience when my baby girl persona wets her nappy. It's not erotic. Unlike the conflicted fetish stage of our identity, it is not a prelude to masturbation. It's comforting. But there's something more…

I feel 'real', and uniquely and distinctively 'me'.

Those are the qualities Winnicott ascribes to the True Self. As a child, I lived with silent unremitting pressures to grow up quickly and be a credit to myself and my family. I was a compliant child.

When Chrissie has the freedom to wet her nappy without shame or reproach, it feels like I get part of my real self – my True Self – back! If you're not AB, this might sound stupid, trite or perverse. It might be a leap of imagination to 'get' it. Trust me, it's very real. If you're AB, you get it.

Winnicott recognized this dimension when he stated –

> *'If by bed-wetting the child is making effective protest against strict management, sticking up for the rights of the individual, so to speak, then the symptom is not an illness; rather it is a sign that the child still hopes to keep the individuality which has been in some way threatened.'*

This recognizes that a reluctance to comply with a demand to be 'dry' can come from a healthy impulse in the child. I think we can also readily accept that bed-wetting can be equated with a reluctance to surrender nappies.

For an AB, that same feeling of getting your real self, your True Self, back, can also be associated with retrieving our comfort in our pacifier, bottle or stuffed toy.

Mirroring

There is the second way in which accepting our baby persona allows ABs to affirm our True Selves - Mirroring.

Remember Winnicott's insight that a baby first discovers and affirms its True Self by looking into the face of their 'good enough' mother. The baby recognizes itself because the mother is attuned to her baby so that her face is a mirror. If the mothering is not good enough, the baby instead sees the mother's preoccupations, whether those are fatigue, frustration, anxiety or depression.

Actual mirrors feature strongly in the lives of ABs, especially if we understand that the cameras of mobile phones and tablets function as mirrors. Look at Twitter and You-Tube. AB's love their selfies. Mirrors and selfies might sound trite, indulgent. Not so!

I believe that for non-conflicted ABs, these also constitute mirroring in the deeper sense that Winnicott understood it. The AB is 'seeing' themselves – meaning affirming their True Self. I can best explain this using my own experience. As a fifty-something, reserved, inhibited man I don't have a relationship with mirrors. I walk past them without looking at my reflection. I have an entirely utilitarian take on my clothing and appearance. There is nothing to see. That's what a child with an insecure attachment sees of their True Self in their mother's preoccupied face - nothing.

That changes completely when I'm dressed as my baby girl persona. I can't walk past a mirror without looking at my reflection. I love it. I don't see the bizarre sight of a hirsute, middle-aged man in baby drag. I see an adorable baby girl toddler. I see Chrissie. Unlike the conflicted fetish stage of our identity, it is not a prelude to masturbation. I see my True Self. That's what a child with a secure attachment sees in their 'good enough' mother's face. Remember my baby persona's nappy and baby clothes are transitional objects – for the non-conflicted AB, they unconsciously recreate the presence of a loving mother. And in that recreated primal drama, the mirror is her loving face, in which I see myself as I am when I feel loved. It is wonderful - deeply affirming.

Inhabiting Our Bodies

Experiencing my child persona helps me feel like I am living in my own body.

An insecure attachment as a child is commonly associated with a lack of nurturing touch. That lack can make you feel that you are a stranger to your own body, as though it was just a bus that you are travelling on. That lack of connection makes people prone to dissociation and to anxiety.

When I put on a nappy, wear a nappy, wet a nappy, I'm conscious of the sensation on my skin, the feel of soft or wet towelling and smooth plastic, the bulk between my legs, and the weight on my hips. The nappy is enveloping. The sensation changes as I move. It's different when I'm sitting, walking or lying down. It's not a sexual experience. It's a grounding, comforting experience. I feel 'here'. I feel 'me'. I don't have to think about it. It just is. For non-ABs, the closest parallel is the way your whole body experiences a comforting restful bath.

When I lie in bed, just before I go to sleep, my whole body is suffused with comforting sensations. There's the texture and shape of my nappy, a soft night-dress or fleecy pyjamas, the soft stuffed toys in my arms on either side, the soft warmth of flannelette sheets, and the comforting silicone bulb of my pacifier in my mouth and the guard against my lips. I'm present in my body, grounded.

Accepting my child persona and being free to wear nappies and baby clothes without guilt or shame, especially when going to bed, has greatly reduced my anxiety. A lot of that is down to the freedom my child persona gives me to inhabit my body.

Innocent Healthy Play

We have already seen that when ABs accept our child persona, our nappies largely return from being fetish objects to being comfort/transitional objects. But that's not the only shift in fetish breakthrough.

I believe that when we accept our child persona, what were formerly conflicted, compulsive fetish behaviours and props give way to healthy play in the way that Winnicott understood play. As for a biological child, it is a means of exploring who we are – for ABs, discovering our child persona, a part of our identity that has hitherto been denied. This innocent play is different from the self-conscious recreation of ABs whose exhibitionistic mannerisms suggest that they are still conflicted about their identity. Winnicott saw such fetishism as incompatible with innocent play.

Rosalie Bent identified the importance of play to the non-conflicted AB –

"Playtimes, in which dolls and toys are pivotal, are a very important element of regression. Regressing to a certain age is one thing, but what do you do when you get there? You play, of course!" [There's Still A Baby In My Bed]

Remember that the capacity for play is the best indication of psychological health in children. Those with an insecure attachment, with dissociated trauma, in childhood, lost part of that childhood. The too-strong False Self impeded the True Self's spontaneous childhood vitality and delight, and that included the full enjoyment and benefit of play.

When we accept our child persona, compulsive sexual behaviour tends to fall away. When we dress in our baby clothes and play with our toys, they aren't fetishistic props. Our subjectively real child persona is inhabiting the creative world of Winnicott's transitional phenomena – it's not objectively real, but it's not a purely subjective delusion either. It's make-believe. And it can be shared with others. It's play!

I can see it in the twitter selfies of AB's innocently cuddling and posing their favourite soft toys – they never fail to bring a smile to the heart of my baby girl persona. When Chrissie wanders about the house in her baby clothes with her treasured soft toy Bunny in her arms, my wife's spontaneous open smile tells me she recognizes and partakes in Chrissie's innocent play. It is marvellously and deeply healing.

My wife brought me a doll's playset for Christmas. It is LOVELY! I will never forget the wonderful feeling when I first picked up and cradled the baby doll. It was a powerful, thrilling, satisfying moment - a spontaneous delight in, and discovery of, self – my True Self. It was instinctive for me to cradle the doll, rock her gently and nestle her close, murmur comfort. It affirmed, in play, the nurturing side of myself that now brings me some of my deepest satisfaction and pride. Would that I could have discovered and affirmed, in play, that side of myself when I was young. Better late than never!

In play, like a biological child, I can make the world as I want it to be. A world where my lovely, shy, innocent Chrissie is happy and safe. And like a biological child, when I return to reality, I carry the world I have made up, in my heart.

Liberating and Completing the Self by Accessing the Identity of Another Gender

An AB's subjectively real child persona can allow them to access the liberating and 'completing' qualities of a gender different from their adult self.

Mostly this seems to take the form of adult male ABs having a female child persona. Rosalie Bent indicates that around half of male ABs have such a persona. I can see no reason why it couldn't work the other way – an adult female AB having a male child persona – if that met the needs of the AB's psyche.

My child persona is a toddler baby girl. She is a deep expression of my psyche. I don't think it would be possible for me to fully 'own' the healing, healthy feelings of being appealingly cute, adorable, lovely – *loveable* - if my child persona was male. All the male modelling in my childhood was unremittingly, emotionally austere. There were no playful, nurturing males. Chrissie overturns all of that. She liberates and completes me. Through Chrissie, my adult self has better access to discover and develop those positive aspects of my psyche linked to my female side which my upbringing didn't give me permission to 'own'.

In my adult self, I don't have sexual dysphoria. I don't need to contemplate being a woman. Why would I? I have my delightful, wonderful Chrissie, always part of my consciousness.

Healing

Jasmin Lee Cori indicates that the wounds of an insecure childhood attachment and dissociated childhood trauma run deep. The healing of those wounds commonly takes lengthy intensive therapy. She states –

> *"Generally, brief therapies and cognitive-behavioral therapies cannot be expected to provide much to those dealing with early childhood wounds. Stated one way, such therapies may affect the neocortex, the thinking brain, but never reach the emotional brain. In most cases, the emotional brain will need to unload its traumas and release its defences, and this happens most easily in a safe, nurturing relationship that develops over time. … what allows the emotional brain (limbic brain) of a person to change is falling into limbic resonance with the therapist and being tuned in by the therapist's emotional brain, just as the baby's brain was originally tuned by the mother's. This generally takes a number of years; there is no quick fix for reprogramming the emotional brain."*

Donald Winnicott worked on this basis – believing that the therapist took the place of the missing nurturing mother in repairing the wounds of insecure attachment and trauma.

The five healing mechanisms described above constitute intensive therapy that changes the 'emotional brain' as Jasmin Lee Cori describes.

They are only fully available to ABs because our child persona is subjectively real. That would not be so if being AB was just role play, a conflicted sexual fetish or an optional 'kink'. None of those has the psychological leverage to heal deep-seated wounds. That's a defining difference between ABs and those for whom nappies and baby play are 'an optional extra' that they can freely live without.

The non-conflicted AB identity is psychologically healthy. Contrast this with the self-medicating behaviour of an addict. Addiction is also a response to a wounded Inner Child. But the addiction is harmful because it masks and denies those wounds. It is true that the behaviour of a conflicted AB is similar – the internal conflict denies the need for nurturing and drives compulsive behaviour. But when we accept our child persona, that changes. That's the difference between addiction and a personal identity. A personal identity might be conflicted. But when that internal conflict is resolved, unlike an addiction, you are left with a healed positive identity.

That's how it is for ABs. The acceptance of a subjectively real child persona within our psyche is the means of healing. We can nurture and heal ourselves. The original wounds to the psyche are unmasked and healed. We strengthen our True Self and feel 'real' and distinctively 'ourselves'. The AB identity and the ongoing need for nurturing don't go away, but we can live with them comfortably and safely. The acceptance of our identity enhances our confidence, resilience and creativity.

Regression?

I don't view being a non-conflicted AB as regression in a psychological sense. That might sound a bit silly. If an adult wears nappies, cuddles soft toys, sucks a pacifier and wears baby clothes, then surely it's regression? I don't think that reflects how it works for non-conflicted ABs. Specifically, it doesn't accurately reflect having a subjectively real child persona as a permanent and healthy part of the AB's psyche.

Regression means returning to something that previously existed. It carries a negative connotation in both its general, and psychological, meaning. For example, when someone involuntarily regresses to a traumatic event in childhood, they are reliving a past trauma as they experienced it as a biological child. If the event is sufficiently traumatic their adult self temporarily 'goes missing inaction', unable to engage with or protect the wounded inner child.

This is not what happens when the child persona of a non-conflicted AB has 'baby time'. Our child personas are not our biological child selves. Sure, those personas are influenced by our biological childhood but they are a creative and healthy product of our subconscious, a redemptive response to the conditions of our biological childhood. The AB's child persona is most definitely not returning to the conditions of the AB's biological childhood. The child persona permanently shares consciousness with the adult self. They are with us in the here and now, we aren't going backward to reach them, in any sense. When a non-conflicted AB has 'baby time' their adult self hasn't disappeared – their Inner Parent and adult self are present, nurturing their child persona. This is self-nurturing, not a neurotic dependency.

Applying the concept of regression to a non-conflicted AB is a legacy of an outdated, erroneous, stigmatizing view of our identity. This is discussed in my book '*The Adult Baby Identity – Coming Out as an Adult Baby*' -

> *"The traditional view of child and personality development is a linear model. Everyone goes through the same sequential stages in childhood, in the same order. Personality disorders in adulthood are thought to be patterned on a personality structure that is normal at some stage of childhood. Adult dysfunction arises because the person has got stuck at that stage and returns to it in stress or crisis. This view originated with the non-empirically based theories of Freud and the first schools of psychoanalysis. It has been carried into psychology more generally. It lends itself to a view that there is a single, majority pattern of personality development and any departure from that is pathological, or at least suspect. ...*
>
> *There is another view, advanced by John Bowlby, the creator of Attachment Theory. He posited a view that personality development isn't a single linear track. Instead, it is a multi-track phenomena where we start out at a similar origin but each point of interaction between the genetic inheritance, the emerging personality and the environment represents a possible branch of development. ...*
>
> *What if being an AB, that is the emergence of a baby/child persona in childhood, wasn't a regression per se, but a diverging branch of personality development? In the same way that other minority, or LGBTQ identities are a diverging, but healthy branch of personality development. It's only a speculation, but in the absence of empirical evidence either way, it is just as tenable as the single linear view."*

This might sound 'academic'. And I wouldn't suggest leading any discussion with non-ABs with this perspective. It will probably come across as denying the 'bleeding obvious'. But if you're AB, it matters. The core, defining feature of the AB identity is having a subjectively real child persona as a healthy part of our psyche. The concept of regression mispresents our identity in ways that buy-into old pathological views of who we are. If we buy-into those views we are continuing to damage ourselves.

Summary

Accepting our child persona lets ABs access healing through five psychological mechanisms –

- self-nurturing using transitional objects;
- reconnecting with the true self;
- inhabiting our bodies;
- innocent healthy play; and
- liberating and completing the self by accessing the identity of another gender.

Through those mechanisms, we can nurture ourselves and accept the nurturing of others. We can heal our wounded Inner Child and ourselves.

10. The Child Persona

The child persona is at the centre of the AB's identity. Accepting the existence of the persona is the most confronting thing about being AB. The persona is rarely discussed directly in on-line AB forums and may be the most misunderstood aspect of being AB. For these reasons, it is important to discuss.

I base the discussion below mostly on my experience of my child persona – a baby toddler girl named Chrissie. To that, I can add some understandings from psychotherapy. In the absence of much public information, that's the best I can do. I hope some of my experience will resonate with other ABs. I hope to be able to shed some light, and provide some reassurance, on our child personas. This is a deeply personal aspect of our identity. Ultimately, every AB is their own best authority and guide.

Character of the Persona

The character of the child persona of each AB is unique, just as the adult selves of ABs are unique. Yet I suspect that there is important common ground in the characters of AB's child personas. They emerge in response to the brokenness of an insecure childhood attachment and childhood trauma. They are a response to the fact that ABs, as children, often felt unloved. And like all children who feel unloved, ABs felt it must have been their fault. They felt themselves to be unlovable.

Our child persona is the antidote to feeling unlovable. Our subconscious created the most lovable child it could. I can best illustrate this from my own life. Chrissie emerged from a temporary traumatic separation from my mother when I was aged three or four. My baby sister and I were left in the care of strangers. My sister was picked up and comforted, but I don't remember being so comforted. Is it any wonder that my child persona is a baby toddler girl? In my eyes, it was my baby toddler sister who got the love. As the elder male child, instead I got expectations to be grown up beyond my years and felt ashamed for not meeting them. In my eyes, I wasn't picked up and comforted because I was an unlovable failure.

Our child personas are a way of affirming to our wounded Inner Child that they are lovable.

Back to Chrissie again –

> *"Dressing to feel authentic is very important. The more I dress in baby clothes that look, and more importantly, feel right for Chrissie the more I feel like a real baby girl. I sometimes say to my sceptical wife that an outfit or piece of Chrissie's clothing is 'cute' – more accurately ,Chrissie feels 'cute' wearing it. There's a world of meaning in that word. It means more than just nice or pretty. It means feeling like a loveable, adorable baby girl – a little princess. That is central to the 'primal drama' in my psyche – I can go back to a time when there should be a secure attachment between baby and mother. Being cute means (this time), I'll be loved and comforted and protected.*

I suspect that for each AB, their child persona, is exactly the baby or child who most melts their heart – who most deserves their love and protection. And because they are loved, we can indulge them and let them have those attributes we feared to have because we were unlovable. Our child personas can be a little spoilt, they can sulk, throw tantrums, knowing they will still be loved.

The child persona is real, permanent, fundamental and healthy.

What do we mean by that? Let take those attributes in turn.

Real

The child persona is subjectively real. That means it's real *within* the psyche of the AB. The child persona experiences themselves and the world through the senses, the feelings and the psychology of a very young biological child. At the deeper levels, this is drawn from the subconscious, not constructed in the conscious mind. The child persona is not 'imaginary'. Their powerful influence plays out subconsciously in ways that we often only discover in retrospect, and which can surprise us because they are very different from our adult selves. They influence us at three levels, that I label –

- nurturing,
- congeniality, and
- play.

Nurturing is the deepest level. The regular need for nurturing, and what creates the feeling of being nurtured, is the most powerful and instinctive way in which our child persona influences our personality. It can't really be turned off. You can only control it by accepting it. If that need is not met or is postponed too long, then that frustration will break through into our behaviour – making us irritable, distracted etc.

The way, our child personas feel nurtured by comfort / transitional objects comes from our subconscious. As we have seen, our child personas derive nurturing from comfort objects via the same psychological mechanisms as very young biological children. Adults, functioning as adults, would not have access to that level of self-nurturing. I didn't fully understand this until I accepted my own child persona. Since then I sleep each night wearing a nappy, soft baby clothes, cuddling a soft toy each side and with a pacifier in my mouth. I really do sleep like a baby, free of adult anxieties.

As an example of the influence of the unconscious at this level, I don't think ABs have unfettered discretion to choose the comfort/transitional objects that satisfy our child persona's need for nurturing. There is an instinct in the selection of which type of objects, or which specific object, will bring our child persona deep comfort and safety. That instinct echoes our subconscious and past associations from our biological childhood. The type of nappy you wear fits into this category. I grew up in the era of cloth nappies and disposables just don't 'cut it' for me in terms of letting me feel nurtured. I suspect that sleeping arrangements for our child persona largely fit into this deepest level. The shades of colour that we find nurturing, is another.

Congeniality is how I label the second level of influence that our child persona has on our personality. I am using congeniality in the sense of *'pleasing or liked on account of having qualities or interests that are similar to one's own.'* Our child personas influence our preferences to align more with their personalities, even in areas which are not directly related to nurturing. For example, I noticed that my taste in movies had changed. I used to love war-movies and had no interest in teen/high school chick flicks. That almost reversed. I also found myself identifying much more with female than male characters in the young adult fiction that I like to read. In my view of society and politics, I found myself identifying more strongly with women, and being more impatient with the intransigence of men in power. These changes, and others, crept up on me. I welcome them, but they were not the product of a conscious decision. They all align with the character of my baby girl persona. The influence at this level is not as compelling as nurturing. It can be more readily over-ridden or postponed by our conscious minds –

when we are aware of it. But it still works at an unconscious level and can subtly and powerfully affect our preferences and behaviour.

Play is the third level of influence. By that, I mean behaviour which is an expression of the young age of our child persona, but which is beyond the most instinctual level of nurturing. This can include our child persona's clothes, mannerisms and recreations (colouring, doll's play, children's TV shows etc). It is the one that is most under our conscious control but can still reflect a significant unconscious influence. Because play is at a more conscious level, the opposing, and contaminating, influences of self-conscious exhibitionism and inhibition are evident. For example, I tried out various recreations that other ABs enjoyed – children's TV, toy trains – but these didn't really 'click' – they felt like self-conscious 'role play/age play'. But when I discovered doll's play, the flashing lights came on. Chrissie loved it. It was instinctive and natural.

This also applies to AB's mannerisms. There is a spectrum between conscious and unconscious control. Sometimes, my baby girl persona is apparent to my wife in my facial expressions, gestures or stance. Those times are not dramatic or self-conscious. This is consistent with my understanding of Dissociative Identity Disorder (DID). With DID, the mannerisms of the parts, and the switching between parts, is commonly more subtle than movie or TV stereotypes. In *'Understanding Trauma and Dissociation'* Lynn Mary Karjala states -

> *"When one part goes completely back inside and another part comes upfront, that's called 'switching'. In old movies switching may be accompanied by some dramatic sign or gesture – the head dropping onto the chest, the face going blank as if the person is suffering a petit mal seizure. In reality, it's rarely that blatant. There may be a subtle signal – a glance downward, an eye blink just slightly longer than usual – or there may be no outward sign at all."*

I'm too inhibited to try and speak as Chrissie in a little girl's voice. I fear that would feel *affected*. Chrissie feels too real and important to me to risk feeling like a self-conscious parody. Some You-Tube videos of ABs seem very natural. Others, where the AB displays extravagant mannerisms seem like they are 'trying too hard'. I suspect that the extravagance of the display indicates a continuing internal conflict about their identity. Every AB is different. I have an avoidant inhibited personality. What might feel self-conscious to me, may be natural for another.

Because so much of Chrissie comes from my unconscious, I have a sense of gradually discovering her character. The key point is that our child persona is subjectively real. It is not imaginary or predominantly the creation of the conscious mind.

Permanent

Our child persona is permanent. It has been there since early childhood. Although often unrecognized or denied for a long time it still made its presence felt by episodically 'breaking through' and driving our behaviour in ways that seemed bizarre and inexplicable.

After we have accepted and healed our child persona, it does not disappear. Some therapists working with 'parts' which emerged from dissociated trauma expect that the 'split' will be reversed; the persona will be reintegrated back into the self as a set of positive attributes available to the self, but not identifiable as persona. This wasn't true for me, nor I think for AB's generally. When I accepted and healed Chrissie, she was very much still there – happy, curious and playful.

In my experience, our child persona does not 'grow up' or 'grow out' of babyish/childish ways. Winnicott had the same view. It feels like my Chrissie will always be a toddler - wanting and needing what a toddler wants and needs – her nappies, soft toys, pacifiers etc.

The Adult Baby Identity
Healing Childhood Wounds

Fundamental

Our child persona is a pervasive and compelling part of our psyche. As Rosalie Bent indicates, the persona is always present in our consciousness 24/7. It can move from the foreground to the background of our consciousness, but it's always there. Unlike uncontrolled DID, there is no present amnesia. An AB's child persona and adult self are fully co-conscious, accessing the same memories.

What does living with a child persona feel like? I can only speak for myself. Chrissie is always with me, separately processing whatever is going on. Most of the time, when I'm my adult-self, she's in the background and I'm not consciously aware of her. In adult spaces, I just 'get on with it'. It's like sharing a house in a long happy marriage; sharing a playground with my best childhood friend, or like a beloved favourite old dog. It's a deeply familiar, companionable presence, where the communication is at a deeper level than the verbal. It feels very natural and normal.

I don't hear Chrissie speaking to me/my adult self, as though we were two different people. That would feel too separate - she is part of me.   But I sometimes sense what Chrissie would say. For example, if my wife and I are out shopping and I see something that I sense Chrissie would love, I'll say *'Chrissie'd love that'* or I might say *'want it'* but only in self-conscious adult mimicry of a little girl - I don't speak as Chrissie.

I am, or can readily become, aware of her feelings, needs and reactions, but these don't overpower my adult self. Sometimes after especially stressful times, I'll 'de-brief' with Chrissie to calm or comfort her. For example, dentists scare me. When I had to go for a particularly scary procedure, I imagined myself beforehand picking up Chrissie and comforting her. It worked. Both Chrissie and my adult-self were less fearful. Understanding when Chrissie is scared or needy, and being able to comfort her, has been a great help in managing my anxiety.

This is what it's like for me. It will be different for every AB. When you have resolved internal conflicts and accepted your identity, stay true to your unique experience of your child persona. Trust yourself. Don't let anybody else – friend, partner or therapist - tell or persuade you to something different.

Having a subjectively real child persona in my psyche does not in any way stop me being a functional adult. Several times recently, I found myself in the middle of a crisis. One was late at night when a domestic violence incident between strangers dropped out-of-the-blue at our front door. Another was a family legal crisis needing immediate action. In both cases, without conscious thought, Chrissie dropped into the background and my adult self-functioned as needed in the moment. In retrospect, the only influence I can see that Chrissie had on matters was, perhaps, in making me better able to comfort the victim of the domestic violence incident whilst waiting for the emergency services. (I should add I normally live a quiet life).

Healthy

Our child persona is a healthy part of the AB's psyche. It is healthy because –

- it is an aspect of our True Self, and enhances our sense of being vital and 'real', of being uniquely and distinctively ourselves - that life is positive and worth living;

- it gives the self, better access to positive child-like qualities of innocent joy, security, contentment, wonder and playfulness;

- it allows us to meet our needs for nurturing and to heal our wounded Inner Child; and

- as for any with a minority identity, self-acceptance, enhances our confidence, resilience and creativity.

Summary

An AB's child persona affirms that the AB's wounded child is loveable. The persona is subjectively real, permanent, fundamental and healthy. It has a benign, pervasive influence on the self and personality of a non-conflicted AB. This is expressed directly through the regular need for nurturing; subtly, through the broader preferences and outlooks of the personality; and through child's play. The character of the child persona of each AB is unique – as is the way each AB experiences their child persona.

11. A Healthy Identity

As ABs, we have looked within ourselves and back into our childhoods. Our guides have been two eminent psychotherapists – John Bowlby and Donald Winnicott.

We did find brokenness.

It was the insecure attachment between mother and child which was broken.

It was the trauma and dissociation which was broken.

We were living with pain and despair long before we become AB. Our Inner Child was wounded long before we became AB. We felt we didn't belong, long before we became AB.

But we found that our child persona, and our AB identity, is *not* broken.

Our child persona is the positive, redeeming response to our broken childhood.

Our child persona is an aspect of our True Self – the self which makes us feel real and alive – what makes us uniquely and distinctively ourselves.

Accepting our child persona is the gateway to healing our wounded Inner Child, and the gateway to psychological health. Through that acceptance we can access powerful psychological mechanisms for self-nurture; to better connect with our True Selves; to inhabit our bodies; to play; and if we need, to access the liberating and completing aspects of a different gender than our adult selves.

We can access those powerful and therapeutic psychological mechanisms *because* our child persona is subjectively real within our psyche. When we were conflicted, the prospect of sharing our consciousness with a child persona was strange and fearful. It felt like a curse. Now we understand it is a blessing.

Even the False Self fetish side of being AB was a means of hiding and protecting our child persona, our True Self, until we were ready to accept and nurture that persona.

Counselling and Integration

The therapist Dr Rhoda Lipscomb indicates that few AB's seek professional counselling. I think we can now better understand the reluctance of ABs to seek counselling. It wasn't just defensiveness.

At some deep level, beneath all the awful internal conflict and confronting compulsive behaviours, I sensed that being AB was an essential and healthy part of who I am. But I didn't have the understanding, and I didn't have the language, to explain it. So that left me powerless and vulnerable in the face of the accepted common and professional wisdom that being AB was a sexual fetish or a kink at best, or a psychosexual disorder at worst.

If I went to counselling, I feared it would confirm the scourging messages of my internal conflict – this is pathological or perverse, you need to give it up, and if you can't you're weak. And the reality, as Rhoda Lipscomb confirms, is that many counsellors aren't equipped to understand the healthy personal identity that lies beneath the AB's conflicts and compulsions.

Many counsellors work with models of psychological health that require a sub-persona or part, which originated with an insecure attachment or with dissociated trauma, to be re-integrated into the self. Effectively this requires the AB's child persona to 'disappear'.

Instinctively, that felt wrong for me. Now I know why. My child persona is an aspect of my True Self – it makes me feel real, and distinctively myself. And it gives me access to powerful psychological mechanisms for self-nurture and healing. As I said in my book 'Living with Chrissie – My Life as an Adult Baby' -

I no longer seek or believe in 'a cure' that will see Chrissie disappear as an alter or sub-personality. I understand that this conflicts with a definition of psychological health based on 're-integrating' my baby side into my broader personality. That doesn't work for me. It's the equivalent of telling a gay man, *'it'll be okay, one day you'll meet the right girl'*. A definition of psychological health that has no rightful place to be comforted by wearing nappies or sleeping with soft toys, or the rest, isn't me. It feels too close to the silent unremitting pressures of my upbringing to grow up quickly, be a mature responsible adult and leave babyish and childish things behind. I internalized that approach and it suppressed real feelings and needs to the detriment of my wellbeing.

Fortunately, there are intuitive therapists and schools of psychology that accept that parts or sub-personalities such as AB's child persona can be a healthy and permanent feature of our psyche.

Seeking professional counselling when you need it is a sign of maturity and psychological health. If I need to, I will undertake counselling in the future. But I will select a suitably experienced counsellor. The right counsellor needs to know about the psyche of babies and young children, and how it feels to the child when their upbringing is broken. They need to know Bowlby and Attachment Theory, Donald Winnicott, childhood trauma and dissociation, and multiplicity in consciousness and parts. And they need the insight and the wisdom to see that a healthy AB identity is a positive, redeeming response to a broken childhood.

The Healthy AB Identity

It is psychologically healthy and valid for ABs to see their child persona as a permanent part of their psyche. (It is more problematic for the AB, if they cling to the False Self, compulsive, fetish side and therefore deny themselves self-acceptance.)

That being said, focusing *only* on our child persona is a dead-end. As Michael Bent indicates, the adult self is the primary personality and the baby or child persona is a sub-personality (see *'The Identity Conflicts of the Adult Baby' in the book 'Being an Adult Baby'*).

Our child persona is not all of our True Self. Our adult self is also part of our True Self. We have discovered many wonderful qualities in our child persona – innocent happiness, tenderness, open joy, playfulness - a loveable side of ourselves. But we cannot vest all these wonderful qualities only in our child persona. They are qualities of our psyche, equally available to, and needed by our adult self. If we own those qualities, we are better, stronger adults as well. Our child persona may not grow up but our identity, our personality, our psyche does grow and develop. In accepting and healing my wounded Inner Child and child persona, I affirmed a deeply protective and nurturing side of myself. Those are properly attributes of my adult self.

Like any vulnerable biological child, our child persona cannot survive and thrive alone in the world. If we invest all of ourselves in our child personas, we put ourselves at psychological risk. There will be times in life when we have to deal with conflict, danger, fear, loss or grief. To do that successfully we need to *see* ourselves as more than just our child persona, we need to *be* more than just our child persona. If not, we will be damaged and traumatized again, just as we were in our biological childhoods. We can't let that happen.

So, our healthy adult baby identity is more than our child persona. It is also our nurturing Inner Parent and a responsible, strong and empathetic Adult. Our child persona feels loved and safe with a secure attachment with our Inner Parent. That relationship is protected by our strong Adult.

There will be many times when our adult self needs to take charge and steer our child persona, for the child's own good. Our child persona is subjectively real. They will have sulks and tantrums – 'hissy fits' – and 'spit the dummy'. There will be times they will be lost in fear or sadness and like any very young biological child not see a way out. That is when our adult self needs to step in, hand our child persona over to our nurturing Inner Parent to be comforted and consoled. To be safe, our child persona needs to know there are parents and adults who can take care of them, shield them because those parents and adults have capabilities that the child does not.

Different and the Same

In understanding ourselves as ABs, we are trying to understand what makes us different from others.

We have spent a lot of our lives feeling alone, feeling different, feeling like we didn't fit.

But reaching a deep understanding of our identity, opens the door to the ultimate healing – to see that, in fundamental ways, we are the same as everyone else.

Everyone has an Inner Child, and many are wounded.

We all need nurturing throughout our lives. We all suffer if those needs are not met, either as children or as adults.

Internal Family Systems (IFS) Therapy says we all have sub-personalities within our psyche. Many people have a conflict between these internal actors, and for some that conflict drives compulsive behaviours.

Many people struggle with self-acceptance.

Many struggle to connect with their True Selves.

As adult babies, we are so different from others, yet in other very important ways we are the same.

Sometimes, it is not so different to be different.

At the deepest level, our humanity is common to all. We do belong.

On-line ABDL forums can be a great resource for peer support and advice – self-help. Understandably, ABs and DLs commonly keep these facets of their personalities, secret or at least private. Feelings of isolation are common. Online forums allow people to reach out to others like them. I have seen many posts attesting to the support and fellowship that ABs and DLs gain from on-line forums. It is also a great way of exchanging information.

But self-help has its' limitations. Cancer peer-support groups are great for moral and instrumental support. But you don't go to your cancer peer-support group to design your chemotherapy and radiotherapy regime.

It's similar to being ABDL.

I am sometimes dismayed at the responses to someone posting on an ABDL forum asking for advice on whether they should seek professional counselling. All too often they are openly or subtly dissuaded from this course of action by others on those forums. The gist of the response is often 'you just need to accept yourself' and it's all good. I didn't need or benefit from counselling.'

There is a lot of denial in the ABDL community, and that includes the people proffering advice. Being a non-conflicted AB is a psychologically healthy space. Being a conflicted AB is not.

Triggering and 'binge and purge' are common in the life histories of ABs. They are both behavioural symptoms of dissociated trauma.

You can navigate healing yourself of an insecure childhood attachment – if you have the emotional resources and/or strong support from a life partner, or friends and family. You don't necessarily need professional counselling, although it's not a bad idea.

Dissociated childhood trauma is different. Living with undiagnosed and unhealed dissociated trauma is an ongoing risk to mental health and predisposes people to anxiety and depression. It subtly warps your perceptions (most notably about yourself), in ways that you do not see. Dissociated trauma can be healed, and that can be life-changing. But it needs the help of a skilled counsellor. It is no-one's place to dissuade anyone from that positive prospect.

An AB or DL thinking about counselling, likely knows turmoil and pain. They probably don't know if they have dissociated trauma or not. The people proffering advice in on-line forums don't know either.

So, if an AB or DL, or anyone, posts on an on-line ABDL forum, contemplating seeking professional counselling the only responsible response is –

- go you! – if you are thinking you need counselling, you probably do
- you will be okay – the turmoil and the pain can be healed with the help of a skilled counsellor
- we are there for you while you are seeking and undertaking counselling
- maybe we can help you locate a skilled and affordable counsellor who regards being a non-conflicted AB as a healthy personal identity.

That is genuine care and support.

References – Annotated List

If you are interested in a deeper understanding of the human psyche, both in children and adults, I recommend the writings of Donald Winnicott. He has a profound understanding, deep compassion for the human condition, an optimism about human nature, and a humility that engenders trust in his insights and motivation. See the annotated list of references for suggested reading.

Ainsworth, Mary & Bell, Sylvia		'Attachment, Exploration, and Separation: Illustrated by the Behaviour of One-Year Olds in a Strange Situation' (1970) Child Development, 41, 49-67. Clear description of the strange situation study. Available free, on-line at - https://pdfs.semanticscholar.org/8272/bd76f36d195023f245735e23e6b5c8b19afd.pdf
Ainsworth, Mary & Bowlby, John		'An Ethological Approach to Personality Development' American Psychologist. Vol. 46 (4) April 1991, pp. 333-341. Useful history of the work and collaboration of the two pioneers of Attachment Theory. Available free, on-line at - https://is.muni.cz/el/1423/jaro2014/PSY103/um/46958257/ainsworth_bowlby_1991.pdf
Bent, Michael		Being an Adult Baby: Articles and Essays on Being an Adult Baby. (2016) (Amazon & Abdiscovery.com.au) A collection of insightful and thought-provoking articles on the AB identity. Notably – 'Identity Confusion in the Adult Baby', 'Finding Balance Between the Baby and the Adult', and 'Binge and Purge'.'
Bent, Rosalie		There's Still A Baby in My Bed: Learning To Live Happily With the Adult Baby in Your Relationship. (2015) (Amazon & Abdiscovery.com.au) A revised version of the 2012 book that first articulated that being an AB was a personal

		identity, not just a fetish. Written by the wife of an AB. Evergreen.
Bowlby, John.		Separation: Anxiety and Anger. Attachment and Loss Volume 2 (1973) (hardcopy: Basic Books. Digital: Amazon).
		Second, and most useful, of the three volumes setting out Attachment Theory.
Cori, Jasmin Lee		The Emotionally Absent Mother: How to Recognize and Heal the Invisible Effects of Childhood Emotional Neglect (Second Edition) (2017) (digital & paperback: Amazon)
		A brilliantly written discussion of insecure attachments in childhood and their effects. Makes Attachment Theory, Bowlby and Winnicott accessible to the lay reader. Highly recommended and inexpensive.
Davis, Madeleine & Wallbridge, David		Boundary and Space: An Introduction to the Work of D.W. Winnicott (1981) Penguin Books. (hardcopy only, no digital copy)
		Very useful and readable coverage of Winnicott's work, organized by topic and with frequent apposite quotations of Winnicott. As a search on amazon will show there is a great deal on Winnicott – some by him and a lot by others on his work. Unfortunately, a lot of the professional literature is expensive.
Holmes, Jeremy		John Bowlby and Attachment Theory. (Routledge. 1993. Reprinted 2005. ISBN 0-415-07730-3). (hardcopy & digital: amazon)
		Recommended. I prefer this to Bowlby's own writing as an exposition of Attachment Theory. It integrates the work of Ainsworth and other later researchers. Unfortunately, both hardcopy and digital are expensive.
Karjala, Lynn Mary		Understanding Trauma and Dissociation. (2007) (digital: Amazon).
		This therapist subscribes to the view that persona/parts disappear upon integration. I prefer Marlene Steinberg's book.
Lewis, Dylan		Living With Chrissie: My Life As An Adult Baby (2018) (Amazon & Abdiscovery.com.au)
		My account of my life as a very late bloomer as an AB ('better late than never').

		Becoming Me – the Journey of Self-acceptance: a Guidebook for Adult Babies Traversing Life (2018) (Amazon & Abdiscovery.com.au) Focuses on self-acceptance and the intrapsychic dimension of identity formation.
		The Adult Baby Identity – Coming Out as an Adult Baby (2019) (Amazon & Abdiscovery.com.au) Makes the case that being AB is a minority personal identity and considers the stages by which the identity is formed.
Lipscomb, Rhoda J.		The Clinical Mental Health Experience of Persons with Paraphilic Infantilism and Autonepiophilia. A phenomenological research study. PhD dissertation (2014). An excellent study of being AB by an informed and sympathetic health professional. Good up-to-date review of literature and research. Available free, on-line at - http://www.esextherapy.com/dissertations/Rhoda%20J.%20Lipscomb%20The%20Clinical%20Mental%20Health%20Experience%20of%20Persons%20withParaphilic%20Infantilism%20and%20Autonepiophilia.pdf
Phillips, Adam		Winnicott A useful inexpensive primer for the lay reader – though I prefer Steven Tuber's book.
Schwartz, Richard		Internal Family Systems Therapy (1995) (Guildford Press [paperback] & amazon) Original exposition of IFS, the school of psychology which may be best suited to counselling ABs.
Steinberg, Marlene		The Stranger in the Mirror: Dissociation The Hidden Epidemic (date) (hardcopy: Harper Collins. Digital: Amazon). Highly recommended. The author is the psychiatrist who developed the leading diagnostic

		questionnaire for identifying dissociative disorders.
Tuber, Steven		Attachment, Play and Authenticity: A Winnicott Primer (2008) (digital: Amazon). Expensive but superb introduction to Winnicott by a talented educator, former head of the doctoral program in clinical psychology at the City University of New York.
Waters, Fran		'Recognizing Dissociation in Preschool Children' by Fran Waters The International Society for the Study of Dissociation Volume 23 Number 4 July/August 2005 Cites an extensive list of references – some linking insecure attachment and dissociated trauma. The context is different than for most ABs, being concerned with DID and child abuse Available free, on-line at - http://www.isst-d.org/downloads/waters-2005-preschooldissoc.pdf
Winnicott, Donald		Winnicott on the Child (2002) (Perseus Publishing) (hardcopy only, no digital copy) A collection of Winnicott's public broadcasts and speeches on child development and parenting for lay audiences. Insightful and very readable. Shows Winnicott's humility, wisdom and compassion.
		'Ego Distortion in Terms of True and False Self' (1960) Winnicott's ground breaking original exposition on the subject. Best read after secondary sources on Winnicott. Written for an audience of psychoanalysts but the fundamentals are still clear to the lay reader. Available free, on-line at – https://www.sas.upenn.edu/~cavitch/pdf-library/Winnicott_EgoDistortion.pdf
		'Transitional Objects and Transitional Phenomena—A Study of the First Not-Me Possession' (1953) International Journal of Psycho-Analysis, 34:89-97 Winnicott's ground breaking original exposition on the subject. Includes concise statement of Winnicott's view of infant psychological development.

		Available free, on-line at – https://pdfs.semanticscholar.org/a56f/ba056a21039574e5b2371f4ad01728b54366.pdf
		'Playing and Reality' (1971) Tavistock Publications. (hardcopy only, no digital copy) Recommended for those with a keen interest in Winnicott. Written for psychotherapists. Best read after reading some secondary sources, or Winnicott's books for laypeople. A seminal book published in the last year of Winnicott's life.
Wikipedia		Attachment Theory Comfort Objects Dissociation (psychology) Donald Winnicott Inner Child Strange Situation True Self and False Self

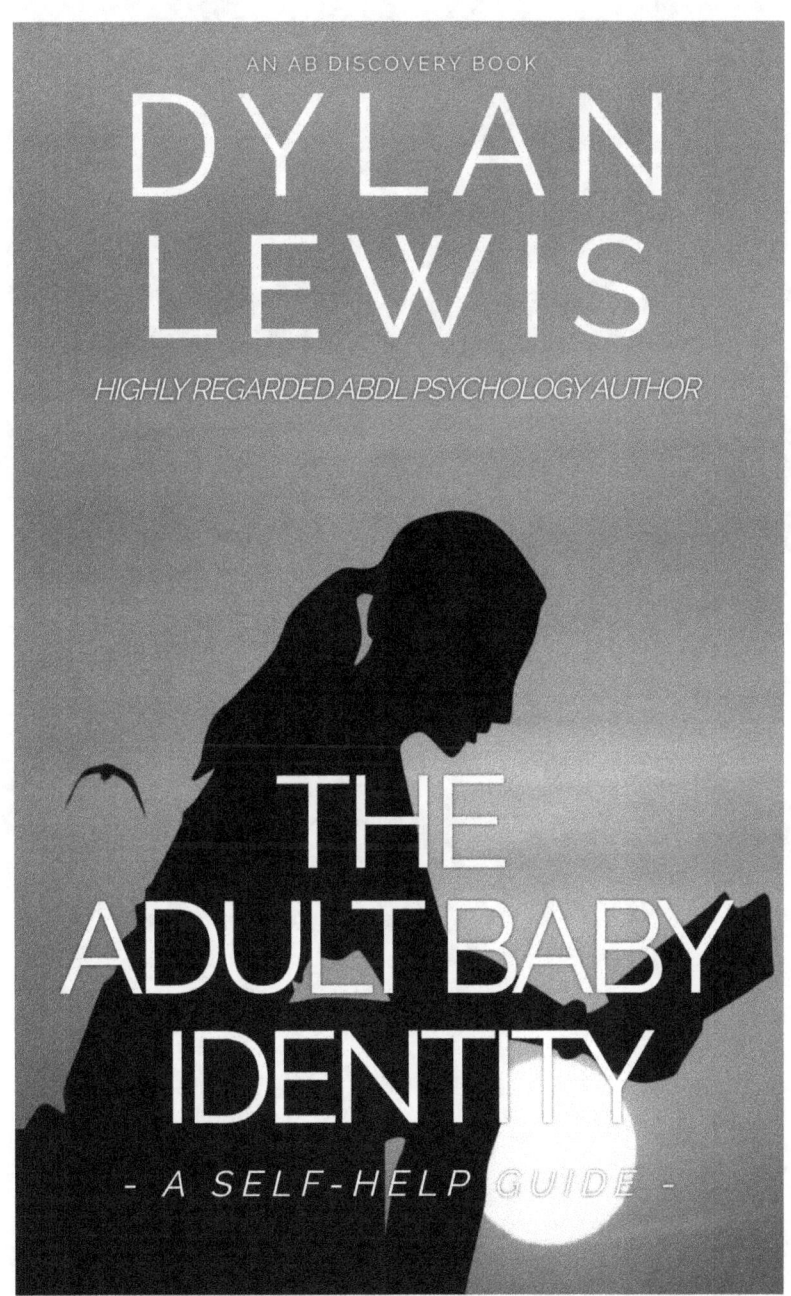

The Adult Baby Identity
A self-help guide

by

Dylan Lewis

Dedication

To my wife, for her constant love and wisdom.

To Rosalie Michael Bent for letting adult babies (and the world) know we aren't mad, bad or alone.

Foreword

Knowing who we are as individuals is the most important journey in our lives and for many, it is the most difficult one. Even for people we call 'vanilla', with no apparent kinks and oddities, it is a herculean task. But when you are an Adult Baby, it is a vastly more complex mission. Add being sissy to the mix and we are already pushing uphill and failing miserably.

But if we don't know who we are, we act as if we are someone we are not. We try to create a personality not fully our own. We create masks and in doing so, we create problems for ourselves and others around us.

This is the true value of books like this and others along the same vein. ABDL is *not* like other identity problems. It is unique, different and requires a perspective all of its own. It is not about gender – although gender issues can be involved. It is not about sexual preference – although that can be involved as well. It is primarily about age and being powerfully driven back to a time of life most have left behind and yet, we still literally inhabit.

And for most, it causes enormous conflicts, both within and without.

The struggle to understand who you are as an adult baby can be immensely difficult and there is no point pretending otherwise, but the benefits at the other end of that journey are indescribable.

Peace

Happiness

Well-being

Satisfaction

Who wouldn't choose all of that?

To the journey…

Michael Bent

1. Introduction

Self-help is all about self-acceptance. And self-acceptance is a huge issue for adult babies.

Being an adult baby can be a roller coaster ride. At its best, there is child-like innocent happiness and security. But at its worst, it is biting shame, tormenting doubt, and compulsive behaviours that can tyrannise your life.

The difference between these best and worst states is one of self-acceptance.

I am an adult baby. I was prompted to write this book after I read an account by another adult baby who said that the answer to the difficulties of being an AB was simply to accept yourself. If only it was that simple!

I realized self-acceptance has hidden depths. If we don't understand those depths, the route to self-acceptance is like a game of snakes and ladders – full of painful pitfalls and demoralizing setbacks. By self-acceptance, I mean living comfortably with the baby side of our personality. It is not the pursuit of 'a cure' that would see our baby side disappear.

Self-acceptance is about resolving our internal conflicts about being AB.

One part of our psyche is fighting with another part. It is a battle within, and against, ourselves. Our wounded Inner Child is opposed by our punishing Inner Parent. It is this internal conflict which drives shame, fear and doubt. It drives compulsive behaviours like bingeing and purging baby clothes.

That internal conflict also causes us to sabotage ourselves and our key relationships. The internal conflict intensifies our craving for acceptance by others, while at the same time sabotaging our prospects of receiving it. Adult babies crave the acceptance of their child persona by others – usually their partner. But paradoxically, the best way to gain a partner's acceptance is to deepen our own self-acceptance.

This book is about finding self-acceptance by resolving the conflict in our psyche. It unpacks what we need to accept about ourselves to live with being ABs without shame and guilt. Its aim is to help adult babies navigate the journey to self-acceptance with fewer hassles. The book uses an approach similar to Internal Family Systems (IFS) Therapy.

There are challenges to finding self-acceptance. For many years I was 'stuck', living with my baby 'side' as a guilty, compulsive sexual fetish. Although the heightened sexual excitement was some compensation for all the turmoil, I wanted something more. But I didn't know what a healthy, stable personal identity as an adult baby felt like, or how to get there. I hope this book helps those who want something more.⬚

Self-acceptance is a journey worth taking. You will discover a wonderful personal identity which is a lot more than an obsession and fetish for nappies. I found that fully accepting my personal identity was profoundly healing. That identity is my saving grace. Self-acceptance holds many benefits beyond the freedom from negative states and conflicts. There are powerful gifts of contentment, security, resilience and creativity.

This is a self-help book.

The key audience is ABs and those who love them. The book is my best attempt to understand our shared identity. It reflects my personal experience as an AB. I have a layman's lifelong interest in psychology. I have no qualifications in psychology. Every adult baby is different, and some will disagree with my views. I do not intend to disparage those whose views are different from mine. Take what is helpful from the book and leave the rest behind.

If you are an adult baby who has no conflict about being AB, then this book is not for you. You have already moved on. But if you have any unease with being an adult baby, then this book might have something of value for you.

This book is based on the pioneering work of Rosalie Bent and Michael Bent in identifying and understanding adult babies as a personal identity. I recommend their books and website www.abdiscovery.com.au . I refer to their insights and understanding throughout the book.

By adult baby, I exclude role players and diaper lovers for whom diapers, baby clothes or baby activities are an optional extra they can freely live without, and fetishists for whom these things are confined exclusively to sexual expression.

This book is the fourth of a non-fiction quadrilogy (After Becoming Me). The second book, *'The Adult Baby Identity – Coming Out as an Adult Baby'*, makes the case that being AB is a minority personal identity and deals with the stages by which that identity is formed. The third book, *'The Adult Baby Identity – Healing Childhood Wounds'*, locates the origin of the identity in an insecure attachment between mother and child, and in childhood trauma.

This book builds on that earlier title, *'Becoming Me – The Journey of Self-Acceptance'*. It is based on the same 'big idea' that self-acceptance comes from resolving our internal conflict, but it is a new book with a more in-depth treatment.

The journey of self-acceptance is not an easy one to undertake alone. You need a confidant who you can trust, and who will be an ally in your healing. If there is no one in your life with whom you can safely share your feelings about your life as an adult baby, seek professional support – preferably from an LGBTQ-friendly therapist who understands issues of personal identity. If you are in crisis or deep distress about being an adult baby, seek professional therapy.

If there is one precept that best guides us through the journey of self-acceptance, it is the words of the poem Desiderata–

"Beyond a wholesome discipline, be gentle with yourself."

2. The Conflicted AB

Being an AB often means living with the push-pull of wanting the freedom to be a young child, and then paying a high emotional price for seeking that freedom. We seek self-acceptance because we want to stop the pain and the turmoil that comes hand-in-hand with being AB. Sure, there are nice moments of comfort: the freedom to set aside the tyranny of potty training by putting on a nappy; cuddling a beloved soft toy that is more friend and protector than a toy; fantasizing about being held, cuddled and soothed. But those moments of comfort are all-too-often preceded by tension and anxiety and followed by guilt and shame. It can be awful.

We have tried giving it all up. Many times. But it always comes back, usually eventually stronger than before. We seem to alternate, sometimes wildly, between wanting to be AB, and wishing we weren't. I call that being a conflicted AB.

We need to begin by acknowledging what life as a conflicted AB is really like.

That covers -

- The Push-Pull of Compulsion and Fetish
- Triggering
- The Binge and Purge Cycle
- Masochistic Fantasies
- Confusion and Turmoil About Ourselves
- Over Compensation
- Problems with Partners
- Isolation and Loneliness

Each of these is discussed below.

Every AB is unique. Not everyone will have all of these problems, and they will have them in differing degrees of strength. I had all of them, bad. But at least I can speak from firsthand experience.

Push-Pull of Compulsion and Fetish

I wanted nappies because they met a deep need within me. I wanted to enjoy the wonderful feeling of freedom, of coming home to myself, that wearing a nappy represented. I was often stressed, tense and anxious. The prospect of wearing a nappy promised at least a brief respite by being able to lose my adult worries and feel comforted and safe. But that goal always got hijacked with me becoming sexually aroused and masturbating while wearing the nappy. A powerful climax was pretty much always guaranteed. But immediately after, I would be filled with feelings of shame and remorse. I would hurriedly fling the nappy aside, put on my adult clothes and quickly tidy everything out of sight. The goal of being comforted in a really deep and satisfying way, always seemed to be just out of reach.

From when I was a teenager until late into middle age, the heightened sexual arousal never failed. When I had the house to myself for a few hours, I would sometimes go through three rounds of putting on a nappy, masturbating, taking the nappy off, putting on my adult clothes and tidying up, and then doing it all again. Each climax was more powerful than the one before. Why didn't I just leave the nappy on? Because the shame after each climax was so strong, I had go through the whole routine of reverting to my proper adult self. But after the shame had subsided, the lure of my nappy powered up again.

When I was a teenager and young adult, I would sometimes masturbate without a nappy, although it was almost always to fantasies of being nappied and babied. But as the years went by, the never-fail, fabulous climax while wearing a nappy eventually meant that I could only reliably climax that way. Sometimes I would promise myself that I would forego or delay masturbating so that I could just enjoy the comfort of wearing a nappy. I would look forward to wearing my baby clothes or exploring baby activities or play for its own sake. Not a chance. It always becomes just a slightly longer prelude to masturbation and was quickly set aside with the nappy after climaxing.

From when I was a teenager, wearing and masturbating in a nappy became my go-to for relieving tension, stress, anxiety, or feeling crap about myself or anything else. It was my drug of choice. Guaranteed relief. It was a compulsion. I couldn't go more than a few days without it. When I was hiding my baby side from my wife, I would twist my mind into knots trying to steal a moment in the day when I could hurriedly masturbate and then stash everything back into its' hiding place. I have some idea of what being a drug addict feels like. I felt furtive and shameful. Even when my wife knew about my baby side and I would take myself off to a closed bedroom to put on a nappy and masturbate, it still felt shameful and guilty. It was the equivalent of a heroin addict being on methadone. Nappies had become a compulsive, guilty, sexual fetish and I was stuck with it.

Triggering

There were times when my need to put on a nappy would be set off by an involuntary 'trigger'. My experience with triggers is described in my book, *'Living With Chrissie – My Life as an Adult Baby'* -

A compelling desire for a nappy could be set off at a moment's notice from any number of visual 'triggers'. It could be seeing a magazine advertisement with a baby in a nappy; anything to do with breastfeeding – especially pictures of women wearing maternity bras; a line of cloth nappies drying on a clothesline would do it every time. For years I couldn't walk down the babies' aisle in a supermarket without 'triggering' the insistent need to get home and put on a nappy. This behaviour was in strong contrast to who I was otherwise – a person of strong emotional control, able to defer gratification.

When this happened, I would feel a compelling need to wear a nappy and masturbate. At its strongest, that need was insistent and could not be delayed beyond a few hours.

Rosalie Bent describes these triggers -

> *"... some attribute about an object that can trigger a regressive episode. It is almost never a generic object, but rather something very specific that triggers a memory or emotion which in turn, triggers the regression. For example, it may be a soft toy, but not just any soft toy. It may be a Care Bear toy, but not just anyone, but rather a pink one, of a specific size and style that clearly has a deep-rooted memory attached to it."* [There's Still A Baby in My Bed: Learning to Live with the Adult Baby in Your Relationship].

This powerful compulsion felt mystifying and shameful.

Binge and Purge Cycle

The most confronting and disturbing aspect of being a conflicted AB is the cycle of binge and purge. That phrase comes from the disease bulimia where the sufferer gorges on food and then, in deep self-disgust and loathing, makes themselves sick until they purge their stomachs until empty. For adult babies, it means something different. The cycle starts with a 'binge' – I would buy a stash of nappies and baby clothes. I was like a drug addict going on a 'bender'. My nappy fetish became stronger and was accompanied by frequent masturbation. The internal conflict also grew stronger. Pleasure was now fighting shame and remorse. The emotional 'let down' after each successive orgasm became more painful and demoralizing. But I was on a runaway train I couldn't stop, even if I wanted to – and I didn't want to. Eventually, the growing internal conflict drove masturbation to a peak. The emotional 'let down' after the final peak orgasm was intensely painful. The disgust, remorse and self-loathing was gut-wrenching.

The only thing that would assuage the intense emotional pain was to 'purge'. I convinced myself that I could completely banish my need for baby things. I would collect every last item of my baby collection and throw it into neighbourhood clothing recycling bins, as a way of making the purge irrevocable. Only then would the painful remorse be soothed. It would be replaced by a new transient kind of 'high'. I had a sense of being cleansed of my weakness and perversity and being free to live a normal healthy life of which I could be proud. I would declare to my wife that I was giving up my 'nappy thing' forever. I meant it when I said it. I would pray for God to give me the strength to maintain my abstinence.

The aftermath of the purge would last a while. My abstinence, at least in terms of physically wearing nappies, would last months, sometimes nearly a year. I would masturbate without nappies for a time, but the comforting fantasies of being babied were always present. Eventually, the unmet needs of my baby side would grow more and more insistent and I would 'binge' again. I was always in some part of the binge and purge cycle. I would have a major/complete purge at least every couple of years, with minor/partial purges in between. With each new binge I would fool myself that, this time, I could keep my baby side under sufficient control so that things wouldn't get out of hand and I wouldn't be driven to purge again. Of course, that was a 'fool's hope'. The internal conflict hadn't gone away or been healed. It was just re-booted. There is that definition of insanity – doing the same thing over again and hoping for a different result the next time. That was me.

I would trigger episodes of purging when I experimented, trying out new types of baby clothes or baby activities. I would develop a guilty fascination with a new facet of being an AB – it could be my first pacifier, feeding bottle or baby dress. I would take weeks to work up the courage to buy it. But then shortly after getting it, my guilt and shame would kick in hard and I would get rid of it. In my thirties, I ordered my first custom made baby dress. After weeks of saving and waiting, the dress arrived. It was lovely. I threw it away within a day because my guilt was so strong. I could not let myself enjoy the dress without paying an unbearable price of shame. It was like holding onto a red-hot fire poker. So, the dress had to go, and with it the rest of my stash of baby clothes. For many years afterwards, I had a guilty fascination with pink, girly style AB clothing, but I would not myself buy any because of the fear of setting off that cycle of guilt and purging.

The binge and purge cycle had a powerful negative effect on my personality and moods. I was tense, anxious, irritable, and had difficulty concentrating on anything other than nappies. At the crescendo of the cycle, just before the final crash and purge, it was like a complete personality change - for the worse. I really hated and despised myself at those times.

I know I am not alone in experiencing the binge and purge cycle. Its prevalence is attested in posts on on-line ABDL forums and in Michael Bent's article *'Binge and Purge: the ABDL Frustration'* (in the book *'Being An Adult Baby'*, or free online at abdiscovery.com.au under the ABDL Articles tab).

Masochistic Fantasies

The fantasy life of adult babies is important and powerful. Whatever baby clothes or behaviours we adopt in real life, these are only a pointer to a much richer repertoire in our fantasies. I suspect most adult babies declare little of this rich fantasy life to anyone else, even their partners.

I had a rich fantasy life which revolved around submitting to attractive, self-assured, capable women who would treat me, though an adult, as a baby. I would be forced to wear nappies and baby clothes and treated like a baby, being fed, changed and disciplined. I was helpless to do anything but comply, although some show of ineffectual resistance or defiance was an essential part of the fantasy. As a day-dream or non-erotic fantasy just before drifting off to sleep, this was a source of comfort. There was as much soothing maternal love and care, as there was coercion or humiliation.

But it was a different matter when it came to the fantasies linked to masturbation. The fantasies were an essential accompaniment to climax. These fantasies quickly came to have a more masochistic character. The coercion was more pronounced, with elements such as physical or chemical restraints. The women would take pleasure in intentionally shaming and humiliating me, including in public. Being forced to wet or mess in my nappy or being made to wear clothes and act like a sissy girl were standard fixtures. These are all tropes of a vast body of erotic AB fiction available on-line, so I know that I was not alone in this fantasy life.

I was like a drug addict who becomes accustomed to a certain dose and no longer gets the same 'rush'. I needed to seek ever stronger masochistic fantasies to guarantee climax. These fantasies were completely at odds with my adult personality which was very much reserved and in control. My guilt and shame at being AB were as much about these masochistic fantasies as it was about actually wearing nappies. At least the fantasies were hidden and private inside my head.

At times I was tormented by these fantasises. The intensity of the imagined submission to a parent substitute figure came from my deep yearning for a secure attachment with my mother which didn't happen in my childhood. In his book *'Arousal: The Secret Logic of Sexual Fantasies'* Michael Bader explains how these fantasies work –

"People prefer to be the subject of negative attention rather than be invisible. In the master/slave relationship, in whatever form it is constructed, an intense bond between the two parties counteracts feelings of insignificance and loneliness."

But the fantasies only made my yearning worse. You can't create, or substitute for, a secure childhood attachment through sexual expression. The fantasies produced an intense sexual climax. That gave me a momentary sense of the impossible, longed-for attachment. But then that moment was quickly gone, leaving me with a deeper sense of loss and pain than before.

So, for me, masochistic fantasies are psychologically unsafe. Wherever the line is drawn between what is psychologically safe and unsafe, adopting psychologically unsafe fantasies is self-sabotaging. They push genuine emotional comfort and safety further away. They make me feel even more ashamed. By identifying with being psychologically harmed I am punishing myself for having genuine emotional needs for nurturing. Fantasies that involve permanently renouncing adulthood are an obstacle to finding a healthy balance between the adult and child in my psyche. Unsafe fantasies intensify our internal conflict.

Even after I stopped the cycle of bingeing and purging baby clothes, my guilt and shame at the masochistic fantasies provoked 'virtual' binge and purge cycles – this time obtaining digital copies of erotic adult baby stories on-line. I would binge by downloading or purchasing a bundle of stories. It was the same cycle, still linked to fetish fantasies and compulsive masturbation. It had the same end result, with me deleting all the digital material I had recently brought.

Confusion and Turmoil

Being a conflicted AB brings a lot of doubt and confusion over our identity – who we are. There were times my baby 'side' felt like a cuckoo in the nest. I was not who I was supposed to be. I was not who I wanted to be. And I was certainly not who everyone thought I was. How do you handle wanting to be a baby – a dependent, vulnerable, wetting baby? It runs counter to everything you are supposed to want, and what everyone else seems to want for themselves. It is like hearing the starting gun in a race, turning around and running in the other direction from everyone else. There are times it feels so WRONG!

I handled it by compartmentalization and denial. I thought of my baby side as quarantined off from the rest of me so that I could 'pass' as normal. It was a separate, hidden, secret 'life'. When I closed the door on it, I maintained to myself that my secret life had no bearing on my 'real', normal life.

But the fear that lurked at the back of my mind was that my baby side was contaminating everything – like the one bad apple that sends the rest mouldy. Even when I succeeded in my education and my career, a part of me felt like a fraud – what if people knew about my secret? What if they knew who I really was? But who was I, really? The man in control of himself and his circumstances or the scared baby who just wanted to have their fears cuddled away? I don't think I really knew, and I was certainly too scared to find out.

And it got worse when I gradually let myself discover my guilty fascination with being a sissy, girly baby. The pictures of pink frilly girly clothes, perhaps even dolls, were forbidden fruit. OMG! Did I really want that? How do you handle being a man on the outside and a baby girl on the inside? I didn't handle it. I just locked the baby girl away in a closet somewhere inside. But I knew she was there, and it doubled up my fears about myself. Was I a sissy? Was I a cross-dresser? Did I want to be a woman? Was I trans-gender?

So, for me, being AB meant I couldn't wholly trust who I was. My deepest fear was that I was a sexual pervert. If I was ever 'outed', people would think I was a paedophile! I never had any sexual attraction towards children. But how do you make sense of a bizarre, confusing fascination for nappies and wanting to be babied? It took me a long while to genuinely trust that I wasn't a paedophile. And I knew that if I was 'outed', I would not be able to convince anybody else I wasn't. I didn't understand myself, so how could I explain it to anyone else? So, for many years the prospect of being 'outed' carried the ultimate fear of disgrace and degradation. I would dishonour myself and those I loved.

Even after I learned to trust that I wasn't a paedophile. I still feared that being AB made me 'damaged goods'. I still had a compulsive sexual fetish that at times made me feel dirty and degraded. At my core, was I broken – irrevocably broken - beyond healing? In retrospect, I think there was a lot of suicidal ideation disguised in my daydreams and thoughts. *(Suicidal ideation is 'psych speak' for thoughts or fantasies of suicide. Suicide is preceded by such thoughts, although these thoughts are common and most of the people who have them do not commit suicide. It is a warning signal, and if you get such thoughts, talk to a friend or a counsellor, or ring a hotline.)*

Over Compensation

Another, insidious effect of my conflict about being AB was 'over-compensation'. That is where I tried 'too hard' in other parts of my life to prove that I was good, psychologically healthy and worthy, because I felt bad about my baby 'side'. At the time, I did not see it. I realized it *after* I had fully accepted myself as an AB.

In my case, the strongest overcompensation was in my career. This is described in my account of my life as an adult baby, *'Living With Chrissie'* –

In hindsight, I can see that every few years I would become a workaholic and eventually pick a quarrel with my superiors. The grounds were always where I was confident, I was standing up for the proper way of doing things. It's likely I caused a succession of superiors some embarrassment at being 'called' on issues they were rather left alone. Things would take their inevitable course and I would end up having to move sideways. At the time, I convinced myself that I was championing 'the right'. In many cases, I was. But that wasn't the whole story. I now realise I was unconsciously setting up conflicts to prove my courage to do the 'right thing'. I needed to prove my courage to offset my shameful weakness in failing to stop my addiction to nappies. It was a recurring cycle that ran alongside the cycle of bingeing and purging my baby clothes.

Over-compensation can be a potent form of self-sabotage. I was never driven to self-harm or open thoughts of suicide directly because of my AB side. But my over-compensation led me to invest all of my self-esteem in my career, to offset my shame at being AB. And that made my psyche vulnerable to setbacks in my career and caused me to once contemplate suicide in a midlife crisis.

There were other ways I over-compensated. My baby 'side' had a guilty attraction to 'sissy' things like dresses, pink clothes and dolls. As a result, I emphasized sides of my personality that 'proved' my masculinity. As an adolescent, I wanted to be a soldier and subsequently served briefly and proudly in the military reserve. Sharing my father and grandfather's interest in military history, was another way of telling myself 'I'm a man. I always loved guns and became a good shot. Having 'come out' to myself as an AB I don't see anything intrinsically wrong with those pursuits. However, I can also see that I was more invested in them than I otherwise would have been – to make myself feel better about a baby 'side' I did not fully understand or accept.

The key point is that while we are living with such a strong conflict about and within ourselves, we are not fully aware of its' effects on our life.

Problems with Partners

Not surprisingly being AB causes lots of problems with our partners. I have been incredibly fortunate. My wife of over thirty years is the love of my life. She is older than I am, and from the start, brought to me and our relationship a warm knowing about life and people. She is also a skilled psychotherapist (we did not meet in her professional capacity, but through mutual friends). But even with all these advantages, being AB caused problems and distance in our relationship.

I told my wife about my 'thing' for nappies before we got married. But I thought of it as an addiction or a sexual fetish, that with therapy and will-power I could renounce. I thought getting married would 'cure' me. This was also the early 1980s, largely before the gay and lesbian liberation movement had taught society about the nature of personal identity.

Of course, being AB did not go away after we got married. In terms of being AB, I was as conflicted about what I wanted from my wife, as I was about myself. On the one hand, I wanted her to recognize and accept my AB side, but on the other, I was ashamed and feared she would be disappointed in me, repulsed or frightened. Hell, it often repulsed and scared me, why wouldn't she be the same? I also didn't want to admit to my wife, my own doubts about being AB. If I recognized that a big part of me still didn't think being an AB was okay, wasn't that just siding with the world against myself?

I am sure my wife picked up very 'mixed messages'. I was saying 'accept my AB side', but at the same time, I was uptight, demanding, and at odds with myself. Only with hindsight, can I see how much anger was generated by the conflict about my denied identity. I now understand that a great deal of displaced anger is one of the hallmarks of the conflicted stages of identity formation. I did not see it before.

No wonder she wanted to keep her distance from my baby 'thing'. I am sure it looked to her a lot more like a harmful addiction or fetish that needed to be contained, rather than a healthy personal identity that could be safely embraced. Like any loving, sane wife, she was protecting herself – and protecting me and our marriage. She was right to do so. In a cruel twist, my conflict intensified my hunger for my wife to accept my child persona, while it was driving her away from doing so. Our conflict is a vicious cycle. It makes prisoners of us all in a jail of our own making, even though the key to the lock is right in front of us.

For the most part, I found it easier to live with being AB, by keeping it away from my wife. ABs are used to living secret lives. We are very, very good at it. Too good. Rosalie Bent indicates that the AB's secrecy is a big problem and risk in a marriage. She is right! In my case secrecy, was not just a habit, it was an ingrained feature of my personality. I said in my book *'Living With Chrissie'* -

> *My wife recently told me that she had no idea about most of my life as an adult baby. I was a lot more successful than I realized in keeping secret my motivations, behaviour and the contents of my collection of clothes. Also, I had largely understood my conduct as an addiction and a sexual fetish. To the extent that I communicated anything to her about my baby side, it was that. With hindsight, I see that I gave my wife no basis to know or understand that being an adult baby was an important part of my identity. For example, she didn't know until much later that my baby collection included dresses, bibs, bonnets, dummies, and so on, which might have given a clue that it was something more than a nappy fetish.*

So even inside my wonderful, loving marriage, I was living in the closet.

Isolation and Loneliness

Of necessity, ABs live a dual life – one life 'out in the open', another life in the closet. Secrecy and withdrawal from others becomes an ingrained part of our personality. So, loneliness is a big part of being AB. As for anyone, that is an ongoing risk to an AB's wellbeing and mental health.

As a conflicted AB, I felt very alone. My psyche seemed to be wired very differently from anyone else I knew – and not in a good way. There are no public role models for healthy non-conflicted ABs. I feared to confide in anyone about being AB for fear of being rejected and judged as a pervert or weirdo. To this day, I have never confided in anyone I have met face-to-face, except my wife and several therapists. Until I wrote my books, my deepest thoughts and experiences of being AB were not shared with anyone, even my wife. Contact on-line with Rosalie and Michael Bent was a turning point for my life as an AB. But it is still not the same as sitting down with someone who knows who you are, face-to-face, eye-to-eye.

I sometimes feel like a fraud with friends and family. There is good reason to keep my AB identity from them. But that is an important part of me that they will never know. And if you don't know that part of me, you really don't know who I am. That leaves a hole. Everyone has a human need to be accepted for who they are. Having to live in secret, often in doubt and shame, gives ABs an intense need to have their identity validated. At its' strongest that need is like hunger. The longer you have spent 'in the closet' the more ravenous that hunger for recognition and validation. Unsatisfied, it can drive adult babies to risky, desperate behaviours.

I discovered well into middle age that I have a propensity for anxiety. Anxiety is an isolating condition. Your own fears and insecurities lock you inside yourself. My anxiety has always been there. Being a conflicted AB made it worse. I suspect that is true for many ABs.

All this might sound very dark. There were times it was, but there were many good times. My reason for being honest about the 'bad stuff' is to let others know you are not alone in having, or having had these doubts and fears.

Summary

Even though we deny it our conflict about being AB reaches into every corner of our lives. The conflict drives -

1. The Push-Pull of Compulsion and Fetish
2. Triggering
3. The Binge and Purge Cycle
4. Masochistic Fantasies

5. Confusion and Turmoil About Ourselves
6. Over Compensation
7. Problems with Partners
8. Isolation and Loneliness

The conflict is so pervasive that it becomes intertwined with our experience of being AB. It is a cruel, bitter irony that we become ABs because we are seeking to comfort a deep need in ourselves, yet the conflict about being AB largely robs any deep comfort from us. Do not despair. The conflict can be resolved and the pains it masked, can be healed.

Rosalie and Michael Bent are the foremost public authorities on the adult baby identity. Rosalie is the wife of Michael, an adult baby. In 2012 Rosalie published the landmark book 'There's A Baby in My Bed' intended for the partners of adult babies. It was the first published work to seriously address adult babies as a personal identity, beyond a sexual fetish. It was updated in 2015 as 'There's Still A Baby in My Bed. Rosalie has also written a book for the parents of teenage adult babies. Michael has published a text 'Adult Babies: Psychology and Practices' and an anthology of insightful articles 'Being An Adult Baby'. Rosalie and Michael are the owners of the website abdiscovery.com.au which is dedicated to helping adult babies understand themselves, and fostering public understanding of the identity.

3. The Internal Conflict

As conflicted ABs, we live with a troubling set of dysfunctions. They are symptoms of an internal conflict. Our psyche is divided, one part is fighting with another. That is what creates the push-pull of being an AB. It is a battle within, and against, ourselves.

The idea of a conflict or dialogue within our psyche is a key feature of psychotherapy. It applies to everybody, not just ABs. We can think of conflicted ABs as having three 'actors' within our psyche –

- A wounded Inner Child
- A punishing Inner Parent and
- A weak anything-to-please Adult.

Our Inner Child is our self as we were as children – our needs and fears before we learned to cover them up. But it is also our child-self in-the-present, remade in our subconscious. For conflicted ABs, our Inner Child is wounded.

Our Inner Parent represents the views of our parents and other authority figures. These may be their actual views, or views that we attribute to them. When we were children our real parents were looking over our shoulder a lot of the time, telling us how to behave. Later our teachers did the same. Long after we left their daily supervision, we still hear their judgements as if they are still there with us.   A conflicted AB's Inner Parent is harsh and punishing.

Our Adult is our grown-up self. They are the one who bears our responsibilities towards our self and others. They are the one responsible for pulling our identity together. A conflicted AB's adult may be functional in other areas of life, like school, work or sports, but when it comes to anything related to being AB, they are weak and uncertain.

For conflicted ABs, the wounded Inner Child and the punishing Inner Parent are at war with each other. The weak Adult is like an ineffective umpire in a very rough sporting match, unable to stop the other two fighting.

Although the conflict about being AB seeps into every corner of our lives, as conflicted ABs we don't know our inner child, inner parent and AB adult that well. To learn more of them we need to see how they are involved in each of our dysfunctions.

The Push-Pull of Compulsion and Fetish

This is about our irresistible need to wear nappies, how that becomes a compulsive sexual fetish, and how our need for deep comfort mostly seems to elude us.

Wounded Child: It is our Inner Child who wants to wear nappies, to cuddle soft toys, suck a pacifier or drink from a baby's bottle. It is a cry to the rest of our psyche, *'I'm here'*, *'I'm real'!* But they don't just want these things – they **need** them. Desperately! And that is the problem. This is a child that has been wounded and damaged. They are hurt, lonely, frightened and angry. No that is not quite true – they are *very* hurt, *very* lonely, *very* frightened and *very* angry. They are simultaneously, desperately needy for comfort, and a behaviour problem who rejects that comfort. This is the traumatized baby/child who will in one moment, cry pitifully for their toy, pacifier or bottle, and the next moment, hurl it across the room. This aligns with our experience of never really getting the deep comfort we seek from wearing nappies and episodes of 'baby time'.

Punishing Parent: Our Inner Parent thinks being an adult baby is absurd. It's ridiculous! It's just plain WRONG! And our Inner Parent doesn't buy this Inner Child crap! It's indulgent, imaginary nonsense! That doesn't stop them having it both ways and berating our Inner Child as willful and ungrateful. Why are we rejecting our toilet training after all the hard work it took the first time around? Ditto with taking up the bottle, dummy and teddy bear again. Our Inner Parent dismisses the notion that our Inner Child needs nurturing, saying harshly, 'Get over it and grow up'. The Parent is disgusted with our weak Adult, and by the sexual fetish and masturbation. It is our Inner Parent that impatiently hurries our baby time along and then rushes to tidy all the evidence of our nappies and masturbation away - 'sweeping it all under the carpet' – out of sight, out of mind.

Weak Adult: Our adult lets our wounded child have their way. They don't know what else to do. Better to give the kid something to keep them quiet, or else they will throw a screaming tantrum and the situation will get out of hand. The heightened sexual arousal is a payoff. At least the adult is getting something out of the never-ending bun-fight between the Inner Parent and Inner Child. Afterwards, the Adult shrugs and placates the angry Inner Parent by sending the Inner Child back to their room and acting like everything is okay.

Triggering

This is about how a compelling and urgent need to put on a nappy can be triggered involuntarily, out-of-the-blue, by sight or another sense.

Wounded Child: This is our Inner Child demanding their nappy and/or baby things. That demand has all the force of a full-on toddler temper tantrum – stamping feet, screaming, howling tears and all. The Child fears our punishing Inner Parent and does not trust our Weak Adult to protect them. The Inner Child knows our Inner Parent doesn't believe the Child is real and doesn't want the Child around. The Child feels alone and uncared for. If they don't take what they need, they won't get anything. The child doesn't know the next time he/she will get to wear a nappy or cuddle a soft toy. And for a child waiting is forever! So, they want it now! We can see the forceful power of our Inner Child in the way that they override our adult selves and compel us to get somewhere and put on a nappy.

Punishing Parent: The insistent demand for a nappy by our wounded Inner Child catches our Inner Parent by surprise. But when they recover, it really pisses them off. Our Inner Child's risky, spur-of-the-moment demand for a nappy, activates our Inner Parent's deepest fear. What if people find out about this freakish perversion? It will be a disgrace! It will ruin our lives! Our Inner Parent sees our Inner Child as a spoiled, whiny brat. Our Parent is ashamed of our Inner Child and afraid of the damage the selfish actions of the child will cause. As with our fetish, our Inner Parent just wants it all over and done with as quickly as possible and back out-of-sight.

Weak Adult: Like the Inner Parent, the adult is caught off-guard. And as with the usual fetish, our adult lets our wounded child have their way. The kid is having a full-on screaming, kicking tantrum. What else can the Adult do? At least if the kid gets what they want, the Adult will get some peace, and they can get back to what they were doing before the Inner Child hijacked everything. And again, the heightened sexual arousal is a pay-off.

At times, when our shame and self-loathing peaks, you can imagine it as a full-on screaming match between our Inner Parent and Child. It is awful – it leaves scars on the psyche. Even after it subsides, it is like the warring pair retire to their own corners, and there is a hostile, sullen truce, while the Adult tries to clear away the mess and broken things.

The Binge and Purge Cycle

This is a cycle of buying a new stash of nappies or baby clothes, or experimenting with new baby activities, building to a crescendo of guilty masturbation, and then discarding everything in a fit of remorse.

Wounded Child: This is our Inner Child at their most demanding. Think of it as going into Toys R'Us with a greedy toddler who wants the whole store and just starts grabbing everything off the shelves. The Inner Child wants nappies, new baby clothes, a new pacifier, baby bottle, new soft toys - everything. Remember, they don't trust anyone will pay any attention to their needs. This feels like their one chance to get everything they want. So, they go for broke! And it works, for a short while. The Child's glee overflows, like a toddler who has too much red cordial at a party. The exhibitionism that risks us being 'outed' in unsafe environments is our Inner Child demanding attention.

Punishing Parent: Our Inner Parent is horrified. Their stern warnings and finger-wagging prove ineffective. It's completely out of control. Everything will be ruined if it isn't stopped now! For good! They come rushing in and shut it all down. They scream at the Inner Child – 'you're bad, you're a freak, you're sick – stop this'! They drag our crying Inner Child into a closed dark room at the back of the house and lock them in alone. The Parent tells our terrified Inner Child they will never be allowed out again, and all their precious baby things will be thrown away. The Inner Child is traumatized all over again. They are left abandoned in the dark.

Weak Adult: As usual, our Adult gives in to what the Inner Child wants. Sure, the heightened sexual arousal is fine, but the extent of the Inner Child's out-of-control woundedness frightens our weak Adult. They don't know what to do. They are grateful to let the punishing Inner Parent take over to sort it all out. But it costs them a lot of self-respect because the Inner Parent makes it clear the Adult can't be trusted to know what is good for themselves. The Parent berates the Adult for being weak and foolishly indulgent towards the Inner Child. From now on, the Adult needs to do just what the Inner Parent tells them. At first, the weak Adult is grateful, but in time, they resent the Inner Parent's heavy-handed control and harsh judgements. The Adult feels sorry for the Inner Child and ashamed they stood by and let the Inner Parent treat the Child so brutally. So, eventually, they let the Inner Child out and try and make them happy. But the Adult only hopes it will be better the next time. They have not learned anything. And so, the cycle kicks off again.

This aligns with the wild emotional swings of the binge and purge cycle - from greedy, gleeful excitement to abject fear and abasement.

Masochistic Fantasies

These are the sexual fantasies about being coerced, shamed and humiliated by a dominant figure.

Wounded Child: This is the Child crying out to be comforted and protected by a strong mother or father. They feel abandoned and unloved. They want to be picked up, cuddled and soothed. They want someone to set boundaries so they will feel safe. They want to feel that someone loves them enough to discipline them with kindness and love. They want to be naughty and know they are still loved and protected. They want to be important to someone who will focus on them, and only them. But they don't trust that anyone loves them, so if there is humiliation and shame it is a price they will gladly pay for the love they desperately seek.

Punishing Parent: Our Inner Parent sees our Inner Child as whiny and demanding. 'Suck it up princess', they tell the Child harshly. Our Inner Parent is frankly disgusted at our weak Adult for getting off sexually on these fantasies. Imagine enjoying thoughts of being babied and dominated? It is demeaning. You should be ashamed! Pervert! From the Parent's perspective, the saving grace is that at least no one else can see. It is all in our heads.

Weak Adult: The Adult sees our Inner Child's constant needs and demands as a nuisance and a distraction. Indulging these fantasies keeps the kid quiet. As before, the heightened sexual arousal is gratifying. And as this is all just in the mind, who's to know, what's the harm? But the Inner Parent's disgust is a stinging barb

167

to the Adult. The element of compulsion and coercion in the fantasies is the Adult's sop to the Inner Parent – *'I don't really want to be babied or submissive, in these fantasies I'm being made to do things I don't want to do'.*

This aligns with the potent appeal and efficacy of the fantasies, as well as the guilt and shame they create.

Confusion and Turmoil About Ourselves

Conflicted ABs live with confusion and doubt about their identity.

Wounded Child: No wonder our sense of who we are is confused and in turmoil. Everything we are striving to be as adults is the opposite of the character of our wounded Inner Child. The latter has the feelings and needs of a very young, scared and wounded child. They don't feel grown-up, independent, capable and brave. The adult world is a big, scary, overwhelming place. They desperately want and need to be feel held, comforted and protected. Also, for me, my masculinity as an adult had a counterpart in an Inner Child who was not only a toddler but a baby girl.

Punishing Parent: Our Inner Parent is terrified that we will 'lose it' in front of others and ruin our lives. 'For God's sake get a grip', they tell our Adult, 'do you want everyone to think you're crazy? And of course, if the Inner Child is a different gender from our adult self, that's just beyond the pale! It is disgusting! Our Inner Parent is angry and afraid of the Inner Child, and ashamed of the doubt and confusion of the adult. To our Inner Parent, it looks like weakness and self-indulgence.

Weak Adult: In terms of our lives as an AB, our Adult is paralysed by confusion and doubt. They can only react, swinging between responding to the demands of our wounded Inner Child, and then to the harsh judgements of our punishing Inner Parent. They have no sure confidence in who they are. Instead, they find what safety they can in following the commands of our Inner Parent - doing what is expected of them, being who everyone expects them to be. The Adult mostly relies on denial. Our conflicted AB behaviours are like a neon light telling us our psyche is wired differently from everyone else, but the Weak Adult is terrified to look deeper. What happens if that just confirms we are damaged, broken beyond help of recovery? So, they just keep telling themselves *'I'm normal'*. But that leaves them feeling deadened and hollow inside. And there seems to be no way forward.

Over Compensation

Conflicted ABs shore up a sense of worthiness by over-investing in some other area of their life, often work or a sport or hobby. This is often unconscious and therefore unrecognized.

Wounded Child: The overcompensation of our Adult self is like having a preoccupied, workaholic parent who doesn't know how to handle their troubled and needy child. The Adult goes off to work each day and ignores the needs of their increasingly unloved child at home. Little wonder that the Inner Child periodically rebels and upsets the apple cart.

Punishing Parent: We have seen that our Inner Parent is deeply disappointed in our Weak Adult. The Parent doesn't trust the Adult to make good decisions or be strong enough. The Parent is disgusted at the Adult's sexual fetish. So, the Inner Parent is like a monkey on the Adult's back, goading the Adult to redeem themselves by succeeding in the eyes of others. Our Inner Parent says, 'you can be an adult baby OR you can be a good person, a successful person, a brave person BUT you can't be BOTH'. And of course, because our Adult can't completely turn their back on the wounded Inner Child, the punishing Inner Parent tells the Adult, 'you're weak, you're a loser, you're a pervert. You need to prove you're a good person!'

Weak Adult: Our Adult is grateful to find a space where they can get away from the incessant fighting of both the Inner Child and the Inner Parent. Sure, it is running away, but it's understandable. It is a space away from the conflict and turmoil where they can feel normal. But they still end up believing part of the Inner Parent's damaging messages. Even in other areas of life, away from the whole AB 'thing', they still feel like a fraud.

Problems with Partners

Being a conflicted AB often brings secrets, underlying tension and sometimes conflict into our relationship with our partner.

Wounded Child: Our Inner Child desperately wants our partner's love. They want our partner to rescue them from our own punishing Inner Parent and Weak Adult. They want our partner to be their fairy godmother, wave a magic wand and make everything all right. But our Inner Child is also wounded and mixed up. They feel left out. They are envious of the love our partner has for our adult selves. They want it for themselves and they want to get in the middle. And they are also afraid our partner will ally with our own Punishing Inner Parent who wants to lock the child in the back room. The Inner Child fears if they get too far out of line, maybe that is what will happen.

Punishing Parent: Our Inner Parent wants to protect our relationship with our partner from the whole messy business of being AB. They are afraid our partner will distance from us or leave us. They don't trust the Weak Adult to do the right thing to keep our partner. The Inner Parent wants to keep all the turmoil, doubt, and especially the disgusting sexual fetish, as far away from our partner as possible. They say, 'better to keep it all in the closet before you lose the best thing you've got going for you.' And they most definitely don't want that spoilt, damaged Inner Child anywhere near our partner.

Weak Adult: Our Adult self doesn't want to damage or lose our relationship with our partner. But at the same time, they have a confused hope that our partner can 'sort us out'. They want to be rescued from our own internal conflict. Maybe our partner can love and heal our wounded Inner Child? Maybe they can get the punishing Inner Parent off our back? It is crazy, it is risky, but where else does the weak Adult have to turn? But mostly, they are too fearful to ask outright, so the Weak Adult, episodically finds backdoor ways to cry for help. But then they get berated by our Inner Parent for dragging damaging baggage into the relationship, and the Adult retreats from our partner.

Little wonder that our relationship with our partner gets complicated. There are three in the relationship, and none is sure where they stand because all are working in the dark.

Isolation and Loneliness

Conflicted AB's often live with deep feelings of isolation and loneliness because of their internal conflicts and the need to keep their identity secret.

Wounded Child: If our Inner Child was a biological child they would have been removed from the family and taken into care by virtue of emotional abuse and neglect. Their needs are not reliably met. They are often left alone and ignored. Perodically the punishing Inner Parent screams abuse at them, makes them feel worthless, locks them alone in a dark room and tells them they are never getting out again. They spend a lot of their time feeling lonely and afraid, and other times terrified and traumatized. This aligns with many of our feelings of isolation and loneliness as an AB.

Punishing Parent: The Inner Parent desperately wants to keep up a pretence to the world that everything is normal. They want to keep others as far away as possible from our AB side and the wounded Inner Child as possible, in case our awful, guilty, dirty secret is discovered and used against us. They don't trust the weak Adult to hold it all together and not let the 'cat-out-of-the-bag.' Isolation and loneliness is a price that has to be paid for safety. If we consider going to counselling our Inner Parent is hoping to win over the counsellor as an ally against our Inner Child – surely the counsellor will see that the Inner Child is the source of all our problems. The Inner Parent hopes the counsellor will agree with the Parent and force our weak Adult to lock the Inner Child away forever.

Weak Adult: Here we can see that our Adult self, is also damaged and wounded. They don't trust themselves. They are living with doubt and episodic turmoil. They are guilty about not caring for the wounded

Inner Child, and ashamed of disappointing the punishing Inner Parent. They feel unworthy and unlikeable. Better to retreat from others than be rejected.

All three internal 'actors' contribute to our feelings of isolation and loneliness.

Never-Ending Conflict

Why does this three-horned-conflict keep repeating, over and over again? Internal or psychological conflict has a healthy function. If it builds up too much, then eventually the pressure becomes unbearable, and we are driven to change. That is not happening. Why?

The conflict is an example of what psychologists call the **Victim-Persecutor-Rescuer triangle**. The three roles in the triangle are –

The Victim – their stance is '*poor me!*' They feel victimized, helpless, ashamed, and unable to make decisions or solve problems.

The Persecutor – They say to the Victim, '*it's all your fault.*' They are blaming, controlling, angry and superior.

The Rescuer – They say to the Victim '*let me help you.*' But they have an ulterior motive. They avoid their own problems by focusing on the victim. Their rescuing keeps the Victim dependent and gives the Victim permission to fail.

Mostly, our wounded Inner Child is the Victim, the punishing Inner Parent is the Persecutor, and the Weak Adult is the Rescuer. But the key thing about the Victim-Persecutor-Rescuer triangle is that actors shift between the three roles.

So, the Inner Child can shift to become the Persecutor - such as when they drive a binge on nappies and blame the Parent and Adult for neglecting them. The Inner Child can also become the Rescuer – such as when they side with the weak Adult being bullied by the punishing Inner Parent.

Likewise, the Inner Parent can become the Victim when they play the martyr – '*I'm just trying to protect us from discovery and ruin, and this is the thanks I get?*'. They can also play the Rescuer, bailing out the harassed Weak Adult by stepping in to 'handle' the Inner Child.

The Weak Adult can play the Victim - such as when they feel bullied by the Punishing Inner Parent or they are driven to distraction by the demands of the Inner Child. The Weak Adult can also be the Persecutor, such as when they hand the wounded Inner Child over to the punishing Inner Parent.

The Victim-Persecutor-Rescuer triangle explains why, despite all the conflict and all the drama - nothing changes.

The Wikipedia article on the triangle sums it up –

> " ... the reason the situation endures is that each gets their unspoken (and frequently unconscious) psychological wishes/needs met in a manner they feel justified, without having to acknowledge the broader dysfunction or harm done in the situation as a whole. ... Each triangle has a payoff for those playing it."

In the Victim-Persecutor-Rescuer triangle, before the pressure becomes too much to bear, and drives change, the three actors shift roles. The Inner Child who mostly plays the Victim, shifts to become the Persecutor, or perhaps the Rescuer. And the same for the Inner Parent and the Weak Adult. And so, the whole drama is re-booted. Now it cycles around again. The re-boots can go on endlessly. The healthy function of conflict is subverted.

But why?

The pay-offs, of course!

Each of our inner actors within our psyche is getting something out of the drama. The Inner Child is damaged and doesn't trust they will ever be genuinely loved and cared for. This is the best they can get. The Inner Parent confirms that their judgements about the failings of the other two are valid – they are proved right, again and again.

The Adult is the one with the power to change the situation. They are the one who pulls our identity together. But the pay-off for them is the guaranteed, heightened arousal of the sexual fetish. The fetish feels like a sure-fire antidote to stress, anxiety and depression. What happens if there is nothing to replace it? That is the reason why the conflict never moves on, never resolves.

Summary

The dysfunctions that harass and bedevil the lives of conflicted ABs are driven by the conflict inside our psyche between our wounded Inner Child, our punishing Inner Parent and our weak Adult. The description of the conflict above reflects my experience of my psyche. Each AB is different. Some aspects of my experience will resonate with you, others won't. The character of these three 'actors' within the psyche, and their interactions, will be different for each AB. But what is true for conflicted AB's is that we are at war with ourselves.

4. Self-Acceptance

As ABs, we have generally learned to live with our 'baby side'. We have lengthened the intervals between cycles of binge and purge. We have learned not to push the boundaries of experimentation with our baby clothes or activities too far, too fast, to avoid triggering deep shame and provoking a purge. We may have moved beyond physical purges of our collections of nappies and baby clothes. We give ourself enough 'baby time' to turn off most of the involuntary triggering. But there will probably still be some cycle of guilt and remorse, even if it is just the occasional purging of digital erotic AB fiction. Deep down, the doubt about ourselves is still there. The over-compensation is still at work, unrecognized. The issues for our relationships are still there. And we still feel very alone a lot of the time.

In short, the conflict about being AB has not gone away or been resolved – we have learned to live with it. We have learned to manage it like a chronic medical condition. We have achieved an equilibrium which is like a truce after a long, exhausting war. But it is not genuine peace, and episodically, guerilla warfare between our wounded Inner Child and our punishing Inner Parent breaks out again. We accept this as the best we can get. At least it is better than going through the ravages of the binge and purge cycle.

This is *not* what I mean by self-acceptance.

By self-acceptance, I mean resolving the internal conflict.

It isn't buried. It is gone. No more guilt and shame. It isn't about being 'cured' of being AB. We are still ABs, we still love nappies, we still have a nappy fetish - but the internal conflict that drives dysfunctions in our lives is gone.

It is not being AB that is unhealthy or harmful.

It is being *conflicted* about being AB that is unhealthy and harmful.

By definition, self-acceptance is accepting something about ourselves.

So, what do we need to accept about ourselves to resolve our internal conflict?

It is simply this:

ABs have a child persona – a 'Little' self - which is real, permanent, fundamental to our psyche, and (when we resolve our internal conflict) healthy. The AB's nappies, baby clothes and baby play can best be understood as a concrete affirmation *to the self* of the existence of the child persona.

The wounded Inner Child we met in the last chapter – or rather, your unique version of them – is a subjectively real part of your psyche. They are not a trick or figment of your imagination. They are not therapeutic play-acting. They are real! A part of your psyche really feels, thinks and behaves like a small child. That child persona is hard-wired into your psyche and has been since you were a biological child.

You have tried pretending they did not exist. You have tried ignoring them. You have tried thinking of them as just a 'side' of your personality. But they are still there, and they won't ever go away. To accept our child persona goes against a deeply ingrained habit of denial. So, if your courage needs to be fortified to embrace this personal identity, ask yourself - has years of denial made you happy? If you are an AB and you are reading this book, the answer is probably no.

You will have questions.

Does this mean I'm crazy?

Why me? Where did this child persona come from?

How do you I live with a child persona in my psyche?

How can I be an adult AND a baby?

What good comes of accepting all this?

Let's take each of these in turn.

Am I crazy?

Fear of thinking of ourselves as crazy, or being regarded that way by others, is one of the main reasons why it usually takes so long to accept that we have a subjectively real child persona.

No, you are not crazy. You are a sane, functional adult. It is simply that you share your consciousness with an innocent child.

Our culture and education does little or nothing to prepare us to think in terms of shared consciousness. For everyone, ABs and non-ABs, it is a deeply ingrained habit to think of ourselves as having one mind or consciousness. But it is no more than an old habit.

Shared consciousness is a norm in many schools of psychology. Dr Marlene Steinberg states –

> *"As diverse as they are, the many theories of identity formation that have been advanced over the centuries have one aspect in common: none of the theorists understood human identity to be a monolithic given. All of the schools of thought were based on the assumption that identity is a construct, built up by the individual from a set of different elements, experiences, capacities, or components. In addition to different layers of consciousness, we have basic instinctual drives and a conscience; faculties of reason, emotion, will and so on; capacities for analysis and logical thought in the left brain and intuitive, artistic and musical capabilities in the right; a predisposition towards introversion or extraversion; characteristics like agreeableness, sociality, conscientiousness, and ambition; and so on."* [The Stranger in the Mirror]

The psychologist John Rowan in his book *'Subpersonalities: The People Inside Us'* shows that ideas about healthy shared consciousness have a respectable pedigree in schools of psychotherapy, going back to Freud and Jung.

Since the 1980s a school of psychology has emerged which views shared consciousness as normal and healthy – applicable to all. **Internal Family Systems Therapy** (IFS) was developed by Richard Schwartz (see his book of the same name, cited in the references). It holds that we all have multiple personas (termed 'parts') lead by a unifying Self. We shall return to IFS later in the book.

You have a subjectively real child persona, and an Inner Parent, both led by your Adult Self. Your non-conflicted adult, child and parent are each aspects of your True Self.

We commonly associate the existence of sub-personalities or personas with Dissociative Identity Disorder (DID), formerly known as Multiple Personality Disorder (MPD). There are many high functioning people with dissociative conditions. A member of my extended family has DID. They are a gifted teacher who has taught special needs children in schools around the world.

AB's share something with Dissociative Identity Disorder (DID) - both identities are defined by shared consciousness – they have subjectively real sub-personalities. And for both identities, problems arise *only* in the conflicted state when the parts act independently of the self. For both the AB and DID identities, when internal conflict is resolved the parts work cooperatively and there is a healthy sense of self. In the absence of dysfunction, the person has a minority identity, not a disorder.

As ABs, we can learn from healthy people with DID. They have learned how to live successfully with shared consciousness. *'Got Parts: An Insiders Guide to Managing Life Successfully with Dissociative Identity Disorder'* tells us –

> *"Parts are never going to disappear or go away; they will always be there, and part of you. Individual parts will always remain separately individual, but the goal of re-integration is to become aware of each other and working so seamlessly and cooperatively together, with shared information and regarding switches, that you can live and function in the outside world with a minimum of distress, without others even knowing about your multiplicity unless you choose to disclose it."*

So, you are not crazy. It may feel a little strange at first to undo a lifetime's habit of thinking of yourself as having a unitary mind. But it is just unlearning a habit. And you have already been living with shared consciousness for most of your life.

Why Me? Where did the child persona come from?

Your child persona is a positive response to difficulties in your early childhood. It was not the cause of those difficulties.

Based on my experience, I believe that there was a time, or times, in your childhood when you felt very frightened and desperately alone. You were a very young, vulnerable child. You felt overwhelmed. That was when the child persona emerged in your psyche. It was the best thing your psyche could do to protect you from despair.

It does not have to mean that you had bad parents. Even with the best will in the world, parents can't always protect their children from the 'ordinary catastrophes' of childhood. Those catastrophes include a young child being very frightened at a temporary separation from their mother or primary caregiver. But whatever it was, at the time, you did not understand what was happening. You felt alone and unloved. And like all children who feel unloved, you felt it was your fault. You felt unlovable. Your Inner Child was wounded. And such childhood wounds stay with us. For some ABs, these wounds may not come from the ordinary catastrophes of childhood, but from abuse or neglect.

Your child persona is a creation of your subconscious. They are not you as a biological child, although you can see *some* influence of yourself as a biological child in your child persona. Your child persona is the most loveable child, the most deserving of comfort and protection, that your sub-conscious could create. Your child persona is your subconscious giving you permission to love and heal your wounded Inner Child. Your child persona is a redeeming feature of your psyche.

The origin of ABs' child personas is explored in depth in my book *'The Adult Baby Identity – Healing Childhood Wounds'*.

How do you live with a child persona in your psyche?

In the last chapter, we met our Inner Child at their worst. They are wounded - scared, angry and demanding. Isn't living with them inside our psyche going to be awful?

No!

Your acceptance that they are real, and their needs for comfort and protection are genuine, is wonderfully healing. It is a game-changer. Over time, your wounded Inner Child will transform into your lovable child persona, who is a delight. The healing and transformation can take a while, but you will see it start to take effect straight away. Imagine being a child who has lived most of their life alone in the dark, denied and unwanted. And one day, someone comes in, opens the curtains to the light, picks you up and cuddles you lovingly, and tells you that you are wanted, and they will never leave you. Yes, the wounds will take time to heal, but now you know there is hope and love.

Your child persona is an intrinsic part of you. As Rosalie Bent indicates, the persona is always present in our consciousness 24/7. They can move from the foreground to the background of our consciousness, but they are always there. They are sufficiently separate to have needs and feelings which are different from your adult self – although these are ultimately your needs and feelings as well. It is not something to be afraid of or embarrassed about. The character of the child persona of each AB is unique, just as the adult selves of ABs are unique.

We will talk more about our child persona in a later chapter.

How Can I Be An Adult AND a Baby?

You are a functional adult with a child persona. You share a common consciousness. When the internal conflict is resolved, your Adult, Inner child and Inner parent work cooperatively. There is a division of labour that all understand. When you want or need to be adult, you are adult, and the Inner Child steps into the background. Your Inner Parent is always there, taking care of your Inner Child so the Child doesn't feel alone and disrupt your Adult doing adult things. When you choose, your Inner Child comes to the foreground to be nurtured and to play – giving you access to child-like innocent happiness, security and contentment.

My child persona is a baby toddler girl named Chrissie. The following is from my book '*The Adult Baby Identity – Healing Childhood Wounds*' –

> *What does living with a child persona feel like? I can only speak for myself. Chrissie is always with me, separately processing whatever is going on. Most of the time, when I'm my adult-self, she's in the background and I'm not consciously aware of her. In adult spaces, I just 'get on with it'. It's like sharing a house in a long happy marriage; sharing a playground with my best childhood friend, or like a beloved favourite old dog. It's a deeply familiar, companionable presence, where the communication is at a deeper level than the verbal. It feels very natural and normal.*

> *I don't hear Chrissie speaking to me/my adult self, as though we were two different people. That would feel too separate - she is part of me. But I sometimes sense what Chrissie would say. For example, if my wife and I are out shopping and I see something that I sense Chrissie would love, I'll say 'Chrissie'd love that' or I might say 'want it' but only in self-conscious adult mimicry of a little girl - I don't speak as Chrissie.*

I am, or can readily become, aware of her feelings, needs and reactions, but these don't overpower my adult self. ... This is what it's like for me. It will be different for every AB. When you have resolved internal conflicts and accepted your identity, stay true to your unique experience of your child persona. Trust yourself. … Having a subjectively real child persona in my psyche does not in any way stop me being a functional adult.

With this understanding of the identity, it has to be admitted that the term 'adult baby' is not ideal, and even counter-productive. In AB, 'baby' is the noun and 'adult' is an adjective. This is misleading and unhelpful in that it suggests the primary identity is the baby or child. That suggests an indulgent or neurotic renunciation of adulthood. For non-conflicted ABs, this is the reverse of reality. As Michael Bent indicates the adult self is the primary personality and the baby or child persona is a sub-personality (see *'The Identity Conflicts of the Adult Baby'* in the book *'Being an Adult Baby', or free online at abdiscovery.com.au under the articles tab*). In preference to the term adult baby, Rosalie and Michael Bent use the term Adult Infantile Regression (AIR). I prefer to say that I am an adult with a child persona. That said, the term AB is now so widely used that I doubt it is amenable to change. It is still important to be clear about the real nature of the identity. Given the issue with the term 'adult baby', I prefer to use the abbreviation AB.

What good comes of accepting all this?

Accepting our child persona as a real and permanent part of our psyche is the start of resolving our internal conflict. The resolution of that conflict will remove the dysfunctions described in Chapter 2.

Accepting your child persona is also the start of accepting being AB as a personal identity. Having a subjectively real child persona is a non-conforming experience of self. Transgender people have a non-conforming experience of self. That makes being AB a minority personal identity, akin to, but not the same as, LGBTQ (Lesbian, Gay, Bisexual, Transgender, Queer) identities. Not a fetish. Not a kink. You can have an identity as an AB and be any sexual orientation - heterosexual, lesbian, gay, bisexual or asexual.

Thanks to the historic struggles of the gay and lesbian community, we now understand personal identity. It is hard-wired in at an early stage in life. As Rosalie Bent says many adult babies can trace the first consciousness of a different sense of self, wanting nappies, back to childhood. You don't consciously choose to be an adult baby – in fact, it is pretty much impossible to consciously choose *not* to be an AB if you are one. We know that identity cannot be 'cured' by psychology, will power or religious faith. It can be denied – at great cost to a person's well being. In denying that our child persona is a real, permanent and healthy part of our psyche we have been denying our personal identity – denying who we are. That can really mess you up. But that is over now. The way to happiness lies in accepting your identity and making what *you* want of that identity. That is what this book is about.

Being AB as a minority personal identity is explored in my book *'The Adult Baby Identity – Coming Out As An Adult Baby'*.

Accepting our child persona is the start, but there is more to self-acceptance. In the next chapters, we will look at –

- the buried emotions that lie underneath being AB;
- building a healthy personal identity with a strong Adult, a nurturing Inner Parent and a happy beloved child persona;
- learning to live comfortably with shared consciousness; and
- improving relationships with partners.

Healing our wounded psyche and self-acceptance, are intertwined. As you move forward you will build a virtuous circle, where self-acceptance fosters healing, and in turn, healing builds self-acceptance.

In my experience, in matters of personal identity, self-acceptance leads to healing. The first steps of self-acceptance are the game-changer. Healing will follow. Self-acceptance removes the internal conflict that comes from denying the subjective reality of our child persona. In turn, the removal of the conflict drains the compulsive energy from the fetish / False Self dimension of the AB identity. The end of the compulsive fetish changes the character of the AB identity. It shifts from masking the pain and despair, to healing it.

This book is largely about self-acceptance. For an exploration of healing the wounded AB psyche see my book – *'The Adult Baby Identity – Healing Childhood Wounds'*.

5. Buried Emotions

O pening up the issues related to our identity is likely to touch on some buried emotions. Some of those emotions are likely to be troubling and painful. I'm telling you so that if this happens, you will know that it is normal and that you will be okay. You can make peace with those hurts.

Every AB is different. I want to understand my emotions because I don't like surprises. But at the same time, deep emotions scare me, and it can take me a long while to find the courage to 'go there'. Some may choose not to open the door to difficult emotions. In some cases, our emotions won't take no for an answer, and do not leave us a choice.

Whatever your disposition, the purpose of this chapter is to provide you with an understanding of the emotional landscape that lies behind being a conflicted AB.

Troubling and painful emotions are likely to come from two sources -

our wounded Inner Child who carries our childhood pain; and

the internal conflict we have carried for many years.

Broken Attachment

I believe that, as very young children, ABs had a broken or damaged attachment with their mothers.

This is based on a well-recognized, empirically based, psychological theory, called Attachment Theory. It was developed by an eminent psychotherapist named John Bowlby. *(Note: Attachment Theory is not the same as Attachment Parenting or Attachment Therapy).*

Studies, replicated in advanced western countries, suggest that around one-third of children have a broken attachment (called an insecure attachment) with their mothers or primary caregivers. ABs keep nappies, stuffed toys and other baby things, very much in view as part of their identity. This suggests unmet needs in infancy. I believe that ABs are part of the larger population with insecure attachments. Patterns of attachment are established very early in life. The empirical studies supporting Attachment Theory show these patterns are well established by the time a child is one year old. Once established, patterns of attachment tend to persist into later childhood and adulthood (although they can be changed).

It does not necessarily mean that our mothers were bad mothers. An insecure attachment happens because a mother was not well attuned to the feelings and needs of her baby. That can happen for all sorts of common reasons – a mother is anxious, feels unsupported, depressed, fatigued or she did not know how to love her baby as she wanted to, because her mother had been the same (insecure attachments tend to get repeated over the generations). In a minority of cases, an insecure attachment can also come from abuse or neglect.

Whatever the reason for it, an insecure attachment means that a child does not fully trust that others will 'be there' for them. They also tend not to trust, either in themselves or their emotions. They believe that they have to earn the love of others. Children with insecure attachments compensate, generally either by becoming reserved and aloof (if they don't trust their own emotions), or dependent and 'clingy' (if they don't trust themselves).

An insecure attachment leaves a legacy of difficult, buried emotions that can last well into our lives as adults. People with insecure attachments often feel alone and uncertain – about themselves and about their place in the world – that they don't belong.

An AB's wounded Inner Child will have a lot of fear and anger. Attachment Theory tells us that a child with an insecure attachment is afraid they aren't loved and safe. For conflicted adult babies, that fear is still there - locked up in the sinews of the personality formed by that insecure attachment.

Attachment Theory tells us of the rage that our wounded Inner Child felt because their needs for safety and comfort were not met. Our Inner Child had to suppress that rage to be the child our mother needed us to be. Conflicted adult babies may not be fully aware of the extent of their anger – but it is probably there, bubbling away deep below and then seeping through the cracks. Ask yourself how angry are you at not having felt as loved and safe as any child has a right to be, and then having to swallow down your anger? How angry are you at being made to feel bad about your genuine needs for recognition and nurturing. If your answer is 'not much', and you have inner conflict and compulsive behaviours, have another look.

There will also be loss and grief - perhaps deep sadness, as you mourn for the lost secure and happy childhood that you deserved and wanted (and perhaps that your loving parents wanted for you). For me, the yearning for the missing childhood attachment was, and sometimes still is, intensely painful. The 'memories' belonging to pre-verbal, pre-logical infancy and childhood are held in the body, not the mind. In airing your buried emotions you need to trust the feelings in your body, as well as memories from the mind.

If you are reading this and recognize that you had an insecure attachment, do not be dismayed. A person who had an insecure attachment as a child cannot 'wipe that slate clean', but they can heal (or at least make peace with) those wounds. Attachment Theory recognizes that an insecure attachment is not fixed. Through various means, adults can change the internal working model that shapes their relationships and move from an insecure to a secure attachment. Those means include self-nurturing, accepting our real identity, a good marriage, a redeeming personal faith, therapy, or a combination of these. In short, healing is possible. An AB's child persona was a response to the insecure attachment, not the cause. When we accept ourselves, loving our child persona is a way of healing the wounds of the insecure attachment.

For a deeper exploration of the childhood origins of being AB refer to my book *'The Adult Baby Identity – Healing Childhood Wounds'*. Therapist's Jasmin Lee Cori's book *'The Emotionally Absent Mother: How to Recognize and Heal the Invisible Effects of Childhood Emotional Neglect'* is a good self-help resource for healing an insecure attachment.

Childhood Trauma

I believe that for many ABs, the effects of an insecure attachment with their mothers, was compounded by trauma in childhood. Children with insecure attachments are more susceptible to being traumatized, both because their psyches are more vulnerable, and because their parents are not well attuned to their needs and feelings to identify or repair the harm. Attachment Theory indicates that young children are very susceptible to being traumatized by even temporary separations from their mothers or primary caregivers. This is especially so when they are too young to understand what is happening. In most cases, this trauma does not relate to abuse or neglect, but to the 'ordinary catastrophes' of childhood. In my case, I was traumatized by a temporary separation from my mother when I was aged three or four. It happened when she took me with her to a sporting club and left me in the care of people I did not know. For a minority of ABs, trauma will be caused by abuse.

Childhood trauma is more than distress. If the trauma is too overwhelming for the child to handle, they dissociate. That means the fear and hurt are quarantined deep in the psyche so that the child can continue to function. Memories of trauma are stored in the brain in a different way than other memories. The components for each sense – sight, sound, smell, touch, the emotions, are split up and each is stored in a different place in the brain. In dissociation, all or most of those memories are buried in the unconscious in what is called repression. You do not even know they are there. In my case, the traumatic temporary separation from my mother was part of family history and I had a visual recollection of the event. But it was only after I talked to a skilled therapist in later life that I recalled my emotional memory and joined it with the visual memory. Only then did I understand how traumatized I had been.

Sometimes if the trauma is overwhelming, a child will split off a separate persona within their psyche. It is the psyche's way of saving itself from giving way to despair. Like the memories of fear and hurt, the dissociation also causes the existence of the split-off persona to be repressed in the unconscious. For many ABs, I believe this is where their child persona originated. It is true for me.

It is common for repression to break down as we get older. Fragments of memory of the trauma return. Also, the split-off persona can episodically 'breakthrough' and influence or drive our thoughts, feelings and behaviours. I believe that for many ABs, their irresistible compulsion to wear nappies and engage in baby activities represents their repressed child persona 'breaking through'. Those behaviours are often completely at odds with the character of the AB's adolescent or adult self. For ABs, the dissociation starts breaking down early, with their child persona often first driving a compulsion for nappies around age ten. After this, unconscious repression starts to shift to denial, which is a conscious refusal not to recognize troubling issues or implications. As ABs, we are aware of many of the symptoms of our internal conflict. We know our adult self is sometimes not in full control of our compulsive behaviour, but we don't want to look 'behind the curtain'.

Some of the symptoms of being a conflicted AB are also symptoms of dissociated trauma. That includes triggering; confusion and turmoil about our identity; and especially, the binge and purge cycle. If you are an AB and you have experienced, or are still experiencing these symptoms, you may have dissociated trauma in your past. Do not be afraid, that trauma can be healed. Dissociated childhood trauma is a serious issue. Living with undiagnosed and unhealed dissociated trauma is an ongoing risk to mental health and predisposes people to anxiety and depression. Speaking from personal experience, I can say that it subtly warps your perceptions (most notably about yourself), in ways that you do not realise. Dissociated trauma can be healed, but it needs the help of a skilled therapist experienced in identifying and treating trauma and dissociation.

If you want to read further about dissociation see Dr Marlene Steinberg's book *'The Stranger in the Mirror: Dissociation The Hidden Epidemic'*.

The Internal Conflict

Each of our conflicted parts – our wounded Inner Child, punishing Inner Parent and weak Adult also have painful emotions from our damaging internal conflict.

Our Inner Child had their original hurts compounded again and again by the harsh treatment of our punishing Inner Parent and the neglect of our Weak Adult. The Child's existence has been denied and their genuine needs for comfort and protection have been ignored. Their trust has been broken. And underneath, they don't feel good about the times when they have been selfish, greedy or hurtful.

Our Inner Parent has been tormented by fear about the harm that would come to us if we were 'outed' as ABs. They feel they got left to 'guard the gate' alone and unsupported. They feel guilt and remorse for the pain they caused by denying the existence and needs of our child persona – all those years of brutal, wounding judgements hurled in anger at our wounded Inner Child simply for wanting what any child wants – to feel loved and safe.

Our Weak Adult feels guilt and shame for abdicating their leadership of our psyche, leaving the protection of our identity to our Inner Parent when the Parent was unsuited for the job, allowing our Inner Parent to be so brutal and for failing to protect our Inner Child.

These harms from our internal conflict are some of the most difficult to confront because this is how we damaged ourselves. Never mind that the world-at-large was unaccepting, this is how we did not 'back ourselves'. We need to forgive ourselves for the war within our psyche. We did not know any better at the time. We do now.

Internal Family Systems Therapy has useful, intuitive methods for identifying and healing wounds, both those of childhood and from the internal conflict between our parts. IFS therapist Jay Earley's book *'Self Therapy: A Step-by-Step Guide to Creating Wholeness and Healing Your Inner Child Using IFS'* is a good self-help resource for this healing.

Conclusion

Recognizing these buried emotions is key to healing. The emotions are real. They have been there a long time, buried deep in our psyche, woven into the fabric of our personality. Do not be afraid of them. Their real sting comes from being unrecognized. That sting will diminish greatly from being validated – recognized as real and understandable. Let yourself feel the buried emotions and release them, knowing that you are building a new, healthy identity, based not on conflict between your parts, but love and support.

Therapist Jasmin Lee Cori states –

> *"Most fields of psychotherapy and programs like the twelve-step recovery movement hold to the notion that you can't heal what you can't feel. Numbing and cover-ups protect the wound but prevent the healing. When we finally break through our self-protections and connect with the lived experience of our childhood, it hurts. There is a well of grief we haven't wanted to touch. This well contains both the feelings that were too powerful to experience at the time and have been stored in 'encapsulated form' somewhere in our systems and the grief we feel now we recognize what we went through and how very much we missed."*

If conflicted symptoms persist or recur, even after you have accepted your AB identity, then it is likely that your conscious self-acceptance is being undercut by buried emotions.

Do not be afraid to seek professional counselling if these buried emotions feel too scary or overwhelming, or if they persist despite your best efforts.

You will be okay.

6. True Self Adult

Accepting your child persona as real is an action of your True Self Adult – your strong responsible Adult. It is a game-changer. That recognition took a courage and clarity that your Weak Adult could never muster.

Remember of the three actors in our psyche – Parent, Adult and Child – it is the Adult who is responsible for pulling our identity together. They are the one who bears our responsibilities towards our self and others. When we were conflicted ABs, our Weak Adult had abdicated their responsibilities. Without strong leadership from our Adult, our Inner Child and Inner Parent ran wild.

With self-acceptance, our False Self, Weak Adult transforms into our True Self strong Adult.

The concept of the False Self and the True Self was developed by the renowned psychotherapist Donald Winnicott. Our False Self is the part of us that lives to meet the expectations of others. As children, it was the part of us that believed we had to earn the love of our parents. We learned to comply with others' expectations to be rewarded emotionally and intangible ways. We all need a bit of a False Self. It lets us survive the demands the world makes on us. It allows us to fit into society, to conform sufficiently with social expectations to 'get by' without being either too vulnerable or too abrasive. But too much of the False Self means we feel like we are 'just going through the motions'. We do not feel genuinely ourselves. Our heart and our spirit feel deadened.

By contrast, our True Self is the part of us that feels spontaneous delight when we discover some new experience of ourselves or the world. It is what makes us feel 'real' and alive - authentically and distinctively 'ourselves'. For someone writing in the secular discipline of psychotherapy, Winnicott's conception of the True Self approaches the notion of a spirit or soul.

Our False Self Adult did not trust our unique personal identity as ABs. That identity was too different from what everyone else expected from us. And we have seen how our False Self adult floundered in our internal conflict. But our True Self Adult understands that we do have a unique personal identity. We have to follow our own road, make up our own minds about who we are and what is right for us. Only then are we really able to share who we are with others. This isn't permission to be arseholes, but it is permission to be true to ourselves.

Winnicott's conception of the True Self is matched by the idea of the Self in Internal Family Systems (IFS) therapy. Remember, IFS is a school of psychology that posits that everyone has multiple sub-personalities called 'parts'. When our psychology is healthy, these parts are led by the Self. Richard Schwartz, the creator of IFS describes it as follows –

> " ... *a major tenet of IFS is that everyone has at the core, at the seat of consciousness, a Self that is different from the parts. It is the place from which a person observes, experiences, and interacts with the parts and with other people. It contains the compassion, perspective,*

confidence, and vision required to lead both internal and external life harmoniously and sensitively." [Internal Family Systems Therapy]

Our strong Adult self is the leader of our AB identity. Our child persona is a distinctive, precious part of our healthy identity as ABs. But like a young biological child, our child persona needs to be protected – they cannot be the leader of our psyche. This is covered in my book *'The Adult Baby Identity – Healing Childhood Wounds'* -

"Like any vulnerable biological child, our child persona cannot survive and thrive alone in the world. If we invest all of ourselves in our child personas, we put ourselves at psychological risk. There will be times in life when we have to deal with conflict, danger, fear, loss or grief. To do that successfully we need to see ourselves as more than just our child persona, we need to be more than just our child persona. If not, we will be damaged and traumatized again, just as we were in our biological childhoods. We can't let that happen. ...

There will be many times when our adult self needs to take charge and steer our child persona, for the child's own good. Our child persona is subjectively real. They will have sulks and tantrums – 'hissy fits' – and 'spit the dummy'. There will be times they will be lost in fear or sadness and like any very young biological child not see a way out. That is when our adult self needs to step in, hand our child persona over to our nurturing Inner Parent to be comforted and consoled. To be safe our child persona needs to know there are parents and adults who can take care of them, shield them because those parents and adults have capabilities that the child does not."

Our True Self Adult is strong, wise and compassionate. They are an example of what is called 'servant leadership'. They lead by protecting, comforting and healing the other parts of our psyche. They understand both our Inner child/child persona and Inner Parent.

The most powerful words in any language are 'I love you'. Some of the next most powerful are 'please, thank you, and sorry'. These are words that our strong Adult is not afraid to say, and to mean it when they say it. When you are ready, those are the words your strong Adult needs to say to both your Inner Child and your Inner Parent.

Our strong Adult loves our Inner Child dearly, they have deep compassion for the Child's wounds, and delight in the Child's happy innocence beneath those wounds. I can hear my strong Adult saying to my Inner Child:

'I am so sorry I didn't protect you.

Thank you for not giving up hope. Thank you for keeping innocent love and joy alive within our psyche. Thank you for being you.

Please forgive me. Please let me protect you from now on.'

Our strong Adult also loves our Inner Parent. They have deep compassion for the Parent's tormenting fear that being unsafely 'outed' would ruin our lives. I hear my strong Adult saying to my Inner Parent:

'I am so sorry I left you alone to guard us from danger when that stopped you being able to love our child persona as you wanted to.

Thank you for bravely sticking to that lonely, thankless duty.

Please forgive me. Please let me protect you from now on and leave you free to lovingly nurture our child persona.'

Our strong Adult is the custodian of our healthy, stable AB identity, and our acceptance of that identity. They guard the boundaries between our child persona and the world beyond – including the world outside our front door. That includes blocking behaviours or fantasies that are psychologically unsafe and safeguarding against being outed in unsafe environments. They safeguard our acceptance of our identity if sometimes, our child persona or Inner Parent unthinkingly fall back into old patterns. Our strong Adult will lovingly bring our child persona and Inner Parent back to the secure parent/child attachment that means everything to both of them. And they protect our relationship with our partner.

Changing False Negative Messages

Remember in our internal conflict, how our punishing Inner Parent gave our Weak Adult terrible messages –

'if you're an adult baby you can't be successful'

If you're an adult baby, you can't be worthy'

If you're an adult baby, you can't be brave'

This is awful, damaging stuff! We heard our punishing Inner Parent saying these things with the force of the whole world behind them – like Moses coming down from Mount Sinai with the ten commandments on the stone tablets.

And because of the wound to our self-esteem caused by our shame, some of those damaging messages 'stuck'. This was true of me. I had a long and fulfilling career. After some ups and downs, the latter stages were successful and rewarding. But through most of that time, I sometimes felt like an imposter. I sometimes looked over my shoulder, waiting for the 'wheels to fall off'. On several occasion,s that was a self-fulfilling prophecy. A part of me had 'bought' the message that I could not be an adult baby and be successful in the other parts of my life.

It is time to fully realise that those messages from our punishing Inner Parent are crap! They are false!

Society used to believe you were one thing OR the other. That message was drummed into us. Women were mothers, Femme Fatales or the girl next door. They could not be law enforcement officers, CEOs, Olympic athletes or fighter pilots. Men are tough and independent. They cannot nurture babies and they cannot cry. Gays were sensitive and flamboyant. They could not be football players, fly-in-fly-out mine workers or combat soldiers. I could go on, but you get it. These are just stupid, false, damaging myths. We are human beings. We have the most complex brains on the planet! We can be more than one thing. We can contain seeming opposites within a healthy personal identity.

I can be an adult baby – an adult male with a baby girl persona – who loves nappies and frilly pink girly dresses –

AND step up to save a stranger from domestic violence;

AND handle important public responsibilities in a career in government;

AND be a loving husband.

Having to choose between your personal identity as an adult baby and your aspirations in the rest of your life is a false choice. Look at the following -

Ben Ingram, author of *'Fear and Joy: A Life In And Out Of Nappies'* learned as a young child and teenager that he liked and was comforted by wearing nappies. He went on to become a soldier and fight three times for his country. He still likes nappies. (available at www.abdiscovery.com.au)

Dr John Marshall, author of *'Australian Baby: A Life of Nappies, Bottles and Struggles'* realized as child and teenager that he was a sissy baby who liked nappies, bottles, dummies and dresses. He went on to get a PhD in Mathematics from prestigious Melbourne University and a prestigious senior statistics job in the capital Canberra. (Available at www.abdiscovery.com.au

Michael Bent grew up wetting the bed and realized he was a sissy baby as a teenager. He went on to create the world's foremost website dedicated to helping adult babies understand their identity, and to help increase public understanding of the identity.

If we could lift the veil of anonymity, I am sure we would see there are many, many more examples.

I can 'hear' my healed Inner Parent saying to my True Self Adult, 'I'm sorry for giving you those awful messages. I was terribly, terribly wrong. I didn't know the strength of our psyche to be uniquely and joyfully ourselves. Please forgive me.'

So, in your healthy AB identity, your True Self Adult leads you to be an adult baby AND successful, worthy and brave (or whatever it is you want to be, or already are)'.

Go you!

Writing Your Own Story

An effective way of putting your True Self Adult in the driving seat is to write an account of your life as an adult baby. This was a powerful experience for me. In writing an account of the ups and downs of my adult baby life, I fully 'came out' to myself, and my wife. I found that writing my story down made it 'real'. The account is best written by your True Self Adult as the story of your whole adult baby identity – including both your Inner Child and Inner Parent. Who else can tell the whole story, being fair and accurate for everyone, including your partner?

Writing our own story can be a big part of self-acceptance, as it allows us to be brutally honest - but at a distance - and then to view – again at a distance – the story of our lives. The act of purging this history onto the page has the effect of putting everything into perspective -both good and bad.

It does not have to be a particular length, long or short. Most people, including myself, seem to find a chronological account the easiest to write – begin at the beginning and see where it takes you. Write it as it comes to you, as you would say it if you were talking a kind and curious stranger you will never see again. Write it for yourself – not with the object of influencing anyone else. When you've written it, keep it, and add to it as you think of more. The key ingredient is honesty. Complete honesty and self-disclosure will open doors to yourself that you didn't realise were there. It is revealing and healing. Being able to tell your own story is both a sign of, and contributor to, psychological health.

After writing his published autobiography as a sissy adult baby, Dr John Marshall stated – 'As a therapy it was invaluable' (see *'Writing Your Own Personal Story'*, free at abdiscovery.com.au under the ABDL Articles tab).

You will want to share your story. It is part of the deep need for validation that all ABs have after living such secret lives. It is important you find a safe place to share it. If you think your partner is ready for it, and you do not have an ulterior motive other than for your AB identity to be recognized, then share it with your partner. If you are a member of an online community and you can safely share it without 'outing' yourself, share it there. Share it with your counsellor.

Not Finished Yet

Now you know your strong True Self Adult, they can lead you through the rest of the process of healing and resolving your internal conflict.

7. Our Nurturing Inner Parent

When we looked at our internal conflict our punishing Inner Parent felt like the evil stepmother in Cinderella or Snow White (or the male equivalent). What possible place can they have in our healthy identity as an AB? Shouldn't they be banished to the outer darkness?

No!

To understand why not, we need to turn once again to Internal Family Systems (IFS) Therapy.

In IFS, our internal 'parts' fall into two categories – Protectors and Exiles. Our wounded Inner Child is an Exile. Exiles carry our hurt and pain. Our punishing Inner Parent is a Protector. The role of Protectors is to 'keep the lid on things' so we can keep functioning as the world expects us to. They are an aspect of Winnicott's False Self. They want to keep hurt locked away inside us so that we do not become overwhelmed. We have seen how in our internal conflict, our punishing Inner Parent tried very hard to keep our wounded Inner Child out of sight, in the background – and at worst, locked in the backroom of the house.

Protectors, like our punishing Inner Parent, are not evil. They are a member of a dysfunctional internal 'family' doing what they think is best because they do not know a better way. IFS has a concept of 'polarisation' to explain what happens when our psyche is conflicted or traumatized. In that state, parts take opposing or competing positions in the mistaken belief that this is necessary to protect the Self. Each part reacts iteratively to the other, taking increasingly extreme positions. We can see this clearly in AB's binge and purge cycles.

Protectors serve an important purpose. They stop our Exiles bringing the Exiles' hurt and pain out in the open when the environment is unsafe, and when our psyche is not yet ready to deal with that pain. This aligns with Donald Winnicott's view of the False Self. Besides letting us navigate society's expectations, our False Self has a second, important role – to hide our True Self until we are ready to accept it. In my case, when I was younger, I can see my False Self/punishing Inner Parent kept my deepest wounds away from further hurt at the hands of my unaccepting family. I would have been too fragile to protect myself from their disapproval. Much later in life, I did not fully come out to myself as an AB until I had retired. My job, and with it my family's financial security, did not need to be protected from me being 'outed'. This is an example of the hidden logic of the False Self or the IFS 'Protectors' at work.

So, if you are an AB and you have read this far, it is likely that your Inner Parent is ready to set your 'exiled' Inner Child/child persona free.

This brings us to another useful concept in IFS – burdens.

Polarised (conflicted) parts often take on extreme ideas, behaviours or feelings derived from damaging situations in a person's life. These burdens lock the part into a conflicted position. In the case of the punishing

Inner Parent, they are burdened by the need to protect our AB identity from being 'outed' in an unsafe environment. The role of safeguarding our identity properly belongs to our Adult self, but in our conflicted state, our Adult was weak, and our Inner Parent did not trust them to do the job. So, our Inner Parent took on this burden. Behind their brutal actions, our Inner Parent was tormented by the fear that our equally polarized out-of-control Inner Child would blow up our lives. Our Inner Parent didn't see that the real harm came from denying our AB identity. They did not know better.

But burdens can be unloaded. Our strong Adult has stepped up to lead and protect our identity with wisdom and compassion. Our Inner Parent can set down that role, trusting that it is in safe hands. That leaves them free to become what they want to be - a loving, nurturing Parent to our child persona.

Our wounded Inner Child needs to be re-parented. They are hurt, angry and mistrusting. You cannot blame them after years of being pushed into the background and left alone. It will take constant, patient love to heal those wounds and build a new trust. And that is what our nurturing Inner Parent is dedicated to doing. Now they can focus all their time and energy to loving and healing our Inner Child. Instead of feeling ashamed and afraid of the wounded Inner Child, our nurturing Inner Parent is their proud, loving carer. In time, their love will comfort our wounded Inner Child so that the Child is no longer traumatized.

I can 'hear' my Inner Parent say to my child persona:

'I love you with all my heart.

I love you when you are happy. I love you when you are sad, frightened or angry. I love you when you are good. I love you when you are naughty.

You are my treasure and my delight.

I am so, so sorry for hurting you.

Thank you for giving me another chance.

Please let me love you as you need to be loved, and as I want to love you.

I will always be there for you. I will always keep you safe.'

Our nurturing Inner Parent is confident of their love for our Inner Child. So, they can be firm and set boundaries when they need to, knowing that it comes from love. Nurturing our Inner Child does not mean spoiling or over-indulging them to the point where they are a selfish, greedy, whiny, tantrum-throwing brat who we would hate if we met in other circumstances. Every child needs boundaries to feel secure and happy, but those boundaries need to be set and kept with love and compassion. It is okay not to give your Inner Child everything they want, or sometimes, demand. Now they have the reassurance and protection of a growing secure attachment with our nurturing Inner Parent. That is what meets their real needs. They do not always have to have that extra dress or soft toy.

Healthy people with DID have learned to re-parent their child parts. 'Got Parts: An Insider's Guide to Managing Life Successfully With Dissociative Identity Disorder' says -

> *"... if your System [psyche] has young parts, and that is not uncommon if abuse or trauma happened at an early age, they need to be afforded the same consideration and respect as any other alter. And, just like 'outside' [biological] kids, whether they are toddlers, they cannot be allowed to run wild and unsupervised doing whatever they want whenever they want. They need manners, rules, guidance and boundaries. They also need love and inclusion, as well as clear, correct, age–appropriate information. Just like every other part, they need to heal from the traumatic incident that caused them to split off.*

... It's also important that they learn and understand and follow the rule that they cannot present ('come out') at inappropriate times or places if the System is to relate in functional and healthy ways in the outside world. ... it will be important for the rest of the System to allow these parts to have some 'body time' (time to be out) at pre-arranged times under pre-agreed conditions.

Remember to love, to cherish, to value these young parts. Just like the rest of you, they have suffered great wounding, and mustn't be neglected, dismissed, or re-abused within the System. That helps no-one; it does not lead to re-integration nor to healing and moving forward.

It can take great patience, finesse and wisdom to deal with wounded 'littles' ... Yet, as they realise the 'bigs' in the System [psyche] will keep them safe, the rewards are well worth the investment of time and effort as they shed layers of fear and distrust and to learn to be open and loving and inquisitive and playful as they do their own healing work."

Re-parenting is a technique everyone can use – not just ABs or people with DID. In his book *'Parent Yourself Again: Love Yourself the Way You Have Always Wanted to be Loved'*, Yong Kang Chan says –

"Even though there's nothing we can do to change what happened during our childhood, we can teach our inner parent to be a better parent for our inner child. Our inner child has unfulfilled needs that are waiting to be satisfied, but we can't assign this responsibility to our birth parents and depend on them. First, you understand what you need the most, and you are the best one who can understand your inner child's deepest desires."

Yong's last comment is especially true for ABs.

If this re-parenting sounds like a parlour game, it is not. I have lived it. It is real and it works. Our Inner Child is a subjectively real part of our psyche. There is a part of us that really does feel, think and behave like a young child. The conflict within our psyche was real, pervasive and damaging. Every part of our psyche was damaged, but none more so than our Inner Child. They and our whole psyche are only going to heal if, this time, our Inner Child feels genuinely loved. That love has to come from within us. If we cannot love ourselves and love our child within, we will find it impossible to heal and to fully accept love from others. Our Inner Child needs to feel loved each and every day. That is what our nurturing Inner Parent does. They can love our Inner Child as we wished we were loved as biological children. They can be the perfect loving Parent.

IFS therapist Jay Earley tells us –

"The reparenting process actually lays down new neural pathways in the brain. That is why your psyche and your life can change so dramatically. You give that child part a new experience of some aspect of your childhood, an experience that heals or replaces the old one. This time, you, as the Self are filling the child's deepest needs, which is exactly what didn't happen in that early situation. While it may look as though you are simply pretending the past was different, what you are actually doing is creating a new, wholesome relationship with the exile [inner child] in the present, which shows her that life can be good and happy. The exile doesn't really exist in the past; she is here right now in the present. ... You are becoming the ideal parent for her. When this happens the exile is transformed. She feels differently about herself and the whole world." [Self Therapy: A Step-by-Step Guide to Creating Wholeness and Healing Your Inner Child Using IFS]

Your experience of your nurturing Inner Parent will be distinctively your own. For some reason, I have not given my Inner Parent a name, like I have my child persona. I think that is because a lot of the time I feel my child persona being parented by Jesus and Our Lady (more on this later). Every AB is unique. If it feels right for your Inner Parent to have a name, go with it.

Visualisation

One way your Inner Parent can lovingly re-parent your Inner Child is visualization. This isn't a substitute for physical 'baby time' for your child persona but is a helpful, calming adjunct to it. If for any reason, you cannot give your child persona their regular physical 'baby time', it will help tide them over until you can.

You can visualize your nurturing Inner Parent lovingly interacting with your child persona. I often visualize my nurturing Inner Parent picking up my baby girl persona, Chrissie, to cuddle and talk to her. Chrissie might be unhappy, tired or throwing a tantrum, but soon I see her smiling and laughing in my (Inner Parent's) arms before contentedly falling asleep. It is healing and settles my whole psyche. In my book *'Living With Chrissie'* I described how this helps me deal with stressful situations -

Sometimes after especially stressful times, I'll 'de-brief' with Chrissie to calm or comfort her. For example, dentists scare me. When I had to go for a particularly scary procedure, I imagined myself beforehand picking up Chrissie and comforting her. It worked. Both Chrissie and my adult-self were less fearful. Understanding when Chrissie is scared or needy, and being able to comfort her, has been a great help in managing my anxiety.

The time before you fall asleep is one of the best times in the day for visualizing nurturing your child persona. Bedtime is an important time of day for your child persona, as it is for a biological child. Through visualization, you can settle your child persona to sleep peacefully. What bedtime routine does your child persona need to go to sleep feeling happy and safe? Visualize it. Add all the details. How would you child persona like to be 'tucked in'? Visualize it. If there are physical things that you want for your child persona but don't have, add them. Most of us don't have a cot. But you can visualize your child persona being put to bed in their cot.

You can visualize a safe space where your Inner Parent can nurture your child persona. Such a safe space is important for people with shared consciousness. *'Got Parts: An Insider's Guide to Managing Life Successfully with Dissociative Identity Disorder'* says –

> *"Everyone in the System [psyche] needs to work together to create a safe space inside where you all reside. This place is sometimes known as the 'Dome'. This is where parts are when they are not 'out', and is a place to get to know each other better, and to do your healing work individually and together. ... Using the creative power of your imaginations, you invent this actual place inside you. It is very important to create the Dome together, and that it is safe. ... [it] can take any physical configuration ... Examples include a Sphere, or Pyramid, or Lighthouse, or Cathedral, or Log Cabin, or Tepee, or Space Station. It could be a beautiful place in nature, like a serene ocean shoreline or wildflower prairie or lush rainforest ... Within these guidelines, your 'dome' can contain within it anything that brings you all comfort, pleasure, peace and security. Do you want a reading area with a fireplace, an area to play or listen to music, a playground for the littles? Would you like to have a perpetual rainbow, or lots of soft, warm blankets and cuddly pillows, or a lake or pool to swim in? Would you like to have unicorns, hummingbirds, butterflies, or a gentle-to-the-System [psyche] but fiercely protective dinosaur? You may have it in your Dome."*

My safe space is a country cottage. It is peaceful, but not isolated. The house has a beautiful nursery with white wooden furniture, including a cot, changing table, and nursing chair; and is decorated in pink and soft pastel colours. There are windows and French doors opening onto a broad shady veranda. Beyond is a soft, soft lawn enclosed in a sturdy white open post fence that keeps wandering toddlers safe inside and everything else outside. In the midst of the lawn, there is a clothesline with lots of fluffy-soft, white cloth nappies drying in the warm breeze. Beyond the fence are wonderful sweeping views of the open countryside. If I need to feel extra safe, I imagine it on a high steep-sided bluff with a wide river winding around - no one bad can get to it. In the day it is always balmy, not hot, and at nights it is cuddly cool – perfect for fuzzy, footed sleepers or pyjamas.

It is lovely to visit when I am in bed falling asleep. It is where I take Chrissie if she gets frightened. Again, it does not take the place of a physical space, but it is an adjunct to it, or a substitute for it if I am away from home.

Visualise your own safe space and put all your love for your child persona into it.

Summary

Self-acceptance releases our punishing Inner Parent from their burden of fear, to become our nurturing Inner Parent. They lovingly and patiently re-parent our wounded Inner Child, building a secure attachment between the Inner Parent and child persona.

8. Our Child Persona

The two most important things about our child persona is that they are a real part of our psyche, and their need for nurturing is real. Getting to know your child persona is a delightful, joyful experience. Earning their love and trust will be one of your proudest achievements. Once you have it, you will never want to lose it.

Gender

Your child persona may be the same or a different gender from your adult self (or not have a fixed gender). Any of those outcomes is okay. As Rosalie Bent says, the fact they have the needs of young child for love and nurture, is vastly more significant than their gender. Child personas, like healthy biological children, have an innocent, not adult sexuality.

Rosalie indicates -

> *'... around half of physically male Adult Babies and Little Ones identity as female infant/toddler, indeterminate or sissy. ... 'Sissy' and 'girl' are quite similar and when determining your Little One's gender, keep in mind the sissy option. It is a subset of the female gender, but for simplicity, I have used it as a separate one.'*

My child persona, Chrissie, is a delightful baby girl. Perhaps one of the reasons it took me a long while to accept my AB identity was that subconsciously I knew my child persona was a different gender from my Adult self. Now I wonder what the problem was? Chrissie and my Adult self, happily co-exist with no issues. My Adult self has no gender dysphoria about being male. I have not personally heard of it working the other way, an adult woman with a boy child persona, but there is no reason why it could not be so.

What's In A Name?

Everything! Should your child persona have their own name? When I asked Rosalie Bent she gave this very good advice –

> *'The vast majority [of adult babies] give their baby persona a name. Sometimes it is simply the addition of 'baby' in front of their adult name as a way of identifying the baby persona from the adult one while others (like my baby) invent completely new names for themselves. I know of only one case where the baby remains nameless. You may find it simpler and less confusing to also use the prefix 'baby' in front of your adult name. An individual needs and wants a name and so your baby persona will as well. Just try it out until something feels comfortable.*

*Being identified as a baby is the single most important driver for a regressed baby and a name is
the single most important attribute of that identification. [Personal Email]*

I believe it is essential to give your child persona a name. Adding 'Baby' to your own name is an option. I favour choosing a separate name. That better reflects that your child persona is not you as a biological child, but a redeeming creation of your sub-conscious. I am sure the name you chose (or have already chosen) will powerfully call to mind the character of your child persona. If they are a different gender from your Adult self it is an even more powerful experience. It was a wonderful, thrilling thing to choose and use my baby girl persona's name.

The daily habit of using their name when you think about your child persona, is a powerful endorsement of your acceptance that they are real.

Getting to Know Your Child Persona

Every AB's child persona is unique. Your child persona is the product of the deepest knowing and yearning in your psyche. They are the most lovable baby or child your psyche can create. They are a delight. Your sense of their personality will develop over time and no one will ever know your child persona as well as you. Rosalie Bent's book *'There's Still A Baby in My Bed'* is a very good guide to that exploration. I find there are times I just 'know' what my Chrissie likes or dislikes. She can be a real 'little miss', and at her worst, a selfish brat. But she's also a shy, easily scared, innocent, loving, affectionate, warm-hearted, fun-loving little girl who melts my heart.

How you think of your child persona behaving and dressing, won't necessarily exactly replicate the attributes of a biological baby or child. ABs will often dress or visualize their child persona behaving in ways that combine elements from different developmental stages that would be unlikely to coexist at the same time in a biological child. That is okay.

To me, my child persona, Chrissie, is a toddler. But I have jackets and knitted bonnets that belong to a very young baby's layette; onesies and baby-suits such as a crawling baby might wear; and two-piece pyjamas and dungarees that you could see on a toddler. I visualize Chrissie being breast and bottle-fed, sleeping in a cot and playing in a playpen – behaviours which are probably most consistent with the 'crawler' stage. But I also visualize her feeding herself (messily), running around (unsteadily), playing with dolls and watching kids' TV shows, attributes which belong to an older age, toddler or beyond.

Let yourself buy presents for your child persona – and feel their delight at receiving them. I find it's not the quantity of such presents which is important – but the few carefully chosen things that your child persona loves dearly.

I find that clothes are another powerful confirmation that my child persona is real. Almost every AB already knows the thrill of seeing a new item of clothing, or outfit, that deeply evokes their child persona - the dress, dungarees, bonnet or whatever, that IS your child persona. Do you think your Adult self could summon up that kind of delight? I don't think so!

Nurturing.

Recognizing your child persona as real is very powerful. But it is not enough.

You need to nurture your child persona – recognize that their needs for love, comfort and play are real. Remember that your child persona is healing for a long time when their needs were stigmatized and disregarded. You are building a secure attachment between your child persona and your nurturing Inner Parent. Ending the damaging internal conflict depends on your child persona learning that they can trust that their needs will be met. If you walk away from that commitment your child persona will see that the other parts of you don't really believe your child persona is real.

You cannot let that happen.

Nurturing our child persona is the best way of healing the painful sadness and yearning for the broken childhood attachment with our mothers.

This self-nurturing is the positive alternative to psychologically unsafe fantasies.

Therapist Jasmin Lee Cori writes about loving your inner child –

> *"Your inner child will help you. A child is like a 'love bank'. The more you put in, the more you get back. Children are innately loving, so as you extend even a trickle of love to the unloved child within you, usually that child will return your love. It may be a little bumpy in the beginning, however. Frequently, an inner child will initially respond with mistrust. Just as a child who has been hurt or abandoned too many times by Mother will not open his arms to her, the inner child may react similarly. If this the case, persist in your efforts to reach out to this child the best you can, realizing that it take time to build up trust."*

Yan Kang Chan in *'Parent Yourself Again'*, gives us a starting point and tells us a child wants to:

Be loved and valued

Be seen and heard

To be themselves and be accepted for who they are

Feel like they belong

Feel safe and secure

Your child persona is unique. Think about the particular nurturing they need. What form your nurturing takes will depend on your circumstances. If you are in a non-accepting environment, it could be something unobtrusive – perhaps a quiet moment where you visualize your nurturing Inner Parent comforting your child persona in their safe space. It could be some quiet moments letting your child persona cuddle their favourite soft toy.

Your child persona's favourite 'stuffie' is in a special category of its' own. It is one of the most tangible signs that your child persona is real. The comfort and safety they experience from cuddling the toy is something that an adult can never fully recapture. But your child persona can! Every day! They might have similar deep feelings for their dummy, or their bottle?

If you are in an accepting environment, your nurturing will, of course, include putting your child persona in a nappy and more. There are a broad range of things you can do to meet their needs. You will learn what regular care creates the greatest security and happiness for them, and what is the daily minimum they need. (See *'Finding Balance Between and the Adult'* in Michael Bent's book 'Being An Adult Baby', or free on abdiscovery.com.au under the ABDL article tab; and the evergreen *'There's Still a Baby in My Bed'* by Rosalie Bent.)

Nurturing a biological baby or child is not a once in a blue-moon 'thing'.

Your child persona needs to feel nurtured on a *daily* basis.

Our child personas really are present in our consciousness 24/7. Like small biological children, their need for comfort and reassurance is pretty constant. We can ignore it but only at a price in anxiety or depression for our adult selves. It is one of the big issues that takes some getting used to in accepting ourselves as ABs. At one time, I was embarrassed by it. Now, I figure it is not much different from the way a very young biological child needs a settled routine.

To feel calm, happy and safe my child persona needs to know –

1. that she will have regular 'baby time' on a daily basis
2. her baby things are physically readily-to-hand.

Now that I am 'out' to myself and my wife, my child persona has her own bedroom. It is 'dressed' as a bedroom if the grandkids visit, so the stuffies on display etcetera, do not attract any unusual attention from visitors. My child persona sleeps each night in her nappy and plastic pants, baby clothes, cuddling her soft toys and sucking her pacifier. Before I retired, I would go off to work and hold down a demanding job. Now that I am retired, my child persona has a wet nappy in the morning if she wants to, and she can freely wander around the house before my Adult self gears up for the day. She usually also has an afternoon nap, nappy and all. My Adult self functions effectively throughout the day and I have a wonderful sense of wellbeing.

Knowing that her nappies, stuffed toys, pacifiers and baby clothes are accessible whenever she needs them keeps her calm and happy. I can handle occasional circumstances where I cannot sleep in a nappy or get ready access to my baby things. I can go a week or a fortnight, but with an increasing level of discomfort.

The point is that my child persona needs the certainty of daily 'baby time', and ready physical access to her baby things. I think that level of need was always there, even when I was conflicted. I just was not fully aware of it, and paid a price in anxiety that I just assumed was a normal part of my personality. I suspect it is the same for many ABs. For some adult babies, Rosalie Bent indicates that going 24/7 in nappies is the level of constant nurturing they need to stop distress and disruption.

As with any biological child, play is an important part of your child persona's happiness. Play is healthy, healing, creative and fun. Give yourself permission to discover what form of play makes your child persona happiest. I tried out various recreations that other ABs enjoyed – children's TV, toy trains – but these did not really 'click' – these felt like self-conscious 'role play/age play'. But when I discovered doll's play the flashing lights came on. Chrissie loved it. It was instinctive and natural.

Whatever the nature and extent of daily or regular 'baby time', what is important is that it is a concrete signal to your child persona that their needs are important and that they will be met. Through commitment and trust, you are building a secure attachment to replace the insecure attachment that created the wounded Inner Child.

I can 'hear' my child persona, Chrissie say to my nurturing Inner Parent (or Jesus, or Our Lady):

I love you.

I'm sorry for when I'm naughty or say bad things. I try my best to be good.

Sometimes I can't help being naughty. Sometimes I like being naughty. Sometimes I need to be naughty.

I know you love me always.

I know you are proud of me.

I know you like me.

Thank you for helping me.

I know you will always be there when I need you.

A Healthy Child Persona

Sometimes, in posts on on-line ABDL forums, or on twitter, I have seen ABs indicate that their child persona is their principal or only personality. They sometimes say that their adult personality is just a 'mask'. This is not the way to go. To renounce a strong adult identity is psychologically unhealthy. It would foster a neurotic dependency on others. We cannot function in the world without an adult identity. To attempt to do so will damage our inner child/child persona, again. This is a cry for help. It is a sign that the person's Inner Child is deeply wounded, and their internal conflict is unresolved. The Inner Child is going to an extreme because they do not trust they will find a safe place, or their need for nurturing will ever be met. That is a dark place to be. If you are in such a place you need to know, you *will* make peace with deep wounds. You *will* find a safe place. You *will* find nurturing. Seek the help of a psychotherapist.

There seems to be something of a fault line in the AB community between those who see being AB as non-sexual, and those who see being AB as including sexual expression. I believe that the child persona of an AB is *always* innocent (yes I know psychologists recognize infantile or childhood sexuality but that is innocent, with a very different character from adult sexuality). To involve an AB's child persona in sexual activity is psychologically unhealthy. Non-conflicted people with Dissociate Identity Disorder (DID) do not involve their child 'parts' or 'Littles' in sex. If you find yourself with any such inclinations seek the help of a psychotherapist. Sexually active ABs must have a safe word that lets their partner know that the AB's child persona has come 'out' during sexual activity, and it is psychologically unsafe for the AB to continue.

ABs are functional adults. They may be sexual or asexual. An AB's sexual behaviour, including their nappy fetish, is a function of their adult self. Because AB's grew up conflicted about their identity, their adult sexuality is commonly expressed as a fetish for nappies, and perhaps some element of BDSM (DDLG or equivalent). Viva la difference! That should not be confused by the AB, or their partner, with the innocent character of the AB's child persona.

Faith in A Higher Power

SPOILER ALERT! The next section is about enlisting your faith in God or a Higher Power in the healing of your wounded Inner Child and building a secure attachment for your child persona. If you are an atheist or agnostic feel free to skip this section – I won't hold it against you. I don't think that it will diminish any benefit you may get from this book. But if you do read the section please don't hold it against me.

My faith is important to me. It is a non-denominational non-church-going kind, based on a relationship with Jesus and Our Lady rather than any close knowledge of scripture. I come from a Catholic fellow-traveller / Anglican-Episcopalian background and accept the faith of adherents of other Christian and non-Christian religions as a real relationship with God. If that is likely to offend your religious or theological beliefs, please feel free to skip this section.

I believe that a loving God / Higher Power / personal saviour is there to be all we need - our father, mother, brother/sister, friend or any such. As ABs with a personal faith we need to be able to take our deepest needs to God. This is not to cure us of being ABs, but to help us live safely and happily with our personal identity as adult babies. God is there for our child persona. He is there to change our nappies, feed us our bottles, pick up the dummy we dropped, tuck us into sleep, hand us our favourite soft toy, soothe our tears and fears, calm our tantrums, read us a story, bathe us, take us for a walk, and play with us. I believe he/she loves our child persona with a deep abiding love. As an AB I treasure the well-known words of Isaiah 49:15 –

'Can a woman forget her nursing child and have no compassion on the son of her womb? Even these may forget, but I will not forget you. Behold, I have inscribed you on the palms of my hands.'

More, I believe that God delights in our child persona in the way that a happy, stress-free, loving parent enjoys the innocent wonder and happiness of their baby or young child. God knows that through the innocence of our child persona we can trust his/her love as a happy secure child trusts their parent's love. I believe that God is incredibly protective and proud of us, our healthy AB identity, and our child persona. As a sign of his protective pride, I treasure the well-known words of Matthew 19:13-14 –

'Then were there brought unto him little children, that he should put his hands on them, and pray: and the disciples rebuked them. But Jesus said, Suffer little children, and forbid them not, to come unto me: for of such is the kingdom of heaven.'

I am not alone in finding special meaning in this verse as an adult baby. Michael Bent in his article *'A Christian Response to Being An Adult Baby'* states –

197

From many years ago I have read that and understood it in a way my fellow believers never could. The sermon might talk about 'coming as a child' to God by adopting child-like responses and faith. However, for me, being child-like is second nature because... I AM A CHILD in so many ways and at so many times.

I have read a children's bible while regressed and simply responded to it as a child would. I have prayed while so very little and the prayers are that odd mix of adult and child that I know God understands so well.

In this respect, being an adult baby can actually bring us closer to God if we allow it; to let our regressive immaturity and wide-eyed wonder to be directed at Him. It was a startling revelation to me that being an adult baby could actually have a positive impact on my walk with Him!

As an AB, the love of Our Lady, Mary the Mother of God is particularly powerful for me. My wife is Catholic, and she introduced me to the love of Our Lady. My wife explained to me how she came to have a personal relationship with Mary. As a single mother in a moment of exasperation when seeking guidance about being a parent, she told Jesus 'what am I doing talking to you, you've never changed a nappy, I need to talk to your mother'. I think any AB is going to 'get' the nappy reference and understand. I can see Mary changing my child persona's nappy and doing all the other things that Jesus does for my child persona. I can also see and feel Mary breastfeeding my child persona with the utmost tender care, with the most secure attachment that any Attachment Theory can envisage. Some might feel that is blasphemy. I don't. I feel it as the love of God.

To visualize and feel God caring for my child persona in all the ways that a father and mother care for a baby or young child is incredibly healing. It brings me to that confidence that I am loved and safe. It feels like it is building the secure attachment that I missed with my mother as a child.

When I was a conflicted AB my avoidant personality leads me to feel that I shouldn't bother God with my baby needs. I sought only consolation from him for the shame, confusion and distress I felt as a result of my internal conflict for being an adult baby. When I purged during the binge and purge cycle, I prayed to Him to cure me of something I experienced as an affliction, a fetish and an addiction. I thought I meant I wanted him to take away the whole adult baby 'thing'. He has answered my prayers. I don't experience my child persona as an affliction, a fetish or an addiction anymore. He has cured me. But in a way I never understood in the depths of my internal conflict, He has left me with a healthy adult baby identity and child persona. It is who I am meant to be. It is who God wants me to be.

SPOILER ALERT! – The end of the God 'stuff'.

9. Shared Consciousness and Internal Family Systems Theory

As adult babies, we have already lived with shared consciousness - whether we wanted to or not. We are discovering that it is healthier to accept our shared consciousness than it is to deny it. It allows us to stop the different parts of our psyche fighting, and to work together. But our culture has not equipped us with the understanding to live comfortably with shared consciousness. It can feel a bit like we are on a car journey to an unfamiliar destination without a satnav or map.

But help is at hand. It is Internal Family Systems (IFS) Therapy.

IFS is the psychological theory which is most suited to meeting the needs of ABs. It provides the concepts and practical techniques for living with shared consciousness. Other psychological theories have useful concepts about the internal dialogue and conflict within our psyche. IFS is unique is being created on the basis that we all have a healthy shared consciousness based on multiple sub-personalities. To return to the car journey analogy, it is like someone just handed you a working satnav system.

IFS was developed by family therapist Richard Schwartz and expounded in his 1995 book *'Internal Family Systems Theory'*. IFS is ingeniously simple. It is an intuitive model of the psyche which gives anyone easy access to the workings of their psyche. It allows people to understand themselves and facilitates healing. Schwartz developed IFS after working with bulimic clients. Like bulimia sufferers, 'binge and purge' cycles are a defining feature of the conflicted AB identity. This may explain why IFS is helpful in understanding ABs.

If you have read this far, you already have a good idea about how IFS works. An AB's child persona, Parent and Weak Adult are examples of IFS 'parts'. Our parts can drive or influence our thoughts, feelings and behaviour. When we are conflicted, we can experience ourselves thinking, feeling and acting in sometimes contradictory ways, at odds with our better nature. We have two types of parts – Exiles like our Inner Child/child persona who carry our pain, and Protectors like our Inner Parent and weak Adult, who keep the exiles in the background, so we are not overwhelmed. Each part has a conflicted and a non-conflicted state. In their conflicted state the parts fight. In their non-conflicted state, they work cooperatively. Our strong Adult is my term for what IFS calls 'the Self', the leader of our psyche.

When I first started writing about the AB Identity, I knew of IFS, but not much about it. In writing about ABs' Child, Parent and Adult I was adapting ideas from other theories. When I got to know IFS, I realized my approach and IFS are parallel ways of understanding AB's shared consciousness.

The IFS way of understanding and working with shared consciousness fits the AB Identity very well. This is a huge benefit for ABs. We are a one-in-a-thousand minority personal identity, mostly living secret lives. It is an uphill climb to reach a shared understanding of our identity, even amongst ourselves. It is an even steeper climb to help the rest of the world reach a positive understanding of our identity. IFS brings a well-developed set of concepts, and language, which are known, or accessible, to a much broader population. ABs can use these concepts and language to better communicate about our identity with other ABs, and with non-ABs.

Shared Consciousness is Safe

Embracing our shared consciousness is the biggest hurdle in AB's self-acceptance. IFS helps ABs understand that our shared consciousness is healthy and safe, because:

Our psyche is led by our higher Self – 'the Self' in IFS terminology. That higher Self embodies the best of us - our spirituality, compassion, wisdom and integrity. Understanding this reassures fears that if we embrace shared consciousness, we will become fragmented into different, conflicting pieces. Instead, our shared consciousness has a solid centre. The 'parts' are like the planets revolving around the sun, and the Self is the sun. Like the sun, the Self is the centre of the psyche and its' most fundamental and defining feature.

The Self is analogous to the renown psychotherapist Donald Winnicott's conception of the True Self – the inner core of our psyche that is the source of our creativity, that makes us feel 'real', and distinctively 'ourselves'. My faith is important to me, and I am comfortable with the IFS conception of 'the Self' as a higher self which acts in a way which is consistent with Faith. We are always responsible for ourselves and our actions.

There are no 'evil' or 'bad' parts. We do not have to fear what is inside us. Parts may be conflicted and sometimes drive or influence us to act in dysfunctional ways. That happens because the parts are acting on a mistaken belief about what is good for our psyche. They always want to act for the good. When a conflicted part gets full information from our Self, and comes to a correct understanding, they will *always* change to work cooperatively with the Self and other non-conflicted parts.

Under the leadership of the Self, our psyche works on the basis of reason, compassion, integrity and trust. When we address our dysfunctions the Self does not bully or coerce the parts. Instead, the Self seeks to compassionately understand a conflicted part, to provide them with full information, and to bring that part to heal. If the conflicted part is reluctant or refuses, the Self finds another way until the part understands that the Self can be trusted. If you like, our psyche is like the perfect democracy with the perfect head-of-government.

It recognizes that the AB's child persona is a permanent feature of their psyche. It does not require the AB's child persona to 'disappear' in psychological health, and be re-integrated into the undifferentiated Self (as some therapists working with dissociation and trauma would expect). In IFS, parts are permanent, they do not 'disappear'. Conflicted parts are transformed when they are healed and surrender their negative emotions, but they remain as healthy, cooperative features of the psyche.

Helpful Concepts

IFS has a set of concepts to help us understand our shared consciousness. These include:

Conflicted Parts are categorized as 'Exiles' and 'Protectors'. This helps to understand the nature and conduct of conflicted parts. Exiles hold the psyche's pain, and in the conflicted state are hidden away by Protectors. Protectors seek to maintain the psyche's capacity to function and fulfil external responsibilities, by stopping it being overwhelmed by the pain held by Exiles. Protectors will only let the 'exiles' out into the light of day when the Protectors feel it is safe to do so. In IFS terms, an AB's Inner Child/child persona is an exile and their Inner Parent is a protector. This categorization fits the AB's Inner Child and Inner Parent well.

Polarization. Conflict or trauma produce a state of polarization within the psyche. In that state, parts take opposing or competing positions in the mistaken belief that this is necessary to protect the self. Each part reacts iteratively to the other, taking increasingly extreme positions. This fits the AB's binge and purge cycle. (I use the term conflicted. This is the equivalent of the IFS term polarization.)

Burdens. Conflicted parts may bear burdens of negative emotions based on past experiences in a person's life. Those burdens keep the parts locked into their mistaken thinking and their conflicted state. The burdens can be lifted/healed, allowing a part to move to a non-conflicted state. This is relevant to the conflicted parts of an AB: the wounded Child, punishing Parent and weak Adult.

Seat of consciousness. This is the vantage point from which we see our own psyche and the world, in real-time. IFS therapist and author Jay Earley uses the metaphor of a big armchair. The seat of consciousness can be occupied by a part or by the Self. If it is occupied by a part, we will be seeing, experiencing and reacting to the world and our psyche from the perspective of that part. Only if the Self is in the seat of consciousness, do we see and act with full information, and with only compassion and wisdom. The Self is the natural 'owner' of the seat of consciousness, and any part will vacate the seat in favour of the Self if the latter asks.

Blending. In IFS, the Self is always calm, compassionate, wise and curious. The Self is detached from negative feeling and has the empathy to understand the emotions of other parts, without criticism. When we are caught up in negative feelings, critical judgements, compulsions or addictions, another conflicted part has 'blended' with the Self. Essentially that means that the part has plopped itself in the seat of consciousness, and we are experiencing and acting based on the desires of that part.

IFS and ABs

ABs have always lived with a shared consciousness. But when we didn't recognize it, there were many times when the workings of our psyche surprised us, and sometimes in a bad way. Now that we accept our shared consciousness, we are in a position to work with the parts of our psyche in more conscious and harmonious ways. Of course, we do this intuitively. But it is unfamiliar territory and it can take a while to learn to trust our way around.

IFS has a 'tool kit' of techniques – simple mental imagery – for anyone to consciously work with the different components of their own psyche. There are techniques for getting to know our parts better, to identify which part is influencing our perceptions and behaviours in real-time, to heal parts and lift burdens of negative emotions, and so on. You don't need IFS to handle your own shared consciousness. It is your consciousness. But I find IFS concepts and techniques helpful, and they provide a common language to communicate about my psyche with others.

No psychological theory can replace your intuition about your own psyche. If there is a conflict between the theory and your own intuition, keep an open mind and be willing to explore. Ultimately, trust your intuition about yourself and your psyche.

I have not seen any writing about applying IFS to better understand ABs, and there are a few areas where I think IFS needs some adapting to better fit AB's shared consciousness. For my own psyche, I take a different view from IFS on several matters -

My child persona is not just another part. IFS does not appear to have a concept for a 'principal' part. There is more to me than my child persona, but it is still a defining feature of my psyche and identity. My child persona's position in relation to my other parts is perhaps 'first among equals'. I have two older male child parts besides my principal child persona, a baby girl toddler. The former emerged from trauma when I was aged nine or ten, one an Exile, the other a Protector. Recognising them is important to the health of my psyche. However, they do not have the strength of presence of Chrissie, and they do not define my psyche and healthy AB identity the way Chrissie does.

I find the simplicity of categorizing parts as either Exiles or Protectors helpful. IFS sub-divides protectors into managers and firefighters. In IFS, in the conflicted psyche, firefighters distract from the pain of exiles by 'acting out' in compulsive behaviours (binge eating/drinking/ shopping etcetera). For me, it is a better fit to think of my acting out behaviours as my child persona / Exile 'breaking through' and seeking to satisfy their unmet needs. This better fits their need and demand for nappies and 'baby time'.

I feel safe with my shared consciousness on the basis of a 'family size' set of parts that I can remember easily. Sometimes, IFS can multiply the number of parts by identifying 'one-dimensional' parts on the basis of a single emotion. I find it more helpful to understand my parts as being multi-dimensional sub-personalities with a range of emotions. For me, that provides sufficient explanation of my psyche without being confusing.

The ingenious simplicity of IFS means it is a great self-help tool and can be learned by anyone as a counselling technique. That virtue can lead to a risk of under-estimating the therapeutic skills need to deal with deep emotional pain, and especially, dissociated trauma. ABs are likely to have both. The creator of IFS, Richard Schwartz, and IFS therapist Jay Earley indicate that people dealing with these issues need the help of a skilled psychotherapist (who may use IFS) to heal safely. See the appendix for a discussion on choosing a therapist.

Conclusion

IFS is the psychological theory which is best suited to meeting the needs of ABs. It views shared consciousness, based on multiple parts or sub-personalities led by a unifying higher Self, as normal and applicable to everyone. The IFS approach provides a reassuring understanding of shared consciousness. It offers ABs an ingeniously simple way of understanding our own psyches and communicating about our psyches with others.

See the end of the references section for a guide to further reading on IFS.

10. Partners

This chapter is about the relationship between ABs and their life partners. I am an AB. I can provide a perspective from firsthand experience as a conflicted and a non-conflicted AB. For an AB partner's perspective, I recommend two books by Rosalie Bent: -

1. the landmark, 'There's Still A Baby In My Bed: Living Happily with the Adult Baby in Your Relationship'
2. *'Coffee With Rosie: Why Does My Partner Want to Wear Diapers'*, which is written as a refreshingly direct imaginary dialogue between two women over coffee.

ABs crave the acceptance of their child persona by their partner. Given that being an AB is necessarily a private identity, where else can we turn? We often focus on our partner's acceptance – dream about it, obsess about it – as the answer to our prayers. I did. I thought if my wife accepts my child persona, then everything will be okay. I will feel okay about myself. My internal conflict will go away.

That is <u>not</u> how it works with personal identity. Don't get me wrong, having the loving acceptance of my wife for my child persona is wonderful. But with hindsight, I can see that my wife only accepted my child persona *after* I fully accepted that persona myself. How could it be otherwise? It is my identity. The empathy and acceptance of others can make the process easier, but we have to make sense of our own identity. My wonderful loving wife is older than I am. At some point, I will be by myself. But I will still have my healthy personal identity as an adult baby. My wife's love has contributed to that identity, but it is my identity.

But, paradoxically, the best way to gain a partner's acceptance is to deepen our own self-acceptance. With this understanding, we can look at how being an AB as a healthy personal identity might fit into a relationship with a partner.

Making Peace with the Past

One of the gifts of a healthy, non-conflicted identity is that we can better see things from our partner's perspective. As ABs, we need to understand what our conflicted identity looked and felt like to them.

For a start it was confusing. We have seen the push-pull towards our partners in our internal conflict. Our Inner Child and Weak Adult wanted to pull our partner in closer. The wounded Inner Child wanted our partner to be the Child's fairy godmother and to rescue the Child from the abuse of our punishing Inner Parent and the neglect of our Weak Adult. The latter also hoped that our partner would 'sort us out', soothe our Inner Child and get the punishing Inner Parent off the Adult's back. But our punishing Inner Parent desperately feared that would drive our partner away from us, either to distance themselves or reject us altogether. They fought hard to keep our

Inner Child away from our partner. So, our partner was getting conflicting messages. On the one hand, 'help, rescue me', and on the other, 'keep your distance, stay away'.

And for our partners, living with our conflicted selves wasn't pretty! Remember, when you are in the grips of a deep internal conflict, you are not fully aware of its' effects on your behaviour or your perceptions. People who are denying their own identity are not always the easiest people to be around. There are times they are fucked up. They can be unhappy, preoccupied, distracted, anxious or depressed. They can flip between these states so that partners don't know who is going to walk in the door (my wife's words). They have a lot of anger, that they are not aware of. But it comes out anyway, in moodiness, in withdrawal, in outbursts. We would have been very, very difficult to live with sometimes. It will have left scars, hurt and anger. We need to accept that our partners will take time to heal, just as we take time to heal.

As Rosalie indicates, it is likely that our partners will have their own fears about our AB identity. I can think of at least four possible grounds –

1. Is there any link to paedophilia? (No, but in the absence of good information, such a fear is understandable.)
2. Over the years it has looked mostly like a not-very-attractive, compulsive sexual fetish? It seemed to make us miserable more often than it made us happy.
3. Is it some twisted sexual Oedipus complex mother-son thing? (or the counterpart father-daughter Electra complex)
4. Is it a neurotic psychological dependency?

The answer to all these fears is that AB's have a subjectively real, *innocent* child persona. A part of an AB's psyche really does think, feel, and at times behave, like a very young child. That child is innocent – not sexual, as per any healthy biological child. An ABs sexual behaviour, including their nappy fetish, is a function of their adult self.

I believe that the best reassurance for our partner's concerns is for them to see in us, and our behaviour, that being a non-conflicted AB is a healthy personal identity. Are we more happy than miserable? - more loving than angry? - more content than unsettled? Our partner needs their own time and space to see that.

Role of the Adult Self

It is the AB's strong Adult self that needs to take the lead in our relationship with our partner – not our child persona. Our Adult respects the most important point in Rosalie Bent's book - to put our marriage/relationship first.

> *"Your adult relationship has to be at all times, more important than your [the AB's]*
> *regressive needs or you will end up having neither."*

Our Strong Adult understands all our partner has been through when we were in the grips of our internal conflict. They are the ally of our partner in protecting our marriage. They want to help our partner understand that our AB identity is healthy and stable and can be safely embraced. Our strong Adult is the ally of our partner in seeking a balance which respects the needs of our child persona AND our marriage. Hopefully, this is something our partner will sense and respect.

As AB's, we are principally responsible for nurturing our child persona – that is the role of our nurturing Inner Parent. It is nice to share the nurturing of our child persona with a loving partner. But that will be sabotaged if we place the greater onus for that nurturing on our partner.

Even when we have accepted our AB identity, there are times when our child persona can't have what they want and throws a sulk or a tantrum. (My wife can vouch for this!) After all, they have the feelings and impulses of a baby or very young child. You cannot expect good behaviour from any child all the time.

Our partner needs to know our strong Adult is on their side in managing bad behaviour by our child persona. There is a distinction between parenting and mothering/fathering. The former is the tough stuff like setting boundaries and discipline. The latter is the 'nice' stuff like comforting, cuddling, play and fun. No-one wants to get left with all the 'crap' parenting stuff. There are no guarantees, but hopefully, the fact that our partner senses that our strong Adult will share the parenting stuff will allow them the space and freedom to do some of the 'nice' stuff with our child persona.

Our Partner and Our Child Persona

I believe that the way forward lies in:

1. Hopefully, our partner recognizing that our child persona is a real and healthy part of our psyche and that to really know our spirit or soul they need to know, and have a relationship with, our child persona (as well as our Adult self); and
2. For ABs to understand that the relationship our partner has with our child persona, is for our partner to determine and that there are many ways in which our partner can show their love and acceptance for our child persona.

That is my understanding of the essence of Rosalie Bent's 2012 book *'There's A Baby in My Bed'* (updated in 2015 as *'There's Still A Baby in My Bed'*). It was, and still is, a groundbreaking 'big idea'.

As non-conflicted ABs, we have come to understand that it is not nappies that are the core of our personal identity – it is the fact that we have a subjectively real child persona. In the same way, we need to understand that our deepest need is for our partners to *'see'* us for who we really are – including our precious child persona – not necessarily to change our nappies.

For ABs to experience, perhaps for the first time, being 'seen' - really seen - by someone who loves us, is life-changing. It is wonderfully and deeply affirming and healing.

In both our identity and our relationship with our partner, don't let our obsession and fetish for nappies blind us. Let your partner know about your child persona – how you experience living with your child persona – the difference that accepting your child persona makes to you. If you find yourself talking mostly about nappies you may be missing the opportunity to help your partner really know you.

For those ABs who think 'great, now my partner will start changing my nappies and feeding me my bottle', I say hold on! That feels like the wounded Inner Child from our conflicted identity. That Child was hurt, angry and demanding. They were saying that the only way they would feel loved and accepted was if our partner changed the Child's nappies and fed them their bottle. That and nothing less. Otherwise, our wounded Inner Child won't trust that they are loved. That was what my wounded Inner Child wanted from my wife. It can sound like emotional blackmail. (If you are AB can't you just hear your manipulative wounded Inner Child saying, 'if you *really* loved me, you'd buy me that pony!') That is not a positive way forward. You already know that demands hurt, not help, a relationship.

It is our partner's choice of how they come to terms with our identity. What is most important is our partner's acceptance of our child persona as real in our psyche.

It is their choice *if* they do that.

It is their choice *how* they do that.

Our partner needs time, without demands, to work through this. As ABs, it took us a good while to accept our child persona as real. Our partner is no different. Very likely, they did not expect to have another child around the house, and 'under their feet'. My wife certainly thought she was done with those days.

If an AB's partner chooses to show their acceptance of the AB's child persona by changing nappies and bottle feeding that is great. Rosalie's book is a wonderful guide to partners who feel comfortable with being a mother to, and physically caring for, their AB's child persona.

It is not the only way that a partner can show their love and acceptance of our child persona. It does not feel right to my wife to be a mother to, and physically care for, my child persona, Chrissie, a toddler baby girl. I respected that but, initially, I was disappointed. I had been living with my conflicted identity and its' thinking for decades. In my experience, it takes a while for an AB's new, deeper acceptance of their healthy personal identity to transform our thinking.

It doesn't mean my wife does not love Chrissie or my adult-self deeply. She does. But some things would feel too wrong for her. She said it would be better if she was Chrissie's aunt. My wife had a wonderful relationship with her beloved aunt, who taught her to have fun and enjoy being a girl so it's a wonderful example.

Gradually, over the better part of a year, a wonderful relationship has developed between my wife and Chrissie. After a tentative start, my wife is fine with Chrissie going around the house in a pink T-shirt, nappy and plastic pants, dummy dangling from a cord and cuddling her beloved softy toy 'Bunny'. My wife interacts with Chrissie as a normal part of our daily life. It is wonderful. She will ask my adult self, 'how's Chrissie'? If we see something pink or fluffy on the TV or when we are shopping, she'll observe 'Chrissie would love that'.

My wife has told me she likes Chrissie. From time to time, she will buy Chrissie presents. On birthdays and Christmas, I'll get my wife a card and present from Chrissie. My wife can laugh with Chrissie. She can laugh *at* Chrissie, especially Chrissie's metaphorical pouts and foot stamping, with a warmth that lets Chrissie know she is loved. I think recognizing Chrissie as real has also been empowering for my wife. She knows who she is dealing with. And she knows how to deal with sometimes demanding or petulant toddlers. Sometimes she will say, "Chrissie is not having THAT", and we both laugh without being self-conscious.

My wife's acceptance of Chrissie has brought me great happiness. It is wonderful! It has been very healing. All of it would have been lost if I had demanded that only changing nappies would show that my wife accepted Chrissie. The key point is that it is our partner's acceptance of our child persona which is fundamentally important, and whatever form that takes is a wonderful gift. That form is up to our partner.

Play

Acceptance of our child persona by our partners, whatever form that acceptance takes, is a healthy form of play for both the AB and their partner. To better understand this, we need to look to the renowned psychotherapist, Donald Winnicott. He understood that play belongs to a unique and important category of human behaviour. When a child at play make-believes that a spoon is an aircraft, that is a creation, an illusion, of the child's mind. Yet in play, the child can share that illusion with another; and in turn, the other person can share their own illusions. Play is neither wholly subjective (within the self) nor wholly objective (the spoon is not an aircraft) – it is transitional between the two. Winnicott understood that all culture belongs to the same category of transitional phenomena as play. When we share sports, political beliefs or religion with others they are neither wholly subjective nor wholly objective – we agree with others to invest shared activities with common meanings which are not inherent in objective forms.

Winnicott can help us better understand how an AB's child persona can fit into the relationship between the AB and their partner. He makes the following statement about transitional phenomena (here called 'intermediate' phenomena) -

> *"Should an adult make claims on us for our acceptance of the objectivity of his subjective phenomena we discern or diagnose madness. If, however, the adult can manage to enjoy the personal intermediate area without making claims, then we can acknowledge our own corresponding intermediate areas, and are pleased to find a degree of overlapping, that is to say,*

common experience between members of a group in art or religion or philosophy." [Playing and Reality]

An AB's child persona is subjectively real – to them. But if an AB insists that anyone else take that child persona as objective reality, ie. the same as a biological child, then people will perceive the AB as mentally ill. However, a non-conflicted AB who is happier, more vital, because they have accepted their own subjective reality, invites a partner to share an intermediate space – where the AB and the partner accept that the AB's child persona is subjectively real. That can be a wonderful, healthy, happy space. For everyone, healthy play (transitional spaces) enriches our lives. The key point is that, as an AB, you can only invite someone to share such a space with you. You cannot compel them. You can appeal, you can explain – although it is far better just to be yourself – but, you cannot demand.

Conclusion

So, if you are an AB remember that your partner's acceptance is what matters. Let your partner find the form that acceptance takes, for them to feel comfortable. Your internal conflict has left a legacy for both you and your partner that takes time to heal. For you, the AB, there are habitual thoughts and perceptions that belong to the wounded Inner Child of your old conflicted identity. That past includes tantrums, sulks, demands and emotional blackmail. Do not let that sabotage your future with your partner. Your partner lived with your conflicted identity for years. They need to experience the difference in you that comes from a non-conflicted identity. I believe that accepting our real identity has a profoundly healing effect and that will be apparent to a loving partner. Give it time.

11. A Healthy Identity

So, what does self-acceptance and a healthy, non-conflicted identity as an AB feel like?

To find out, we need to revisit the symptoms of the conflicted AB.

The Push-Pull of Compulsion and Fetish

This was our irresistible need to wear nappies, how that became a compulsive sexual fetish, and how our need for deep comfort mostly seemed to elude us.

Astonishingly, after I fully accepted myself as an AB and 'came out' to myself and my wife, my compulsive behaviour *completely* disappeared. I am no longer driven by impulses that I can't control. The shame is gone, and so has my compulsive masturbation. After living with this demoralizing tyranny for many years, it is wonderful to be free of it. Don't get me wrong – masturbation is fine. The compulsion was the problem. The heightened sexual excitement has gone too. I don't need it anymore, and it came at too high a price. I still have a nappy fetish, and always will have. Nappies are essential to my sexual arousal.

My child persona, Chrissie feels happy and safe. Now I often take comfort and security from wearing a nappy and baby clothes, sucking a dummy and cuddling a soft toy and don't feel sexual or the need to masturbate. In fact, those are the times I feel most content. The regularity of wearing a wet nappy has made it normal – a reliable source of security and comfort. It is no longer something edgy and exciting, instead it is just 'nice', just 'right'. My 'baby time' is now so routine that I am not thinking of a new dress but instead, more nappies to rotate through the wash, and a nappy bucket, so I am not washing every day.

Triggering

This is about how a compelling and urgent need to put on a nappy can be triggered involuntarily, out-of-the-blue, by sight or another sense.

I don't experience triggering any more. There is no involuntary compulsive need to put on a nappy or baby clothes. Chrissie knows that she will be cared for each day by my nurturing Inner Parent, and that my strong Adult will see that space for nurturing is protected. I sleep like a baby each night and have regular baby time when Chrissie needs it.

The Binge and Purge Cycle

This was the cycle of buying a new stash of nappies or baby clothes, or experimenting with new baby activities, building to a crescendo of guilty masturbation, and then discarding everything in a fit of remorse.

I had stopped the binge and purge of physical baby items years before I fully accepted myself. But there were other ways in which cycles of compulsive purchases followed by shameful remorse regularly featured in my life. All those cycles of compulsion and remorse have gone. No more guilt and shame. None! Before I fully accepted myself, I had accumulated a large collection of baby clothes. But it was never enough. I always wanted more because each new item was a statement to myself that my child persona was real. Now I have fully accepted my Chrissie, I'm quite happy with my existing collection of clothes. My shopping addiction is gone. I'd rather spend the time playing as Chrissie.

Masochistic Fantasies

These were the sexual fantasies about being coerced, shamed and humiliated by a dominant figure.

I have made my peace with being a submissive in my fantasies, sexual and non-sexual. I like fantasies or daydreams of being supervised and gently but firmly disciplined by 'mummy' and safely 'outed'. I don't feel ashamed about that. How could it be different being a heterosexual adult male, with an insecure attachment as a child, and a child persona as an integral part of my psyche? For me, fantasies of being under the supervision and control of a loving mother figure are enjoyable and safe. Fantasies including the kind of discipline appropriate to a loved small child of a previous generation (spanking or being made to sit on the 'naughty step') are a psychological reassurance that I'm important and loved.

I have learned to avoid masochistic fantasies. Mostly they no longer hold the same compelling fascination. My Chrissie knows that she will be kept safe by boundaries kept with firm love by my nurturing Inner parent. But old bad habits take time to heal, and those fantasies continue to be psychologically unsafe for me. They still have the power to trigger the yearning and pain of the missing childhood attachment.

Confusion and Turmoil About Ourselves

Conflicted ABs live with confusion and doubt about their identity.

For me, this is the best bit. The doubt, confusion and turmoil are gone. I know who I am. I am an adult male with a baby girl persona. I am an adult baby, and I'm proud of who I am.

The end of the internal conflict feels like peace after a long war. It doesn't feel like one part of me is fighting another part. I feel much more relaxed and freer to be myself. I like myself a lot more. I feel better about the world – it seems like a kinder place with more possibilities than risks.

A lot, indeed most, of my anger has disappeared. I experience that difference on a daily basis. I still have an anxious disposition, but my anxiety is a lot easier to manage than before.

Self-acceptance brings two other valuable gifts - resilience and creativity.

Resilience doesn't come from living an easy, comfortable life. ABs have not had it easy - from starting life with an insecure attachment with our mothers, and then a long struggle to understand and accept ourselves. But coming out the other side we have a deep knowing of who we are; we have found a strength to persevere and believe in ourselves; we have learned to replace anger and hurt with love and gentleness; and we have learned to withhold judgement and extend compassion to others, giving to others what we seek for ourselves.

I have also found that accepting my real personal identity has unchained a great amount of creativity. For me, that's writing. It will be different for each AB. In my experience, it is like tapping into a formerly hidden, clear flowing stream within my psyche. It makes life fresh and hopeful.

Over Compensation

Conflicted ABs shore up a sense of worthiness by over-investing in some other area of their life, often work or a sport or hobby. This is often unconscious and therefore unrecognized.

I still have an obsessive streak to my character (ask my wife). But the compulsive, driven, need to prove myself worthy or okay is gone. With the internal conflict gone, the overcompensation has, in a way, reversed. My baby girl child persona has influenced the outlook of my adult self in ways that are not directly related to being AB. For example, I found myself identifying much more with female than male characters in the young adult fiction that I like to read. In my social and political views, I found myself identifying more strongly with women, and being more impatient with the intransigence of old men in power. I welcome these changes. I feel renewed and released from a burden to be someone else.

Problems with Partners

Being a conflicted AB often brings secrets, underlying tension and sometimes conflict into our relationship with our partner.

We covered this in the last chapter. Suffice to say, I cherish the openness and ease with my wife about my child persona and adult baby identity. She likes and interacts with my child persona daily, so that both my child persona and my Adult self feel loved and accepted. My wife feels safe with my adult baby identity. I don't have to hide who I am. It is a wonderful freedom.

Isolation and Loneliness

Conflicted AB's often live with deep feelings of isolation and loneliness because of their internal conflicts and the need to keep their identity secret.

In my experience, this is the one aspect where there isn't a transformation between the conflicted and the non-conflicted states of being an AB. Isolation and loneliness is still an issue.

Self-acceptance is first-and-foremost about an AB 'coming out' to themselves, and perhaps a life partner. After that, there is a question about disclosing to a wider range of people. Being AB is an identity centred on a vulnerable young child persona – and like a young biological child, that persona needs to be protected from unsafe environments. Ours is still a largely misunderstood and stigmatized minority personal identity. As a society, I believe that we are on the journey that will turn that around. But at the moment we still have a long way to go. So, there are no easy answers to the issue of disclosure. Extreme caution is advisable. The threat of harm is real, and disclosure cannot be taken back. See my book '*The Adult Baby Identity – Coming Out As An Adult Baby*' for a discussion on the way forward for the AB identity.

So, for most of us being AB is going to be secret or, at least, private part of our lives, fully shared with only a carefully chosen few, perhaps only our life partner. That is a big issue. Because everyone has a human need to be accepted for who they are. To stay psychologically healthy, non-conflicted ABs need to find safe and positive ways to make contact with other ABs. Online and social media environments seem to offer a good prospect, allowing contact and trust to build up slowly without risk of identity being disclosed prematurely. Caution is essential. There are enough posts and stories on-line about those with ulterior motives, or simply people falling out, attesting to that.

The quality of the contact matters. Many ABs are in the conflicted stages of identity formation and are focused only on the fetish side of being AB. That is not going to 'feed the soul' of a non-conflicted AB. You are seeking contact where you can share your experience of your personal identity, not just an obsession with nappies. It is also natural to want face-to-face contact with people who know and accept that you have a child persona. That doesn't necessarily mean that you need to share your child persona in full technicolour with someone to enjoy their acceptance of your AB identity.

Hopefully, society is changing for the better, but in the meantime isolation and loneliness will continue to be issues for most ABs, even those who have fully accepted their own identities.

Give It Time

In my experience, it takes many months, even years, for the virtuous cycle of self-acceptance and healing to fully transform how ABs experience and express their identity. That is not surprising, given that we lived for many years with our conflicted identity. The positive changes from self-acceptance start straight away and make a big difference. But the full change, flowing into the depths of our psyche, takes a while. The journey of self-acceptance never really ends. It just gets smoother.

When we have accepted our child persona as real, our experience of 'baby time' meets our need for nurturing and heals our wounded Inner Child. That is the equivalent of intensive therapy. As therapist Jasmin Lee Cori indicates, it goes much deeper than the 'thinking' brain and reaches into the emotional ('limbic') brain. That is where the real healing is happening. Your Adult, Parent and Child are learning to trust the healing power of self-acceptance. That will heal your hurts and transform your experience of yourself. Give it time.

In the interim, sometimes we will 'relapse' and fall back into old conflicted patterns of perception, thinking and behaviour. The source will usually be our wounded Inner Child. Like a wounded biological child, they are learning to trust and will test safe boundaries. Do you really love me, or will you reject me again if I am rebellious or make a mistake? Will you enforce new boundaries with love, or will it be harsh like before?

Our wounded Inner Child may drive exhibitionistic impulses that risk us being 'outed' in unsafe environments. Understand this for what it is – a sign that the wounds are still hurting, even as they heal, and a test to see if they can trust you. Be cautious of overconfidence or 'false' self-acceptance, in the form of these exhibitionist impulses. You may be 'trying too hard' to give your child persona everything they missed out on. There is a real danger to our new self-acceptance in being unsafely 'outed'. As I say in my book *'Living With Chrissie'* -

I have a hair-trigger for feeling shame. I've had more than enough of it in my life. I don't need any more. Chrissie doesn't need any more. In her pink tutu skirt, only those who look with the eyes of love, see Chrissie. Everyone else would see something different – something wrong. I don't want to see Chrissie through their eyes. But driven by shame, I couldn't help but do so.

Such a setback may flip our Inner Parent back into reacting harshly. It is only habit, not a bad intent, but it will harm the trust we are building with our child persona. This is where our strong Adult steps in to prevent exhibitionism, and the harm and setbacks it might cause.

In my experience, it takes a while, years, to *fully* accept our own reality of shared consciousness. Old habits of denial die hard, and there is little in our culture that validates the experience of people living with shared consciousness. There will be occasions when doubt creeps quietly into our thoughts. Despite the benefits and relief that self-acceptance has brought us, there will still be times when we question if shared consciousness, if our child persona, is real? Perhaps we might question the wounds of our long-ago childhood? Others with identities defined by shared consciousness have also faced these doubts. *'Got Parts: An Insider's Guide to Managing Life Successfully with Dissociative Identity Disorder'* tells us -

> *"There may be times when you may begin to wonder, or doubt whether your traumatic experience ever happened, or if it was really 'that bad'. There may also be times when you may question, even go into denial about whether or not you really are DID [AB]. This is very normal. ... Don't get stuck here or let this de-rail you. ... Sometimes it comes down to intuition, faith, trust*

and deciding that even though you don't have all the answers, or don't know everything you long to know ... you can still move on in reclaiming your life."

Doubt is normal, and not something to be feared. Step back from the doubt. You have lived being AB, the bad, and the good. You can trust your own daily experience of shared consciousness. It is a real part of your healthy psyche.

A Healthy Psyche

Self-acceptance is being proud of your identity. As ABs, we have a shared consciousness - we are functional adults with a subjectively real child persona as part of our psyche. Our adult baby identity includes our child persona and our nurturing Inner Parent, both led by our strong Adult Self.

Your child persona is free of fear and hurt. They are a source of innocent happiness, contentment and wonder. The comfort and happiness they can take from the simplest things, a wet or fresh soft nappy, their favourite dress or onesie, their soft toy, their dummy – delights and grounds you. They have a secure attachment with your nurturing Inner Parent (and if you have a faith – with God or whatever higher power you conceive). They feel safe knowing that their feelings are recognized. They still have the occasional tantrums and sulks of course – after all, they are a young child. But they are readily calmed and comforted by your Inner Parent (and perhaps your partner). They accept boundaries that keep them and our adult baby identity safe. They are loving as well as loved.

Your Inner Parent is nurturing and proud of your child persona. They are attentive and loving, constantly aware of the feelings and needs of your child persona – a doting parent. They are happy to spoil your child persona a bit – but not too much so that they become greedy and selfish. They are not afraid to set and keep boundaries that will keep your child persona contented and safe. They can take the occasional tantrums and sulks happily in their stride, being firm but not harsh – and find the humour in your child persona's frowns and pouting. And they are rightly proud of the happiness and security they have been able to bring to your child persona, healing the wounds of your childhood.

Your strong Adult is responsible and compassionate. They safeguard your hard-won and much-treasured self-acceptance. They are proud of having resolved the inner conflict that tormented you for so long – and they won't let it reappear. They will firmly step in if your child persona slips back into the hurts of the wounded Inner Child and throws a stinker of a tantrum, or your Inner Parent falls back into fear and reacts harshly. They will bring both your child persona and your Inner Parent back to the secure attachment that means everything to both of them. They keep you safe from fantasies or practices which are psychologically unsafe, and from unsafe public disclosure. They understand all your partner has been through when you were acting out your inner conflict. They are the ally of your partner in protecting your marriage. They want to help your partner understand that your adult baby identity is healthy and stable and can be safely embraced.

Self-acceptance is indeed a goal worth the journey.

A Personal Identity

How do you know if being AB is important enough, deep enough, to be part of your personal identity?

You just *know*.

Even after all the struggles and doubt – when you listen to the small, still voice inside you – you know.

For me, fully accepting myself as AB was like coming home to myself – after a long and difficult journey.

It lets me be who I am.

Not who I am supposed to be.

213

Not who everyone else expects me to be.

Not even who I wanted to be.

Who I am.

In the depth of my spirit. My True Self.

That is a freedom worth having.

Appendix - Choosing a Therapist

ABs are generally reluctant to go to a therapist. Dr Rhoda Lipscomb is a therapist and the author of the best writing on ABs by a health professional that I have read (her 2014 PhD thesis, available free on-line and cited in the references). She writes that few ABs seek psychotherapy. She also indicates that the psychotherapy profession has a mixed track record in terms of showing empathy for ABs.

So, this appendix has two purposes:

1. to encourage ABs to consult a therapist if personal issues are stopping them living the happy, psychologically healthy lives they want to live
2. to assist ABs to choose a therapist who will help the AB freely determine their personal identity for themselves.

What do I bring to this task? I have consulted professional therapists or counsellors in six instances in my adult life – some have been helpful, some have not, but the net benefit was very positive. I have no qualifications in psychology. I have a layman's lifelong interest in psychology. My wife is a psychotherapist.

Why go to a therapist?

Most personal issues we can work out for ourselves – often with the support of partners, or friends or family. That is how it should be. But sometimes there are issues or situations which overwhelm us - even with the best will in the world, and a supportive partner or friends. Or the same troubling issue or situation keeps coming back to bite us.

The truth is, mostly we go to a therapist as a last resort. That is especially true if we haven't been to a therapist before. We are reluctant to see a therapist because it can seem like an admission of failure. We are afraid of handing control over our lives to someone else. Iit costs money, and sometimes we know we've been avoiding something we would prefer not to deal with. All of that is understandable. What overcomes those concerns is emotional pain. We might be afraid of dentists, but if the toothache gets bad enough, you go to the dentist.

Once people have had a positive experience of therapy these concerns fade. Seeing a therapist is not an admission of failure, but a sign of psychological health and maturity. You are not losing control over your life – you take from therapy what you choose, it is your choice, not the therapists. Therapy is an investment in your life. There is nothing within us we haven't already been living with. As a result, people who have had a positive experience are generally more likely to go to a therapist in the future.

My view is that it is human nature to initially regard seeing a therapist as a last resort. That is a lot better than no-resort. The worst alternative is to numb, or distract ourselves from, the emotional pain. Then the pain, and the issues that cause it, become a chronic condition. We learn to live with it. In the meantime, we aren't living the life we want to live. Emotional pain has a healthy function. It is an alarm – a signal we need to change something. Ignoring the signal just means the next time the pain will be worse.

Speaking from firsthand experience, ABs have more need than most to see a therapist at some point in their lives.

Being an AB is a largely misunderstood, stigmatized, minority personal identity. For most of us, our psyche is hard wired differently from everyone we know. Most of us live secret, double lives with a valid fear of how others in our lives would react if they knew about us.

Many ABs have denied their personal identity for many years. That really fucks us up. Issues about personal identity reach into the deepest parts of your psyche – including your childhood and your closest relationships.

Being an AB most likely originated as a response to difficulties in our childhood, namely a broken attachment with our mothers, and trauma.

All of that is a lot to handle.

So, it is understandable if going to a therapist is the last resort, provided you do go when you need to.

'Right' and 'Wrong' Therapists

Choosing the *right* therapist is essential.

Therapists have different levels of skill and take different approaches. At best, choosing the wrong therapist is a waste of your time and money. At worst, it is a lost opportunity and may cause you harm when you are vulnerable. The harm comes if the therapist is not sufficiently skilled, or suited to help you with your specific issues, and mistakenly reinforces negative experiences and messages you have received from others or given to yourself. That can set your journey of self-acceptance back by years.

You are most likely better with a psychotherapist, rather than a counsellor. Counselling generally deals with alleviating or managing troubling symptoms. Psychotherapy is concerned with identifying and resolving the issues that create those troubling symptoms. Matters of personal identity fall into this latter category. For ABs troubling symptoms will often be linked to the AB's conflicted and denied personal identity.

A good psychotherapist is a doctor for the psyche. They are rightly proud of their professional skills. They know their way around the psyche – how to accurately locate pain in the psyche's strained and torn ligaments, and how to help you heal that pain. Good therapists see you as an equal. They respect that you are in charge of your own life. There are times they may bring up questions you may find difficult, but they do not talk down to you.

The 'Wrong' Therapists

The conventional psychological and psychiatric opinion is that being AB is a paraphilia – a compulsive sexual fetish or perversion, and if you experience any distress in relation to being AB, then it is a psycho-sexual disorder. This is how it is defined in the Diagnostic and Statistical Manual of Mental Disorders (the DSM), the standard diagnostic tool published by the American Psychiatric Association (APA).

A health professional who works from this perspective is not going to see being an AB as a healthy minority personal identity. They are not going to look beyond compulsive behaviours and internal conflict. That is sufficient proof to them that being AB is a disorder. They will not consider that, if these conflicts are resolved, underneath is a healthy personal identity. Instead, they will regard being AB as a pathological condition, which cannot be 'cured' but has to be 'managed' like a chronic disease. They regard an AB's desires to wear nappies and fantasies of being babied, as symptoms of an unhealthy addiction (like alcoholism) and that like an addiction, abstinence is the solution. Likely they will get an AB to use cognitive behaviour therapy (CBT) to maintain this abstinence by attempting to change habits and responses to 'triggers'. Refer to my book *'The Adult Baby Identity – Coming Out As An Adult Baby'* for a case study from a psychological textbook describing this damaging treatment approach.

Essentially, this is the same approach psychologists and psychiatrists took to being gay or lesbian before society understood that being homosexual was a healthy minority personal identity. As late as 1980, the DSM labelled being homosexual as a psychological disorder. The fact that people were conflicted about being gay or lesbian (in large part because society stigmatized those identities) was taken as evidence that these were disorders. This was a self-fulfilling diagnosis and a vicious cycle. There was no valid empirical evidence that being gay or lesbian was harmful, it was simply that it was unacceptable to many in society. Even today, there are still a few non-mainstream therapists who offer 'gay conversion therapy' which purports to 'cure' people of being gay or lesbian. This is now generally regarded by health professionals and the public as ineffective, harmful, and professionally unethical.

An AB going to a therapist who subscribes to the conventional view of being AB in the DSM, essentially risks being subject to the contemporary equivalent of 'gay conversion therapy'. It is harmful and should be avoided in all circumstances.

It is also a good idea to avoid 'formula' therapists. These are health professionals, who may have degrees and be registered, but who are rigidly committed to one psychological theory. They are going to fit you into their theory whether that works for you or not – like playing every shot in golf using a nine-iron because that is the only club you've got. Typically, a 'formula' therapist will use CBT. That focuses on changing perceptions and habits rather than identifying and healing buried emotions. CBT has its' place. That place is not addressing issues of personal identity. In the context of being AB, CBT is predominantly used to manage the dysfunctional symptoms of a conflicted identity, while ignoring the sources of those symptoms in the denial of that identity.

The 'Right' Therapist

Fortunately, there are many therapists who disregard the pathological view of being AB in the DSM. They take the view that being AB is a fetish or a kink, and provided it is not causing distress to the AB, they regard it as a benign feature of the personality. The therapeutic focus is resolving the person's internal conflict so that they can live without distress. This is an improvement over the approach in the DSM, and over CBT.

The best therapists for ABs will be open to recognizing that being AB can be a healthy minority personal identity. The therapeutic focus is on resolving internal conflicts and healing buried emotions so that a person can determine their own identity free of fear and pain.

I believe that ABs need an intuitive therapist. They are the opposite of a 'formula' therapist. An intuitive therapist is flexible and can use a range of psychological theories and approaches. No psychological theory fits everybody all the time. Sure, there are patterns, but the permutations of the human psyche are infinite. An intuitive therapist will mix'n'match between approaches, to get the best fit for you and your issues (ie. they fit the theory to you, not the other way around). They are more committed to the wellbeing of their clients than to a theory.

Remember being AB is a rare, 'one-in-a-thousand' trait. Most therapists will not see many ABs in their practice. The professional literature is of little help. What little there is, is often misleading, or outdated and harmful. There is little empirical evidence guiding the best way to provide therapy for an AB. So, the therapist will have to work out most of their approach for themselves – with your help. The therapist needs to be able to trust their own intuition.

The empathy of the therapist is as important as their therapeutic skill. To be an ally in your healing you need to feel that the therapist is sincerely trying to understand what it is like to 'walk a mile in your shoes'. This is particularly important for ABs. We have spent a lot of time feeling, and fearing, being judged harshly by the world at large. With good reason. To heal you need to feel safe. And to feel safe you need to feel that you are not being judged. A therapist may have a different take on the issues that you are tackling. That's part of the professional skill you are paying for. You can take that in your stride if you know the therapist is genuinely trying to look at the world through your eyes.

So how do you choose the right therapist?

The best way to choose a therapist is word-of-mouth recommendation – knowing someone you trust, who has seen a therapist, and you can see it has made a positive difference in their lives. Unfortunately, most of us aren't in that situation.

Searching on-line will probably be the way most of us find a therapist. Go to the websites of the professional associations. Read the reviews. If possible, make a shortlist, and telephone or email their office and ask questions.

Good therapists are usually in demand. A lot of their caseload will come from returning clients and referrals from existing clients or health professionals. There is often a long wait to get an appointment. That can be a problem if you are in crisis. A good therapist is worth the wait. If you are in crisis it may be an idea to book your preferred therapist, even if the appointment is some way off, and see another counsellor in the interim. If the interim counsellor turns out to suit you well, you can cancel the appointment with the other therapist (before the deadline when you have to pay if you cancel).

There are questions you can ask a therapist to determine if they are suited to you.

Are they experienced in counselling people about issues related to their minority personal identities (ie. LGBTQ)?

All-things-being equal, yes is better. It suggests that the therapist will not be judgmental if you have, or may have, a non-conforming identity (ie. AB). They will have an understanding of how identity runs deep in the psyche; how a conflict about identity can produce symptoms such as anxiety, anger and depression; and the feelings of isolation and alienation that can arise with having a minority personal identity.

Are they experienced in counselling people in relation to broken childhood attachments and trauma?

All-things-being equal, yes is better. It is important for ABs, because the likely origin of the AB identity is a broken attachment with our mothers, and dissociated childhood trauma. Preferably, the therapist will have a good knowledge of the psyche of children and what it feels like when a child's upbringing is broken. Trauma and dissociation is a specialist field with its' own expertise. We are at our most vulnerable when we are dealing with issues of attachment and trauma. You need to know you are in safe hands.

Can they conceive of being a non-conflicted AB as a healthy minority personal identity?

They may not have thought about it. The key issue is are they open to the idea? This is a pointer to whether the therapist will have empathy, see you as an individual and avoid pre-conceived judgements. If not, then they probably belong to the category of therapists who subscribe to the perspective in the DSM - that being AB is intrinsically unhealthy. Potentially, they would have proceeded without being honest about that view. This is a deal-breaker. If the answer is no, find another therapist.

What psychological / psychotherapeutic theories or approaches do they use?

Preferably, the therapist uses a range of different theories or approaches, that they can customize to suit the needs of each client. If they only use one theory/approach, be cautious. If their only, or main, approach is Cognitive Behavioural Therapy (CBT) they are unlikely to be suited to help you with the deeper issues of personal identity. Find another therapist. If they can't name the approaches they use, or they're vague, be cautious, it is basic professionalism.

It is an advantage if the therapist uses Internal Family Systems (IFS) therapy. But the therapeutic skill and empathy of the therapist is the most important factor. Some other psychological theories can accommodate shared consciousness. To insist only on a therapist who uses IFS would potentially eliminate therapists with high levels of skill and empathy.

Did their training, and does their professional development, include reflecting on their own psyche?

All-things-being equal, yes is better. A therapist who knows their own psyche is less likely to step on their own issues in working with yours. That is important. This is basically asking 'do you practice what you preach?' If they don't, underneath they may have a superior attitude, and be less likely to respect that, ultimately, you have the answers for your own life.

Do they have professional supervision?

All-things-being equal, yes is better. Professional supervision involves the therapist regularly meeting with another professional therapist to talk through issues that arise for them, in their work with their clients. Again, it's a way of making sure the therapist doesn't step on their own issues in working with yours. It suggests they don't assume they are perfect and have a commitment to continuous improvement and professional development.

The therapeutic skill and empathy of the therapist are what is most important. The questions are largely a guide to help you make an intuitive decision about whether you and the therapist are a 'good fit'. Apart from the two make-or-break questions, the others are flexible.

If you can't get the answers to the questions before, then ask them at the first session. If the answers don't sound promising, ask for the therapist to refer you to another therapist better suited to you. It will cost you the price of a session, but it's better than persisting with a therapist who turns out later, not to be suited, and you've wasted a lot more time and money.

Getting the Most from Therapy

One of the things a therapist will usually ask you in the first session, is what do you want to get out of therapy? Your answer forms the basis for 'the contract' between you and the therapist that will guide your therapy over multiple sessions. Give this some thought before the first session.

Set your goal based on what you want to achieve from 4 to 6 sessions. You can make a lot of progress understanding and healing yourself with 4 to 6 sessions with a good intuitive therapist. That is enough for many people. If you get to the end of that schedule of sessions, and think that you need more sessions, ask for another 4 to 6 sessions and make a new contract with your therapist about what you want to achieve. You can keep extending if you and your therapist agree. Some types of psychotherapy are based on weekly sessions that last for a much longer time, even years. The therapist is there to equip you to live your own life, independently, 'under your own steam'. If you are in therapy over the long term, both you and the therapist need to be mindful of the risk you will become dependent on the therapist.

Work on your issues between sessions with your therapist. In each session with the therapist, you will discover new insights into your own psyche and the issues you want to work on. Think on these in between sessions. You will discover more insights to discuss with your therapist at the next session. It's like doing homework. It will help you make more of each session. It's your dime/ten cents.

The following is to assist readers, or potential readers, who have questions about the relationship between the books of the quadrilogy.

The quadrilogy consists of –

Becoming Me – the journey of Self-Acceptance

The Adult Baby Identity – A Self Help Guide

The Adult Baby Identity – Coming Out As An Adult Baby

The Adult Baby Identity – Healing Childhood Wounds

[subsequent to this book is a fifth book – Adult Baby: a identity on the dissociation spectrum. Editor]

The purpose of the quadrilogy is to outline that being AB is a complex, healthy, minority personal identity, originating as a positive response to difficulties in early childhood. This corrects the mistaken view that it is a kink, a sexual fetish, a paraphilia or a psychosexual disorder.

Each book is an in-depth treatment of a different 'big idea' about the AB Identity –

Becoming Me	This is a preview of the issues covered in the later three books.
A Self Help Guide	self-acceptance of our AB Identity is based on resolving our internal conflict between our Inner Child, Inner Parent and Adult
Coming Out As An Adult Baby	being AB is a minority personal identity, similar to LGBTQ identities, and the identity is formed through a sequence of stages
Healing Childhood Wounds	an AB's child persona is a positive response to; a broken attachment between mother and child, and dissociated childhood trauma

A full understanding of the AB Identity rests on all three 'big ideas'. Each supports the others.

Why not just write one larger book? Taking one 'big idea' per book seems like the best way of making the content accessible to ABs, the primary audience.

An important aim of the trilogy is to illuminate the nature and origin of the AB Identity using recognized psychological theories. In part, this is intended to prompt health professionals to discard existing inadequate and pathologising approaches to a complex personal identity. The theories are shown below-

A Self Help Guide	Internal Family Systems (IFS) Therapy, developed by Richard Schwartz
Coming Out As An Adult Baby	Cass Theory of Lesbian and Gay Identity Formation, developed by Vivienne Cass

References – Annotated List

Bader, Michael	Arousal: The Secret Logic of Sexual Fantasies (2003) (Virgin Books) (ISBN 0 7535 0739 0) Paperback only. No digital copy. Highly recommended for anyone wanting to understand troubling sexual fantasies. Finds the emotional meaning of fantasies with compassion and insight. The author is a gifted intuitive psychotherapist.
Bent, Michael	Adult Babies: Principles and Practices (2015) (Amazon & Abdiscovery.com.au) The first text taking an analytical approach to the AB identity, written by an AB.
	Being an Adult Baby: Articles and Essays on Being an Adult Baby. (2016) (Amazon & Abdiscovery.com.au) A collection of insightful and thought provoking articles on the AB identity. Notably – 'Identity Confusion in the Adult Baby', 'Finding Balance Between the Baby and the Adult', 'Binge and Purge', 'A Christian Response to being an adult baby'
Bent, Rosalie	There's Still A Baby in My Bed: Learning To Live Happily With the Adult Baby in Your Relationship. (2015) (Amazon & Abdiscovery.com.au) A revised version of the 2012 book that first articulated that being an AB was a personal identity, not just a fetish. Written by the wife of an AB. Evergreen.
	Coffee With Rosie: Why Does My Partner Want to Wear Diapers. (2017) (Amazon & Abdiscovery.com.au) An imaginary dialogue between two women over coffee about ABs. Written by the wife of an AB. Great for a wife's perspective. Refreshingly clear and direct.
Chan, Yong Kang	Parent Yourself Again: Love Yourself the Way You Have Always Wanted to be Loved. (2018). (digital & paperback: Amazon) A very good self help book on re-parenting. The author is from an Asian background where the emphasis is on achievement rather than nurturing or self fulfilment. Recommended. Digitial copies are inexpensive.

Cori, Jasmin Lee		The Emotionally Absent Mother: How to Recognize and Heal the Invisible Effects of Childhood Emotional Neglect (Second Edition) (2017) (digital & paperback: Amazon) A brilliantly written discussion of insecure attachments in childhood and their effects. Makes Attachment Theory, Bowlby and Winnicott accessible to the lay reader. Highly recommended and inexpensive.
Earley, Jay		Self Therapy: A Step-by-Step Guide to Creating Wholeness and Healing Your Inner Child Using IFS, A New Cutting-Edge Psychotherapy. Second Edition (2012). (digital & paperback: Amazon) IFS is the psychological theory most suited to meet the needs of ABs. This is the best introduction to IFS. It walks the reader through IFS ideas and methods with helpful examples. Highly recommended. Digitial copies are inexpensive.
		Self Therapy, Volume 2: A Step-by-Step Guide to Advanced IFS Techniques for Working With Protectors. (2015). (digital & paperback: Amazon). A useful adjunction to the first volume, but not essential. Digital copies are inexpensive.
Lewis, Dylan		Living With Chrissie: My Life As An Adult Baby (2018) (Amazon & Abdiscovery.com.au) My account of my life as a very late bloomer as an AB ('better late than never').
		The Adult Baby Identity – Coming Out as an Adult Baby (2019) (Amazon & Abdiscovery.com.au) Makes the case that being AB is a minority personal identity and considers the stages by which the identity is formed. References the Cass Theory of Lesbian and Gay Identity Formation.
		The Adult Baby Identity – Healing Childhood Wounds (2019) (Amazon & Abdiscovery.com.au) Explores the origins of the identity in an insecure attachment and trauma in childhood. References John Bowlby and Attachment Theory, and Donald Winnicott.

Lipscomb, Rhoda J.		The Clinical Mental Health Experience of Persons with Paraphilic Infantilism and Autonepiophilia. A phenomenological research study. PhD dissertation (2014). An excellent study of being AB by an informed and sympathetic health professional. Good up-to-date review of literature and research. Available free, on-line at - http://www.esextherapy.com/dissertations/Rhoda%20J.%20Lipscomb%20The%20Clinical%20Mental%20Health%20Experience%20of%20Persons%20withParaphilic%20Infantilism%20and%20Autonepiophilia.pdf
Rowan, John		Subpersonalities: The People Inside Us (1990) (Routledge) (digital & hardcopy: Amazon). Useful history of shared consciousness in psychology going back to Freud and Jung but can be obscure/dense to read. Expensive in both digital & hardcopy.
Schwartz, Richard C.		Internal Family Systems Therapy (1995) (Guildford Press) (digital & hardcopy: Amazon) The Original exposition of IFS by its creator. IFS is the school of psychology which is best suited to counselling ABs. Moderately priced. Recommended.
Steinberg, Marlene		The Stranger in the Mirror: Dissociation The Hidden Epidemic (2010) (hardcopy: Harper Collins. Digital: Amazon). The author is the psychiatrist who developed the leading diagnostic questionnaire for identifying dissociative disorders. Highly recommended.
W, A.T.		Got Parts: An Insider's Guide to Managing Life Successfully with Dissociative Identity Disorder. (2005) (digital & paperback: amazon) A good self help book, recommended to me by a family member with DID. It is relevant to anyone with mulplicity of consciousness. Digital copies are inexpensive.
Winnicott, Donald		'Ego Distortion in Terms of True and False Self' (1960)

		Winnicott's ground breaking original exposition on the subject. Best read after secondary sources on Winnicott. Written for an audience of psychoanalysts but the fundamentals are still clear to the lay reader. Available free, on-line at – *https://www.sas.upenn.edu/~cavitch/pdf-library/Winnicott_EgoDistortion.pdf*
		'Playing and Reality' (1971) Tavistock Publications. (hardcopy only, no digital copy) Recommended for those with a keen interest in Winnicott. Written for psychotherapists. Best read after reading some secondary sources, or Winnicott's books for laypeople. A seminal book published in the last year of Winnicott's life.
Wikipedia		Attachment Theory Dissociation (psychology) Donald Winnicott Internal Family Systems Model 'Karpman drama triangle' (for the victim, persecutor, rescuer triangle) True Self and False Self

IFS References

The following references are for those with a further interest in IFS.

The best introduction to IFS is Jay Earley's 2012 book 'Self Therapy: A Step-by-Step Guide to Creating Wholeness and Healing Your Inner Child Using IFS, A New Cutting-Edge Psychotherapy'. The author is a talented educator and the book is very readable. It is available in digital and paperback from Amazon. The digital copies are inexpensive.

There is a useful Wikipedia article titled 'Internal Family Systems Model' (as at April 2019, it has been flagged for review since 2012 on the basis that it doesn't present a balanced critique of IFS).

Richard Schwartz's 1995 book 'Internal Family Systems Therapy' is the original exposition of the theory. It is clear and comprehensive, and available in digital and paperback from Amazon for a moderate price.

Both Jay Early and Richard Schwartz have written other books on IFS which will come up in any search on Amazon.

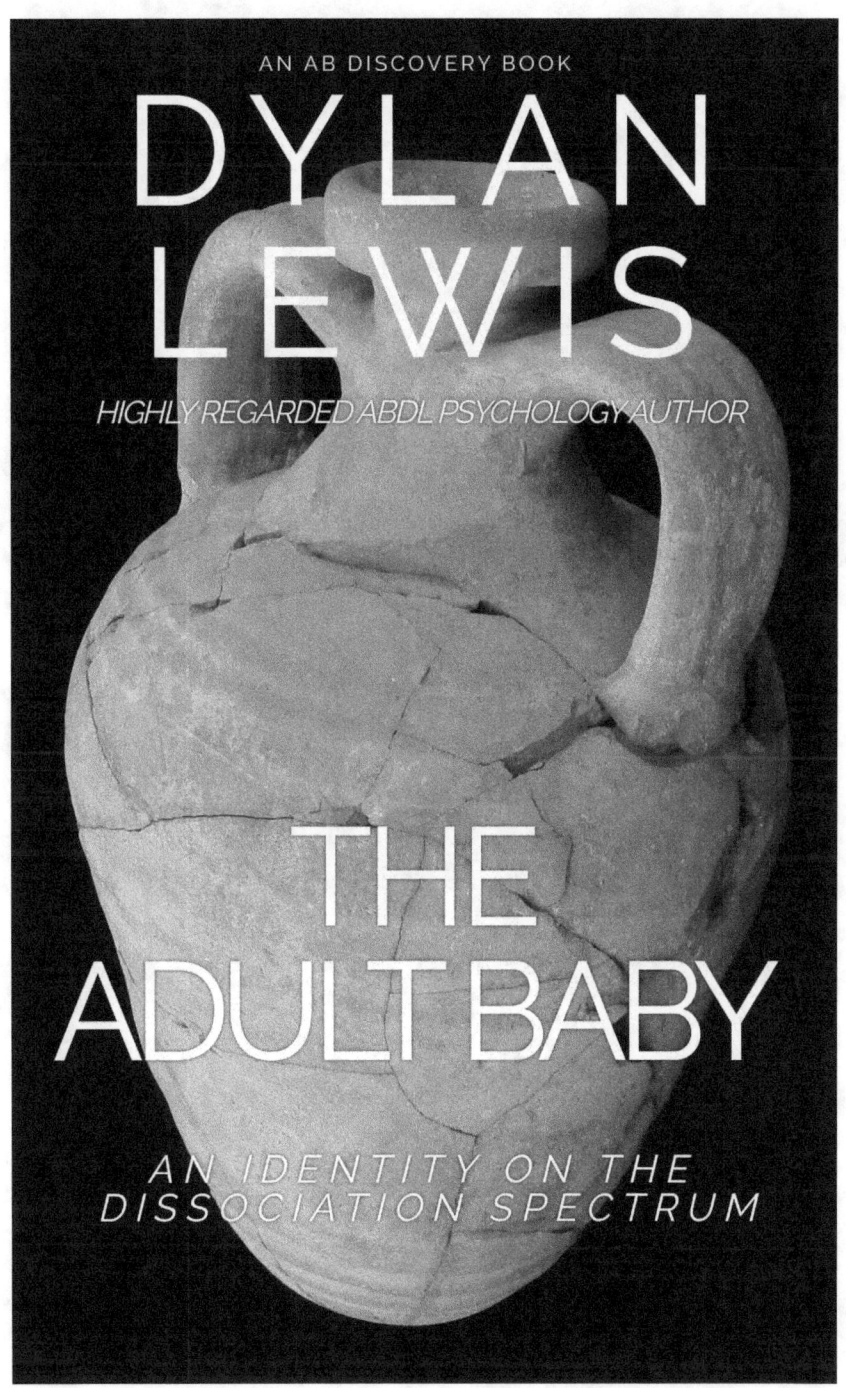

AN AB DISCOVERY BOOK

DYLAN LEWIS

HIGHLY REGARDED ABDL PSYCHOLOGY AUTHOR

THE ADULT BABY

AN IDENTITY ON THE DISSOCIATION SPECTRUM

The Adult Baby –
An Identity on the Dissociation Spectrum

*By Dylan Lewis
with Dax Jordan*

Dedication:

To my wife for her constant love and wisdom.

To Rosalie Bent and Michael Bent for letting adult babies (and the world) know we aren't mad, bad or alone.

Foreword

I n 2011, Rosalie and I set out to write a book about Adult Babies.

Initially, we were unsure about exactly what to write and the scope of the topic. This was because the amount of non-fiction material available about ABs was appallingly small and much of it was of little to no value. Being an adult baby and wearing nappies was considered just a sexual fetish and as someone who has wanted nappies since I was three years old, I knew that to be nonsense. So, we spent a lot of time researching and interviewing other adult babies and we fell upon a definition that we perhaps had known all along. Adult Babies are subjectively *real* babies and toddlers. It is not a sexual fetish but, it is is in fact, a viable *personal identity*. And so the book, *"There's still a baby in my bed!"* was born, not in small part out of personal pain and a desire to help others avoid or mitigate that pain.

We now understand a lot more and accept that the adult baby is a complex, almost incomprehensible person that is both adult and infant, often at the same time. The causes, the structure of this is only just now being slowly revealed. PhD candidates are now looking at the detail of AB life having finally – and long overdue – recognising that it is not a sexual fetish at all, but a genuine regressive identity that both needs – and demands – acceptance.

Our book was never intended to be the final word. Rather, we hoped that others would take up the mantle and continue the task of discovering more about who we are and how we can deal with it. Dylan Lewis is one of the foremost authors and researchers in this field and this latest book is his crowning achievement.

The notion of dissociation is a scary one. It certainly scared me, even though I suspected it to be true from my very early years. I am sure it scares you too, but this brilliantly-crafted book removes the fears and replaces it with facts, understanding and a comprehensive 'aha!' moment of finally putting the pieces into place.

This book is *the* next step in understanding the complexities of the adult baby and opens windows that let light and fresh air into a soul that may be stale and listless because it stands alone and hidden. But we stand alone no longer because we know that who we are and who we can become, is both real and refreshingly healthy.

Dylan Lewis is to be applauded for taking his own experience of being an adult baby and enlightening us all about who we are.

It is okay to be an adult baby. And now we know why.

Michael and Rosalie Bent

1. Introduction

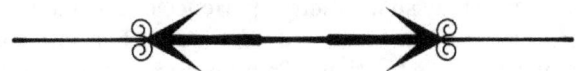

Being an adult baby is a big deal.

It is a mind-blowing, one-in-a-thousand identity.

I am an AB – an Adult Baby. At some point, each of us realizes our psyche is hard-wired differently to everyone else we know.

We are sane, functional adults. Yet we have a compelling need to wear nappies. They comfort something deep inside us. We need to see ourselves in nappies. We want others to see us wearing them (whether we act on that or not). Many of us at least wet them. Many of us fantasize about being babied – cuddled, changed, fed, disciplined etcetera. And that's without all the rest – stuffed toys, pacifiers, baby clothes, bottles etc.

WTF!

It is no wonder coming to terms with being an AB isn't simple.

This is a book for ABs who are ready to understand that nappies are the tip of the psychological iceberg. It is about understanding ourselves so that we can live happily and safely as ABs.

Accepting being AB is a permanent and central part of my psyche and sent me on a journey to understand exactly why that is true. I'm the kind of person who hates not knowing. I can (eventually) handle difficult truths, much better than I can handle not knowing.

I discovered being AB is an identity on the dissociation spectrum. That's the same spectrum as Dissociative Identity Disorder (DID) - which used to be known as Multiple Personality Disorder (MPD).

For some ABs, that information may be unwelcome. I can imagine the internal dialogues – "shit! It's tough enough already accepting or explaining being AB, and you go and dump being crazy on top!"

Hear me out. Forget the movies. Dissociation does *not* equal crazy. There are many high-functioning people with some form of dissociation. It forms a broad spectrum. Everyone on the spectrum has an individual 'footprint' with its own unique experience of self and life. DID is at the further end of the spectrum, and being AB is akin to *next door*. Dissociation is common. It is estimated ten per cent of the population has substantial levels of dissociation. That makes it as common as mood disorders like depression and anxiety. As with ABs, people with dissociation do not disclose and commonly hide amongst us in plain sight.

I believe dissociation is the most valid way of explaining being AB. Let's face it, the hard wiring in our psyche is pretty different and rather deep. You know that because, like most ABs at some time or other, you have tried giving it up. Any valid explanation for being AB is going to have to go pretty deep into the psyche. There is no clear empirical or clinical evidence backing any explanation. We are left to make up our own minds based on our logic, reading and self-reflection. The other explanations for being AB are shallow ('it's a kink') or fall into the category of 'bad or mad' – it's a fetish or a psycho-sexual disorder. Dissociation not only offers a better explanation, it also shows how being AB can be a healthy and stable personal identity.

This book explores 'being AB' as an identity on the dissociation spectrum. It does that through a comparison between being AB and DID. You may be an AB who finds a comparison with DID confronting. That is understandable. I ask you to set aside preconceptions and prejudice about DID – the same way, as ABs, we ask others to set aside their preconceptions and prejudice about us.

The Adult Baby – An Identity on the Dissociation Spectrum

***TRIGGER WARNING**: If you are in the initial stages of understanding your identity, either with DID or being AB, a comparison with another misunderstood minority identity may be over-loading and confronting. You may wish to put this book aside for a later time.*

What is the benefit of the comparison? There is a compelling similarity between the two identities. Both have alternate personalities which powerfully shape their experience of self and life. For ABs, it is our child alters who need nappies and all the rest, to feel recognized, nurtured and safe. For both identities our reality is subjective. It is invisible and incomprehensible to others. There is no way of directly proving the existence of alternative personalities to a doubting person. They are visible only through behaviours which are otherwise inexplicably at odds with the personality we present to the world.

I liken being AB to finding out you are adopted. Adoptees are confronted by the fact they do not share DNA with those around them. That's like ABs realizing our psyches are hard-wired differently than everyone else's. For me, realizing I shared some of my hard-wiring with people with DID was like an adopted person finding their only close living relative. At last, someone who really gets what it's like to live with the subjective reality of an alter which is compelling to me, but incomprehensible to others. Someone who can help me understand the wiring in my psyche. Some people with DID refer to themselves as 'multiples'. ABs often refer to themselves as having a 'Little' and an adult side. We are multiples too – a different kind from people with DID – but still multiples.

The comparison is largely between one AB (myself, Dylan) and one person with DID – Dax, my co-author. Dax is a member of my extended family. He is high functioning, a teacher who taught special needs children around the world. I also read autobiographies, case histories and the published work of four psychiatrists who know DID. Each AB or person with DID is unique. No one individual can be representative, but I hope Dax and myself exemplify some of the key traits and issues for our respective identities.

The book shows what it feels like to live with DID and being AB – when it feels similar and when it feels different. There are compelling similarities between the child alters of ABs and people with DID. It also demonstrates being AB is not DID. There are clear differences. The comparison pinpoints what they are.

Why did I think of this comparison? Let me explain. Until my early fifties, I experienced being AB largely as a conflicted sexual fetish – nothing to do with identity, dissociation or DID. Then Dax visited from overseas and stayed with my wife and myself several times over two years. My wife is a psychotherapist. She suggested that like Dax, I too might have alternative personalities. The thought fell on fertile ground – a few years before I had read Rosalie Bent's ground-breaking book *'There's a Baby In My Bed: Living With the Adult Baby in Your Relationship'*. It viewed being AB as an identity, not a fetish. Therapy confirmed I had child alters. It was an epiphany that revolutionized my understanding of my AB identity. My need to wear nappies, wear baby clothes and all the rest, was not the product of a sexual fetish, but having a subjectively real alternative personality, a very young child.

That discovery caused me to change my view of dissociation. I could be 'messed up' at times, but I am a sane and functional adult. I have a long happy marriage and I am happily retired from a successful career. That didn't fit with the uninformed view of dissociation as crazy and debilitating.

Understanding that ABs are multiples also helps us understand our complicated sexuality. A later chapter shows the unconscious logic behind our sexual needs and compulsions.

This book is a collaboration between Dax and myself. I asked lots of questions about DID, and advanced hypotheses about the similarities and differences between the two identities. Dax sent me lengthy emails explaining his experience of DID and responding to my hypotheses. On this basis, I prepared the text which Dax reviewed. Dax's grasp on DID is insightful and articulate. I believe the most compelling understanding of DID comes where I have quoted directly from his emails.

This is a self-help book. The key audience is ABs and those who love them. It assumes you know a lot about ABs and where you fit on the ABDL spectrum, but know less about dissociation and DID. The book is my best attempt to understand our shared identity. I have no formal qualifications in psychology, but I have a layman's lifelong interest in the subject. Every AB is different, and some will disagree with my views. I do not intend to disparage those whose views are different from mine.

The Adult Baby – An Identity on the Dissociation Spectrum

As adults, we all construct our own identities, based on what we choose to believe about ourselves. Those beliefs can change over time and our identity changes with it. At any point in time, our identity represents what we need to believe to feel safe and okay, with ourselves. In terms of our personal identity, no one has the right to tell us what we should believe about ourselves. So, if after scanning or reading this book, you want to think of being AB as a kink, or a fetish, and/or being AB has nothing to do with subjectively real alters or childhood trauma, that's okay. That's you, defining you. This book is about offering people information based on my best honest understanding, and giving them a choice about what they believe. Take what is helpful from the book and leave the rest behind.

The other intended audience is mental health professionals, who I hope will be prompted to think more deeply about the AB identity. The health professions' present ways of understanding 'being AB' are just labels that explain little or nothing. How can the obvious pointers to fundamental issues in AB's early childhood be ignored? How can being AB be thought of as just a paraphilia or sexual fetish? Sure, it is often a fetish as part of its expression. That's a symptom, not the cause. It doesn't explain why ABs seek and derive emotional comfort from their nappies and fantasies of infancy. How long can the involuntary character of many AB behaviours (triggering etc) - so at odds with the AB's adult personality - be viewed simply as a compulsion or addiction? These symptoms require dissociation and repressed childhood trauma be included in any competent differential diagnosis.

This book is based on the pioneering work of Rosalie Bent and Michael Bent in identifying and understanding ABs as a personal identity. I recommend their books and website *abdiscovery.com.au* . I refer to their insights throughout the book.

By adult baby, I exclude role players and diaper lovers for whom diapers, baby clothes or baby activities are an optional extra they can freely live without, and pure fetishists for whom these things are confined exclusively to sexual expression.

This book follows my *'The Adult Baby Identity'* trilogy – *'Coming Out as an Adult Baby'*, *'Healing Childhood Wounds'*, and *'A Self Help Guide'*.

The journey of self-discovery is not an easy one to undertake alone. You need a confidant who you can trust, and who will be an ally in your healing. If there is no one in your life with whom you can safely share your feelings about your life as an adult baby, seek professional support – preferably from an LGBTQ-friendly therapist who understands dissociation and personal identity. If you are in crisis or deep distress about being an adult baby seek professional therapy.

2. Preview

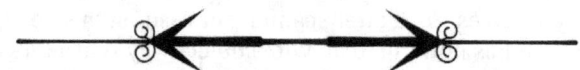

There were times when researching this book was a revelation for me. I was very surprised to see the similarity between the child selves of AB's, their 'Littles', and the child alters of people with DID.

Below are two accounts of a 'Little' or child alter written by the person's partner. See if you can pick the one that belongs to an AB, and the one that belongs to a person with DID. I have edited out identifying text but otherwise, the accounts are quoted verbatim.

Account 1

[Chrissy's husband says] "Chrissy [was] so excited to be out and about with me, seeing all of these wonderful new sights. … We had barely walked half a block when Chrissy yanks me into a charming shop with a variety of handmade wooden toys, puzzles and dolls. Chrissy is quietly sharing with me her delight and excitement of this wonderful world of toys. … With much exuberance, she pulls me up the stairs to a wall loaded floor to ceiling with stuffed bears. … Pink bears, green bears, and rainbow bears. The pleasure Chrissy feels in seeing the princess and ballerina bears light up her sparkling eyes. … no one pays much attention until I push a button hidden in the first dancing bear's paw. The music starts and the graceful bear spins around and around. Before I can comprehend the implications of this one bear, Chrissy waltzes her way to five more paw-activated bears. Now they're all singing, laughing and talking while Chrissy cries out in joy and claps her hands. Soon even more of these once-cute but now loud and obnoxious bears are gyrating and convulsing, with Chrissy laughing all the way.

I soon feel that the situation is out of my control. I glance down the stairs and notice the shop owner scowling up at me. … I don't want Chrissy to sense my discomfort. She is truly just experiencing what any child would the very first time in a toy store or even on Christmas Day. You wouldn't want to stifle a child then, but I am feeling anxious.

Sadly, I am unable to prevent Chrissy from noticing my discomfort, and what began as a splendid adventure of wonder turns into her feeling confused and ashamed. … She sheds many tears while apologizing for embarrassing me. I hold her tight, trying to reassure her that she didn't embarrass me, the situation did."

Account 2

[Joanne's wife and mother says] "Joanne was happy and content and her needs were being well met. Then one overnight there was a storm. My little three-year-old is terrified of wind and storms at night and so we had night-time tears, fear and when morning came, there was just a scared little infant in bed and the adult was as far away as he has ever been. Joanne was thoroughly and irredeemable regressed and she would not and could not grow up. We had plans for that day. Adult plans. They were cancelled as there was no adult there – just an infant behaving at her youngest age level of 12 months old.

It was a difficult day. It was difficult to communicate with her beyond limited baby talk or gestures. By evening she was communicating better but the following morning there she was again, very little and quite regressed. I felt like we were still back in the nursery level.

It took two full days for her to really return back to her place of balance and peace and I am reminded again that just as in the parenting of physical children, you can do all the right things and still get bad things happen. Joanne is normally a delightful and happy child and it is an exciting and happy time for her and for me. But those two days were difficult for us both because for at least one of those days, we had lost control."

Account 1 is from Christine Pattillo's autobiography *'I Am We: My Life With Multiple Personalities'*, and is narrated by her husband who is the father of six-year-old alter Chrissy.

Account 2 is from Rosalie Bent's on-line blog (cited in the references). She is the wife of her AB husband, and mother to his 'Little', baby Joanne.

You may have picked correctly, you may not. But I think the similarity in the character of the two accounts is compelling. The similarity is not a one-off. I chose these two out of a larger sample cited in Chapter 9. Compare Rosalie Bent's account with another description of a similar night-time incident by Christine Pattillo.

> *"Well, last night there was a small windstorm in our neighbourhood … We were all snoozing soundly when a power transformer, less than a mile away, shorted out. The sound was like a gunshot and startled Chrissy, even though she was asleep inside Cita's [Christine Pattillo] mind. Chrissy's fear was so acute she burst into tears and shifted right out, waking Christopher. Christopher immediately began to comfort her and calm her down."*

The similarity represents the two closest points in the experience of DID and AB. Christine Pattillo's account of her DID is unusual in the warmth and openness with which she and her family have embraced her child alters. Rosalie Bent's husband is a regressive AB. The latter term is one used by Rosalie to describe ABs who have a powerful need to express their 'Little'.

Many people with these two identities would not have this degree of commonality in their experience and expression of self. But even where the overlap is not so strong, I believe it is still there. The rest of this book is about exploring the origin and nature of that commonality.

Rosalie and Michael Bent are the foremost public authorities on the adult baby identity. Rosalie is the wife of Michael, an adult baby. In 2012 Rosalie published the landmark book 'There's A Baby in My Bed' intended for the partners of adult babies. It was the first published work to seriously address adult babies as a personal identity, beyond a sexual fetish. It was updated in 2015 as 'There's Still A Baby in My Bed. Rosalie has also written a book for the parents of teenage adult babies. Michael has published a text 'Adult Babies: Psychology and Practices' and an anthology of insightful articles 'Being An Adult Baby'. Rosalie and Michael are the owners of the website abdiscovery.com.au which is dedicated to helping adult babies understand themselves, and fostering public understanding of the identity.

3. Dissociation

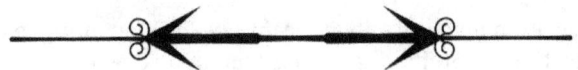

I believe dissociation is key to understanding ABs.

To help guide an understanding of dissociation, this book references the published writing of four psychiatrists.

Marlene Steinberg is an American who developed a key diagnostic questionnaire for dissociative conditions, the *Structured Clinical Interview for Clinical Disorders* (SCID-D), sometimes cited as the gold standard for such identification. Her excellent 2010 book *'The Stranger in the Mirror: the Hidden Epidemic'* demystifies dissociation and DID. Contrary to the prevailing wisdom she focused on dissociation from the beginning of her career in the early 1990s.

David Yeung is a Canadian who retired in 2006 after a forty-year career. He worked with about one hundred DID clients in the latter half of his career. He was concerned at the scarcity of mental health professionals willing and able to work with DID clients. After retirement, he wrote a set of case studies and therapeutic guidelines for mental health professionals *('Engaging Multiple Personalities' Volumes 1 and 2)*. His approach is notably empathic and client-centred.

Colin A. Ross (b. 1950) is another Canadian. He is a widely published authority on trauma and dissociation, and the author of a key textbook on DID, *'Dissociative Identity Disorder: Diagnosis, Clinical Features, and Treatment of Multiple Personality'*. He developed another key diagnostic questionnaire for dissociative disorders, the *Dissociative Disorders Interview Schedule* (DDIS). His grounded approach emphasizes working with the internal logic of DID. He has powerful insight but understates the subjective reality of alters. I draw most on his recent (2018) book *'Treatment of Dissociative Identity Disorder: Techniques and Strategies for Stabilisation'*.

Jeffrey Smith is an American. He was the therapist of Robert Oxnam, one of the most high-profile people who have 'come out' with DID. The latter is known for his 2013 autobiography *'A Fractured Mind: My Life With Multiple Personality Disorder'*. Dr Smith does not claim to be an authority on DID/MPD. However, his epilogue to the above autobiography, *'Understanding DID Therapy: The Case of Robert B. Oxnam by Jeffrey Smith MD'*, is outstanding for its insight and clarity.

What is Dissociation?

In essence, dissociation means detachment or disconnection - detachment from external factors (others, the environment), or detachment from the self, or both. Dr Colin Ross states –

> *"Dissociation basically means disconnection. A person can be disconnected from thoughts, feelings, memories, sensations or any aspect of the mind and body."*

Dissociation is a common and functional coping mechanism for dealing with a range of situations. It can be voluntary, such as when there is a compelling need for intense single-minded focus, or involuntary, such as in a car accident or a heart attack.

Dr Yeung gives an example of a common, functional example of dissociation –

> *"Dissociation is not always pathological. For example, a surgeon in the midst of a nasty divorce must remain able to concentrate in the operating room. The act of separating the ordinary stream of divorce-related thoughts from the task of surgery at hand requires effective dissociation." [Engaging Multiple Personalities (Volume 1): Contextual Case Histories.]*

Colin Ross comments:

> *"... every woman who has given birth has been in an extreme dissociative state."*

In sudden trauma, dissociation involuntarily quarantines incapacitating fear or pain in one part of the psyche so we can continue to function. Dr Steinberg defines traumatic dissociation as -

> *"...an adaptive defence in response to high stress or trauma characterized by memory loss and a sense of disconnection from oneself or one's surroundings". ... To help us survive, certain perceptions, feelings, sensations, thoughts, and memories related to the trauma are split off from full awareness and encoded in some peripheral level of awareness. Miraculously, dissociation alters reality, but allows the person to stay in contact with it in order to help himself." [The Stranger in the Mirror: Dissociation The Hidden Epidemic]*

There are many misconceptions about dissociation. I discovered it –

1. is a broad spectrum ranging from mild forms through to clinical conditions;
2. is a lot more common than people think;
3. need not prevent a person from being functional and successful;
4. has five components which may be present in differing combinations and strengths depending on the individual, so everyone with dissociation has their own unique 'footprint'.

Let's look at each of these.

Spectrum

The spectrum ranges from -

- mild dissociation which can take such forms as an intense single-minded focus, or 'zoning out' from disturbing or confronting situations;
- sub-clinical dissociation which involves altered states of consciousness, which may have a significant effect on a person's experience of self and life, but does not trigger medical intervention; and
- clinical conditions which trigger medical intervention and include separate streams of consciousness, identity and/or self. These can include a sense the self or the world is unreal (depersonalization and derealization), fragmentation of identity, such as DID, or complex post-traumatic stress disorder.

More Common Than You Think

The Wikipedia article 'Dissociation (psychology) states –

> *"... in the normal population, dissociative experiences that are not clinically significant are highly prevalent with 60% to 65% of the respondents indicating that they have had some dissociative experiences."*

A recent meta-analysis of around one hundred other studies indicated around 10 per cent of the population would meet the criteria for a dissociative disorder (see *'The prevalence of Dissociative Disorders and dissociative experiences in college'* by Mary-Anne Kate in the references). Dr Steinberg's 2010 book cites a survey which estimates that 14 per cent of the US population experiences *substantial* dissociative symptoms. These figures indicate the prevalence of dissociative conditions is on a par with the better known and accepted mood disorders such as depression and anxiety.

DID, the most extreme form of dissociation, used to be thought of as very rare. That's no longer thought to be true. Within the broader population with substantial dissociation symptoms, Dr Steinberg estimates up to one per cent of the population may have DID. Wikipedia, in the article on DID, cites a figure of two per cent. The International Society for the Study of Trauma and Dissociation's (ISSTD) 2010 Guidelines for Treating Dissociative Identity Disorder in Adults cite estimates that one to three per cent of the population have DID.

Doesn't Stop People Being Successful

There are many high functioning people with dissociative conditions. Dr Steinberg states that they –

> *"… run the gamut from PhDs to prostitutes and are generally highly intelligent, creative, brave, articulate and likeable. Many are accomplished professionals, married, raising children, holding down responsible jobs."*

People with DID work successfully in many walks of life. Dr Yeung states –

> *"Without conscious effort, many DID persons utilize their dissociative abilities to enhance their work. Teachers with DID can be exceptionally perceptive and sensitive to their students' difficulties because their young alters easily attune to their students' needs. Similarly, a therapist with alters can be readily attuned to their patients in therapeutic work."*

Amongst the autobiographies of people with DID I read, one person was a high powered US Department of Justice lawyer (Olga Trujillo), another a prominent international academic (Robert Oxam), and another a very high profile sportsperson in the US NFL (Herschel Walker).

Because of fear of being thought crazy people with dissociative conditions commonly do not disclose. Friends, colleagues and acquaintances are mostly not aware the person has a dissociative condition. Given the prevalence indicated above, it is very likely one or more of the people you interact with on a weekly basis have, or have had, substantial dissociative symptoms (in the same way you interact with people who have depression or anxiety).

Components

Dr Steinberg identifies five components of dissociation. These are -

1. Amnesia – gaps in memory or 'lost time';
2. Depersonalisation – a feeling of detachment from your emotions or your body, or looking at yourself as an outsider would;
3. Derealization – a feeling of detachment from your environment, such as feeling the environment or other people aren't real, or familiar people are Strangers;
4. Identity confusion – a feeling of uncertainty, puzzlement or conflict about who you are - perhaps a continuing struggle going on inside you to define yourself; and
5. Identity alteration – a shift in role or identity, accompanied by such changes in your behaviour that are observable to others – you may experience the shift as a personality switch or loss of control over yourself to someone else inside you.

Each individual on the dissociation spectrum has a different 'footprint'. They may have all five components or only some, and in different strengths. Each different 'footprint' produces a unique experience of self and life. Your footprint is *your* footprint. Accepting that you are on the dissociation spectrum doesn't mean your experience has to conform to anyone else's.

Identity Alteration

It is the fifth component - *identity alteration* - which is most important to understanding DID and being AB. People with identity alteration have one or more subjectively real personas, distinct from the host-birth personality. The depth of those personas can vary. With moderate levels of identity alteration, the personas maybe only two dimensional, feeling states – barely personas. With stronger levels of identity alteration, the personas have a repertoire of thoughts, emotions, capabilities, and needs that represent a fully formed alternative personality.

Dr Steinberg states -

> *" ... research has found that identity alteration, as with all the dissociative symptoms, occurs along a spectrum of intensity: mild levels in the general population; mild to moderate levels in people with nondissociative psychiatric disorders, but also with people with dissociative disorder not otherwise specified (DDNOS); severe levels of identity alteration in people with dissociative identity disorder (DID).*

A person with moderate levels of identity alteration may act as if he or she is like two (or more) different people, but it's not clear whether these identity alterations assume complete control of a person's behaviour or represent separate personalities. ...

Severe identity alteration, the *sina qua non* of DID, involves a person's shifting between distinct personality states that take control of his or her behaviour and thought. These alter personalities are more clearly defined and distinctive than the personality fragments that characterize moderate levels of identity alteration. Each alter has its own name, memories, traits and behaviour patterns.

Identity alteration differs from identity confusion in that identity confusion represents the internal dimension of identity disturbance, whereas identity alteration represents the external dimension. A person with identity confusion, in other words, has thoughts and feelings of uncertainty and conflict related to his or her identity; a person with identity alteration manifests the uncertainty and conflict **behaviourally**.

Trauma and Splitting

Alternative personalities emerged as the psyche's response to trauma, typically in early childhood. To understand that phenomena we need to recognize trauma can have deep and lasting effects on the psyche.

Dr Ross describes the nature of trauma –

> *"The impacts of trauma on a person can be profound, and multiple. Trauma could affect a person in terms of the cognitive, behavioural, emotional, interpersonal and even physiological aspects of self. Why?*
>
> *Trauma may make a person feel like the world is dangerous and unpredictable.*
>
> *Trauma may make a person think that no one can be trusted.*
>
> *Trauma may make a person believe that he/she is not loveable.*
>
> *Trauma may make a person feel very angry, depressed or frightened.*
>
> *Trauma may make a person try hard to avoid any similar situations and anything that could remind him/her of the traumatic event.*
>
> *Trauma could profoundly affect one's body (eg. Amygdala, hippocampus, autonomic nervous system). After trauma, a person may become very sensitive and hyperaroused; his or her*

stress response systems are also affected, and he/she may have difficulty in relaxing or getting to sleep.

Trauma leaves a person with unprocessed memories and unaddressed emotions, which may become nightmares or lead to flashbacks." [Be a Teammate with Yourself: Understanding Trauma and Dissociation]

Trauma is a challenge for someone at any age. But it is particularly challenging for a child who's psyche is still dependent on the care and support of others. Trauma can be caused by abuse. It can also be caused by more mundane events - the 'ordinary catastrophes' of childhood such as accidents, temporary separations from caregivers, or bullying. It can happen in any situation where a child experiences great distress or fear, and feels themselves to be physically alone, or feels unprotected by those to whom they might look to for protection.

In the face of overwhelming fear and distress, a child's psyche may 'split off' a distinct alter. This is a sub-conscious process. Dr Steinberg indicates the younger the child, the more susceptible they are to 'splitting'.

Dr Jeffrey Smith describes the process of traumatic 'splitting' -

Multiple personality begins with dissociation. When we note that adult victims of disaster seem to be in 'a daze', we are referring to dissociation. There is the dissociation of feeling from fact. Trauma survivors will often remember the moment they dissociated. For example, a child who was molested, focused on a spot on the ceiling. Soon she began to experience herself looking down dispassionately from the ceiling as if the girl below were someone else.

Where there is complete amnesia, the dissociation is more extensive, involving memory as well as feeling. ... what makes a particular trauma severe enough to trigger loss of memory? The first and foremost factor, in my view, is aloneness, the lack of a safe person to share the event. The need for human connection, especially in times of stress, begins very early in life. A six-year-old girl in the process of being abused by her drunken step-father was able to keep from being overwhelmed by hoping that her mother would soon return. When her mother did come back, the girl quickly realized that her mother was no more able to stand up to her abuser than she was. Suddenly aware that her hope was illusory ... she ran out of the house into the night. Years later, the only thing she remembered was the image of headlights shining in her eyes. Aloneness makes traumatic events much more damaging, and dissociation much more likely. [A Fractured Mind: My Life With Multiple Personality Disorder – Epilogue]

Splitting quarantines incapacitating fear and pain so the rest of the psyche can continue to function. It can also preserve attributes or capabilities that might otherwise be damaged or lost due to the trauma. Dr Smith states –

"... when events overwhelm emotional defences, the damage is less when it can be encapsulated in dissociation. Trauma survivors who are not able to dissociate often sustain greater damage than those who are able to split. The harm to self-esteem and to the sense of safety affects their entire being. By contrast, multiples often have parts that are entirely spared the effects of trauma. There may be joyful, innocent children existing side by side with those personalities that have been most damaged."

Dr Yeung describes this response to trauma as the psyche's 'self-triage'. Splitting can occur multiple times as dissociation becomes the pattern for responses to trauma.

Repression and Denial

In cases of traumatic dissociation in adults, the memory of the traumatic event is commonly either never lost, or returns shortly afterwards. Dissociation linked to childhood trauma is different. It often has lasting effects on the psyche, effects which persist into adulthood. Yet despite those effects, the memory or full experience of the trauma may be hidden in the unconscious for many years and decades.

Both the original trauma and the resulting alter are initially buried in the sub-conscious in what is called repression. When the alter and memories are repressed we genuinely don't know they are there. It is amnesia.

Repression is key to understanding dissociation.

Based on my personal experience, I think of repression as a high wall. It was erected quickly in an emergency. It was not so much built, as 'thrown up', using whatever materials and labour were at hand. In places, the wall is made of big concrete blocks, well-mortared and on deep foundations, and will never come down. In other places, the wall is just house bricks, sometimes poorly mortared and without a solid footing beneath. In those places, the mortar ages and crumbles and eventually the bricks tumble down, leaving gaps in the wall.

The memories of trauma, and trauma-related experiences, such as the splitting of alters, are not only buried in the unconscious, they are stored in a way that makes their retrieval complex and uncertain. They are not stored as useable, accessible memories (explicit memory). Dr Smith explains the difference between explicit and implicit memory -

> *"Explicit memory is processed for storage in a structure [in the brain] known as the hippocampus, while implicit memory is more diffusely spread out in the brain. Simply stated, **explicit** refers to that which is in the foreground of our consciousness and accessible to language, while **implicit** refers to the background, or context, and is nonverbal."*

Dr Steinberg indicates that –

> *"the amygdala shapes and stores traumatic memories in the limbic part of the brain, which processes emotions and sensations, but not language or speech. As a result, survivors of childhood abuse may carry implicit physiological memories of the terror, pain, and sadness generated by the abuse but may have few or no explicit factual memories to explain their flashbacks and the feelings and sensations they arouse. They live with the repercussions of the event without having a narrative – this is what happened at this time or place – to provide a back story. Memories of traumatic experiences are not retrieved so much as they intrude. They pop up in jagged impressionistic fragments overloaded with sensations and emotions that can distort the details."*

This pattern of memory is applicable to any repressed trauma, not just abuse.

Over time repression breaks down - fragments of memory return. The buried, split off alter 'breaks through' and influences a person's thoughts, feelings, perceptions and behaviours, even when the source of that influence is unrecognized. Repression can start breaking down early. For example, ABs commonly start acting on their desire for nappies around age ten, or sometimes even earlier. That desire is compelling, but incomprehensible because it represents the first breakthrough of repressed unconscious needs.

After that has been happening for a while, repression can start to shade into denial. Unlike repression, denial is a product of the conscious mind. Therapist Lyn Mary Karjala explains -

> *"It [denial] happens when there's some aspect of the external world that's simply too painful for us to face, so we can't allow ourselves to see it. The classic example is the alcoholic who admits that he drinks but vehemently denies that he has a drinking problem, in spite of the mounting evidence that's increasingly apparent to people around him. He's not knowingly lying when he says he doesn't have a problem – he's genuinely unaware of it. In other words, he's kept the knowledge of his behaviour in his conscious awareness – he knows that he drinks – but he's dissociated the significance and the danger of the behaviour." ['Understanding Trauma and Dissociation: A Guide for Patients and Loved Ones']*

The Adult Baby – An Identity on the Dissociation Spectrum

For this book, the reader might replace the reference to an alcoholic and drinking with an AB and their compulsive need for nappies. We might imagine hearing an AB say, *"its just a kink or fetish, nothing to do with deep issues in my psyche and my childhood ... "*

Dr Steinberg states –

" ... people suffering from a dissociative disorder often have a huge amount of denial. ... Their worst fear is that if they talk about their symptoms to a therapist, they'll immediately be labelled as a freak or a crazy person.

Very often, people who have separate parts of themselves keep them hidden, because they don't think of them as well-defined personalities, but more as 'aspects' of their own personalities or different internal voices or puzzling 'sides' of themselves with which they are not in touch with all the time."

"One of the trickier aspects of dissociation is that the more chronic some symptoms are, the less stress they may cause because you've adapted to them and they have become as normal to you as breathing."

As a result of repression and then denial, it can take decades for the unconscious to release its' secrets. I mean decades! To change analogies, the way repression releases its grip on memory is like the front of a glacier where it meets the sea. Mostly it just melts, releasing the meltwater so slowly that it's imperceptible. But at other times, great blocks of ice will crack and fall off the glacier and crash into the sea throwing up a shower of spray. Then we will have blocks of memory suddenly return. Even years after self-acceptance and therapy, the unconscious continues to release new insights and memories.

Only those who have lived long enough to see the unconscious repression in their own early life break down and be revealed, understand its power. Trying to explain that to others, especially those in the first half of life, can be a bit like trying to explain colour to the colour-blind. Recognizing the power your unconscious has had over your life is confronting. It humbles our pride that we are the ones in conscious control. The first decades of adolescence and adulthood are about establishing that control. It is not a time of life well suited to recognize some of that hard-won control is illusory.

Dissociation Becomes Dysfunctional

We have seen that dissociation is functional when a child is faced with overwhelming trauma. It quarantines fear, hurt or pain within one part of the child's psyche so they can continue to function after the trauma. It protects resilience. Dissociation is a creative, subjective denial of objective reality.

However, continued reliance on dissociation when we are adolescents and adults can become dysfunctional. Denying objective reality becomes a two-edged sword. Some denial might not cause too much harm. But denying objective reality too much, or the parts of it that we need to heed to be safe and functional becomes dysfunctional and harmful. It reduces our resilience and makes us more psychologically vulnerable. That is what happens for people with severe uncontrolled DID.

If you have dissociated trauma in your childhood, the problem is that you don't pick and choose rationally when to use dissociative coping strategies as an adult. Those choices are being made in your sub-conscious and driven by the unhealed childhood trauma. And coming from that fearful and hurt place some of the choices will be bad ones. That's why it's important to identify and heal childhood trauma. Only that allows a person to make conscious and rational choices about how they cope with the difficulties they encounter.

The Adult Baby – An Identity on the Dissociation Spectrum

Now that we are armed with a greater understanding of dissociation we can revisit the dissociation spectrum with greater precision. Dr Ross states –

> *"The spectrum of dissociation is often portrayed as: no symptoms at the left-hand end – symptoms but no diagnosable disorder – dissociative amnesia – depersonalization/derealization disorder – other specified dissociative disorder (OSDD) – DID at the right-hand end." [Treatment of Dissociative Identity Disorder: Techniques and Strategies for Stabilisation"]*

ABs who are confronted by the idea they are on the dissociation spectrum might find it easier to think of it as an 'inner child spectrum'. Dr Ross continues -

> *"... a good conceptual framework for the spectrum of dissociation is the inner child spectrum. The inner child is therapeutic lingo for unresolved feelings from childhood. The only question is: are these just feelings, or are they contained in an inner structure that has some degree of separateness from the adult self?*
>
> *The inner child spectrum goes: no inner child – a metaphorical inner child – a sense of an inner child – a definite knowledge that there is an inner child inside – the inner child is visualized internally – the person and hear and talks to the inner child (DID)."*

For ABs, the inner child is at the DID end of the spectrum. We may not hear the voice of the child in our heads, but their infantile needs result in persistent behaviours like wearing nappies, using pacifiers and baby clothing.

Summary

Dissociation means detachment from the self, or from the external environment, or both. Dissociation falls on a broad spectrum, ranging from common every-day, voluntary mental states through to involuntary, clinical conditions. Dissociation has five components. Every person on the dissociation spectrum has a different footprint, a unique combination of some or all of the five components, and in differing strengths. Each individual dissociation footprint produces a unique view of self and life.

Identity alteration, having distinct personalities or alters within the psyche, is one of the five components of dissociation. It comes from childhood trauma, where in response to overwhelming fear or pain, the psyche splits off an alter. That alter serves to quarantine the fear or pain to allow the rest of the psyche to function. It can also preserve attributes and capabilities within the psyche which would otherwise be damaged or lost. The memory of traumatic childhood dissociation is buried in the unconscious is what is called repression.

4. Dissociative Identity Disorder (DID) and being an Adult Baby (AB)

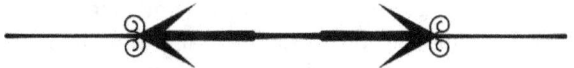

This chapter looks at DID and being AB and their respective places on the dissociation spectrum.

Concepts

To understand people with alternative personalities we need to use some concepts from DID.

A person who has an undivided, unitary psyche is called a 'singleton'. Anyone who has at least one alternative personality is called a 'multiple'. I use the term psyche to describe the whole person, whether a singleton or a multiple. When I use the term psyche for a multiple, it refers to all their parts (people with DID often use the term 'the system'). The 'host' is the personality who is out front most of the time. The host may, or may not be, the original personality from whom all the others sprang, directly or indirectly – the latter is the 'birth personality'. Each personality is called an 'alter', short for alternative personality (people with DID sometimes use the term 'parts').

For people with DID who's psyche is fragmented by amnesia, the total stock of memory is compartmentalized within different personalities. If fragmentation is reduced and personalities share memories, they are 'co-conscious'. A personality may be co-conscious with one or more other personalities, but not necessarily all.

The personality who is in executive control of the person's body is 'out', and others are 'in' (meaning inside). When the personality in executive control of the body changes, that is referred to as 'switching'. If the two personalities involved in the change are not co-conscious, switching can be very abrupt. If the two personalities involved are co-conscious, the change may be smoother and is termed 'shifting'. If more than one co-conscious personality simultaneously shares executive control of the body, they are referred to as being 'co-present'. (*Shifting* and *co-present* are terms which seem have originated with psychiatrist Colin Ross).

What is DID?

People with DID have multiple alters, who have distinct characters which may be similar or different to the host personality. Alters can be adults or children. In a fragmented state, the alter in control of the person's consciousness – their perceptions, thoughts, feelings and actions – can switch unpredictably. Switching can be triggered by a range of factors, for example, stress, anxiety, a set of terms or raised voices. Also in a fragmented state, these alters do not share memories, so the person can find clothes in their wardrobe they don't remember buying or wake up with injuries they don't remember sustaining. The common origin of DID is severe, repeated abuse in childhood.

The experience of each person with DID is unique. Behaviours linked to DID typically manifested early in life, commonly in adolescence. Some people are diagnosed and accept their identity in adolescence. Others are not diagnosed until mid-life, and before that developed coping mechanisms to navigate life while hiding their identity. A parallel is the way in which adults who are illiterate have developed effective and subtle ways to conceal the fact. Unless they are in acute distress, many people with DID go about their lives without acquaintances, colleagues or even friends being any the wiser. There are people with DID in many walks of life.

The goal of treatment of DID is to reduce the extent of fragmentation of the psyche. The success of treatment varies depending on the individual and the severity of the childhood trauma. At its best, the fragmentation can be healed or greatly reduced.

What about being AB?

Like DID, the experience of every AB is unique. It covers a large range. Some identify as diaper lovers (DLs) who wear diapers/nappies but do not acknowledge any other attraction to the trappings of infancy or early childhood. Adult babies are attracted to nappies, and to the trappings and fantasies of infancy – with a repertoire of baby clothes, stuffed toys, pacifiers, bottles etc, that varies with each individual. ABs often refer to their baby or child side as their 'Little' and to inhabiting their baby side as 'little space'. For either DLs or ABs, the attraction can be exclusively sexual, exclusively for emotional comfort without a sexual dimension, or a combination of both.

The attraction to nappies commonly first manifests at an early age, even before adolescence. There is a strong involuntary dimension to the attraction. It is a deep need. Attempts to suppress it for any period commonly result in the involuntary triggering of an urgent and compelling need to put on a nappy.   Attempts at suppression also create a 'binge and purge' cycle with sharp, tumultuous and involuntary shifts in mood and behaviour. Conflicted ABs are typically adept at disguising these attractions and behaviours, even from those closest to them. The behaviours and fantasies are commonly incomprehensibly at odds with the adolescent or adult personality of the AB, and a source of deep shame and confusion that seeps into many aspects of the AB's life.

Some DLs and ABs come to terms and accept this side of their personality in adolescence (particularly after the advent of the internet and social media age). Many, especially those who grew up in an earlier age, remain deeply conflicted well into mid-life. There is often a high level of denial amongst ABDLs – of the amount of space their 'Little' occupies in their psyche, its' origins and its' implications.

DID on the Dissociation Spectrum

DID is the most extreme form of dissociation.

Dr Steinberg indicates people with DID typically have all five components of dissociation, and to a high degree. Amnesia, not just for past trauma, but for the activities of different alters in the present, is a defining characteristic of DID.

The DSM-5 is the current version of the Diagnostic and Statistical Manual of Mental Disorders - the standard diagnostic tool published by the American Psychiatric Association (APA). It states the following criteria must be met for an individual to be diagnosed with DID:

1. The individual experiences two or more distinct identities or personality states (each with its own enduring pattern of perceiving, relating to, and thinking about the environment and self). Some cultures describe this as an experience of possession.
2. The disruption in identity involves a change in sense of self, sense of agency, and changes in behaviour, consciousness, memory, perception, cognition, and motor function.
3. Frequent gaps are found in the individual's memories of personal history, including people, places, and events, for both the distant and recent past. These recurrent gaps are not consistent with ordinary forgetting.

The symptoms cause clinically significant distress or impairment in social, occupational, or other important areas of functioning.

The differential diagnosis for DID excludes symptoms directly caused by other medical conditions (ie. seizures) or substances (ie. a drug of abuse or medication).

Essentially, the DSM-5 definition says DID is a combination of identity alteration and amnesia. For the purposes of the DSM-5 definition, these two components also subsume the other three identified by Dr Steinberg (identity confusion, de-personalisation and de-realization).

Dr Smith makes clear the link between identity alteration and amnesia –

"The term 'multiple personality' does refer to the most striking feature of the disorder, but it also misplaces the emphasis. The key to making sense of dissociative identity disorder is to look not at the personalities but at the memory barriers between them. We could describe a house in two ways, either as a collection of rooms or as a collection of walls. Both are true, but one cannot construct a house out of rooms. Only walls can be constructed, and rooms are the result. When we first confront multiple personality, we see dramatically different personalities before our eyes. We see rooms, and it is easy to forget that their existence is really a consequence of there being walls – that is, dissociative memory barriers resulting from trauma. As memory barriers become fixed and are maintained over time, the personalities on opposite sides develop separate histories, values, allegiances, possessions and relationships. ... A consequence of the development of memory barriers is the development of sharply different personalities that diversify even more over time and are capable of vying for control over the body they inhabit."

Even with DID, denial is common. The ISSTD's 2010 Guidelines states -

"Clinicians should bear in mind that some persons with DID do not realize (or do not acknowledge to themselves) that their internal experience is different from that of others. In keeping with the view that dissociation may serve as a defense against uncomfortable realities, the presence of alternate identities and other dissociative symptoms is commonly denied and disavowed by persons with DID. This kind of denial is consistent with the defensive function of disavowing both the trauma and its related emotions and the subsequent dissociated sense of self."

Overlap Between DID and AB

The DSM-5 criteria let us see clearly the relationship between DID and being AB. There is a strong overlap. A conflicted AB matches three of the four DSM-5 criteria for DID.

ABs fit the first DSM-5 criterion for DID - *"two or more distinct identities or personality states (each with its own enduring pattern of perceiving, relating to, and thinking about the environment and self)".*

ABs fit the second DSM-5 criterion, notably the change in behaviour – *"The disruption in identity involves a change in sense of self, sense of agency, and changes in behaviour, consciousness, memory, perception, cognition, and motor function."*

ABs do **not** fit the third DSM-5 criterion – *"Frequent gaps are found in the individual's memories of personal history, including people, places, and events, for both the distant and recent past."*

Conflicted ABs *can* fit the fourth DSM-5 criterion – *"The symptoms cause clinically significant distress or impairment in social, occupational, or other important areas of functioning."*

We need to look further at the four criteria.

Conflicted DLs and AB's may consider they don't have a distinct child alter – it's just a 'side' of their otherwise adult personality. That may be true. In an earlier quotation, Dr Steinberg refers to moderate levels of identity alteration involving 'personality fragments' rather than distinct personality states with persistent traits and behaviours.

Conversely, for many ABs, I suspect the non-acceptance of a child alter represents unconscious repression, conscious denial, or the early stage of coming to terms with their confronting identity. For people with DID or ABs, often the personality of alters doesn't emerge from the sub-conscious until after self-acceptance (refer to Chapters 8 and 10 on alters). Before that, the alters influence behaviour, but largely from the sub-conscious. There are parallels with other minority identities where people don't accept their non-conforming sense of self until mid-life. That can happen even where they have kept secret over a long time, behaviours and thoughts which pointed towards that non-conforming sense of self.

Behaviour may be a more objective indicator of whether an AB fits the first two DSM-5 criteria for DID (an alternate personality, manifested behaviourally). For ABs, the extent of persistent involuntary behaviour commonly includes –

- a frequent irresistible compulsion to wear nappies - often triggered involuntarily;
- a deep need for non-sexual emotional comfort from nappies, pacifiers, bottles or the like;
- strong behavioural and mood swings linked to the 'binge and purge' cycle;
- a rich fantasy life deriving emotional comfort from identifying as a helpless or dependent baby, and being babied by caregivers and substitute parents.

We need to focus further on the 'binge and purge' cycle because it is the clearest indication of identity alteration for ABs. The phrase comes from the disease bulimia where the sufferer gorges on food and then, in deep self-disgust and loathing, makes themselves sick until they purge their stomachs empty. For adult babies, it means something different. It means bingeing on a new or extra stock of nappies and often other baby clothes and paraphernalia. Sometimes the binge is downloading digital AB erotic fiction.

The binge prompts recurring bouts of increasingly compulsive masturbation, perhaps fueled by psychologically unhealthy, masochistic AB fantasies. Like the bulimic, the binge causes initial euphoria and then deep self-loathing, which in turn results in a compulsive purge. The AB disposes of their entire stock of nappies and other AB supplies and vows to give up being AB forever. They may delete the digital copies of AB erotic fiction. There is an initial euphoria at being 'cleansed' of something bad. But after an interval, the AB's unmet needs for the comfort of nappies and baby fantasies kicks off another binge and the cycle reboots. The cycle is emotionally wrenching and exhausting.

Both the binge and purge are involuntary. Having been through the cycle before, the AB's adult self is fully aware, but their executive control of decision making and physical action is over-ridden. In the *binge*, the over-ride is by a part of the psyche that is desperate for the comfort of nappies. In the *purge*, the over-ride is by an opposing part of the psyche that is terrified and repelled by these infantile needs and behaviours.

The binge and purge cycle and other involuntary AB behaviours fit Dr Steinberg's definition of "severe identity alteration, … [which] involves a person's shifting between distinct personality states that take control of his or her behaviour and thought." That suggests a distinct child alter, whether acknowledged or not. Such behaviours fit the first and the second DSM-5 criterion for DID.

In terms of the third criterion – amnesia – ABs do not lose memory in the present or the recent past. They only have amnesia in terms of the repression of old childhood trauma and the origin and existence of the alter(s) which split during the trauma. Any alters which do emerge are fully co-conscious. Thereafter, sharing memories, the alters and the birth personality influence each other's traits and behaviours.

In terms of the fourth criterion – distress or impairment – conflicted ABs are intermittently tormented by the involuntary behaviours described above. The see-saw conflict between their adult and child selves constitutes 'identity confusion', one of the five components of dissociation. At its worst, such as the height of the binge and purge cycle, it represents distress and impairment.

The affinity between DID and being AB is illustrated in Dr Steinberg's statement -

The Adult Baby – An Identity on the Dissociation Spectrum

"In the most basic terms dissociative identity disorder, or DID, formerly called multiple personality disorder, is what happens when your 'inner child' or some other hidden part of yourself operates independently, seizes control, and makes you act inappropriately or impairs your ability to function."

As an AB I can certainly recognize a lot of myself in Dr Steinberg's description. I suspect many other ABs would also.

I believe being AB is similar to DID, but without the amnesia.

It is interesting that women are far more likely to be diagnosed with DID than men, while ABs are far more likely to be male than female. The DSM IV-TR, the penultimate version of the Diagnostic and Statistical Manual of Mental Disorders, indicates DID is diagnosed three to nine times more frequently in adult females than adult males. I suspect the prevalence of the genders in both identities is more evenly balanced, and gendered patterns of behaviour conceal this. Women are more likely than men to seek assistance from mental health professionals, and less likely to disclose in often fetish-orientated AB forums and groups.

Being AB on the Dissociation Spectrum

I believe being AB is next door to DID on the dissociation spectrum. Let me explain.

I completed the diagnostic questionnaires for each of the five components of dissociation in Dr Steinberg's book. It indicated, in my conflicted state as an AB, I had moderate levels of identity confusion and identity alteration. I also had moderate levels of depersonalization in the form of detachment from my emotions and my body, and a sense of being a witness as much as a participant in my own life. But these latter sensations are not uncommon for emotionally avoidant, inhibited males. I have no significant derealization (experiencing the environment or others as unreal). Importantly, I have no amnesia. All my alters are co-conscious, they share present memory. In the absence of amnesia being AB is a sub-DID part of the dissociation spectrum.

The fact that some of the intermittent turmoil related to my conflicted AB identity did not ever result in medical intervention and a clinical diagnosis is, to some extent, a fortunate accident. In less advantageous circumstances, it might have been different. If I had been accurately diagnosed with a dissociative condition using the current DSM-5, it would likely have been *Other Specified Dissociative Disorder* (OSDD). I would fit the traits described by Dr Ross –

"Many people with chronic, complex dissociative disorders do not have full DID. In DSM-IV they had DDNOS [Dissociative Disorder Not Otherwise Specified], while in DSM-5 they have OSDD (Other Specified Dissociative Disorder). These are partial forms of DID in which the parts are not so distinct and separate, there is no full amnesia, or there is more co-presence [shared sensation and control of the body] than full switching. Sometimes the person has full DID, but the whole picture hasn't emerged yet, in which case OSDD is used until the picture does become clear." [Treatment of Dissociative Identity Disorder: Techniques and Strategies for Stabilisation]

"... a patient may have several distinct personality states, but not have dissociative amnesia." ['Be a Teammate with Yourself: Understanding Trauma and Dissociation.']

The Wikipedia article *Dissociative Disorder Not Otherwise Specified* indicates "DDNOS is the most common dissociative disorder and is diagnosed in 40% of dissociative disorder cases."

The ISSTD's 2010 Guidelines state -

"A substantial proportion of the dissociative cases encountered in clinical settings receive a diagnosis of DDNOS. Many of these DDNOS cases are well described by the DSM–IV–TR Example 1 of DDNOS: "Clinical presentations similar to dissociative identity disorder that fail to meet the full criteria for this disorder" ... There appear to be two major groupings of such

DDNOS-1 cases: (a) full-blown DID cases whose diagnosis has not yet been confirmed (via the unambiguous manifestation of alternate identities) and (b) complex dissociative cases with some internal fragmentation and/or infrequent incidents of amnesia ... Patients in this latter group of DDNOS-1 are "almost-DID." DDNOS-1 patients are typically subject to DID-like disruptions in their functioning caused by switches in self-states and intrusions of feelings and memories into consciousness. Because these latter phenomena are often more subtle than cases with florid DID, it may require more skill and expertise on the part of clinicians to discern their presence."

ABs fit in category (b). As we have seen above, ABs have distinct personality states that manifest intermittently in behaviours which persist over a long period and are consistent in their character. But ABs do not display amnesia, except for the repression of the original trauma.

Blogger Rob Spring on the website PODS (Positive Outcomes for Dissociative Survivors) suggests OSDD/DDNOS can be distinguished from DID by a lesser level of trauma and lesser number of alters -

"In terms of other differences, it seems that as a general rule the degree of the trauma or attachment difficulties leading to DDNOS will be less severe than people who are diagnosed with dissociative identity disorder ... People with DDNOS may, for example, have had some 'good enough' attachment experiences or other mitigating factors. ... "

According to Van der Hart et al's structural model of dissociation (The Haunted Self, 2006), dissociative identity disorder is a case of tertiary dissociation with multiple ANPs [Apparently Normal Personalities] and multiple EPS [Emotional Personalities], whereas DDNOS is a case of secondary dissociation with a single ANP and multiple EPs. ['DID or DDNOS: does it matter?' cited in the references]

The last paragraph is saying something important, but the wording is a bit obscure. It is saying DID is the third, highest level of dissociation with multiple adult/functional personalities and multiple child/dysfunctional personalities. OSDD/DDNOS is the second, next level of dissociation with one adult/functional personality and multiple child/dysfunctional personalities. The latter characterization fits ABs.

To consider ABs' place on the dissociation spectrum, we can look at the size of three populations.

1. The first is people with substantial dissociative symptoms – they are estimated to represent 10% of the total population.
2. The second is people with DID – they are estimated to represent 1% of the total population (a subset of the first group).
3. The third group is ABs – they are estimated to be one-in-a-thousand or 0.1% of the total population.

The estimated size of these populations does not prove but is consistent with, ABs being a subset on the sub-DID part of the dissociation spectrum. (If these orders of magnitude were reversed it would prove being AB could not be on the dissociation spectrum).

The Psyche is Wired Differently

I said in the introduction ABs that realize at some point their psyche is hard wired differently from everyone else they know. When I started this book, I thought of that in terms of the psychology of ABs. But I found several expert medical references which open the possibility it may be literally true, in terms of key structures in the brain. The two articles are from 2006 and 2008, the former from the American Journal of Psychiatry. They are cited in the references and discussed in greater detail in appendix 1.

The articles indicate when the brains of people with DID were imaged with magnetic resonance imaging (MRI), they show discernible differences from 'healthy' people. The 2008 article found people with DDNOS, those next door to DID on the dissociation spectrum, also had discernible differences when their brains were imaged. As discussed above, I believe ABs fall into the DDNOS/OSDD category. On this basis, it may be literally true the brains of ABs are hard-wired differently from singletons.

The articles are concerned with several key structures in the limbic (emotional) system in the brain – the hippocampus and the amygdala. The hippocampus has important roles in relation to memory - spatial memory that enables navigation, and decision making in uncertain circumstances (according to the Wikipedia article of the same name). It seems the size of the hippocampus can be affected through life by factors such as trauma and stress, medication and perhaps long term psychotherapy. The amygdala has a primary role in memory, decision-making and emotional responses (including fear, anxiety, and aggression) (again, according to the Wikipedia article of the same name). There are two of each structure, one on each side of the brain.

Smaller hippocampal volume has been reported in several stress-related psychiatric disorders, including post-traumatic stress disorder (PTSD), borderline personality disorder with early abuse, and depression with early abuse. The causal relationship between trauma and the size of the hippocampus is unclear. Is the smaller volume caused by trauma, or are people born with a smaller volume more vulnerable to trauma? The relationship between early stress and accompanying psychiatric disorders to amygdalar volume is even less clear.

The two articles suggest the people with DID had 19-25% smaller volumes in the hippocampus. This compares to a study of Vietnam War combat veterans with PTSD which showed a 20% reduction in volume compared with veterans having suffered no such symptoms (cited in Wikipedia). Other studies have suggested people with Borderline Personality Disorder have a 13-21% smaller volume for the Hippocampus than healthy people.

The 2008 article indicated people with DDNOS had 14% less hippocampal volume than healthy people. This would put them about midway between the people with DID, and 'healthy' people. It indicated otherwise the DID and DDNOS groups were similar, with both having 10-12% less volume in the amygdala, and 19-20% less volume in another key structure, the parahippocampal gyrus (which serves as an interface between structures in the limbic brain), than the healthy control group.

We need to be cautious about what we infer from the above. Both articles indicated when they were written in 2006-8, they were amongst the first research into the neurobiology of DID. They are based on small study populations. We don't know if the symptoms of the DDNOS study group resembled those of ABs (identity alternation rather than amnesia). I have no knowledge of neuroscience. I don't know how significant the differences in brain structure between the three populations are in terms of influencing cognition and behaviour. For ABs, I am not inferring any kind of behavioural determinism from those differences, or any diminution of personal responsibility. We need to acknowledge ABs share the vast majority of their psychology with everyone else. What I do take from the articles is a tentative basis for the idea the different wiring in AB's psyches may be neurological rather than just a matter of psychology.

It is important but confronting to realize that people with DID have never had a 'normal' unitary psyche as adolescents and adults. The childhood trauma which gave rise to their DID generally occurred at a young age, before the teenage years. From that point on their psyche has taken a divergent track. The ISSTD's 2010 Guidelines for Treating Dissociative Identity Disorder in Adults states -

> *"In short, these developmental models posit that DID does not arise from a previously mature, unified mind or "core personality" that becomes shattered or fractured. Rather, DID results from a failure of normal developmental integration caused by overwhelming experiences and disturbed caregiver-child interactions (including neglect and the failure to respond) during critical early developmental periods. This, in turn, leads some traumatized children to develop relatively discrete, personified behavioural states that ultimately evolve into the DID alternate identities."*

The 2006 article cited above states –

The Adult Baby – An Identity on the Dissociation Spectrum

"Accordingly, the disorder [DID] has been conceptualized as a childhood-onset posttraumatic developmental disorder."

I suspect this description is also largely true for ABs.

Childhood Trauma

So, if being AB is a form of identity alteration, there must have been childhood trauma where an alter split within the psyche. My book '*The Adult Baby Identity – A Self Help Guide*' describes the likely scenario for such trauma -

"Based on my experience I believe that there was a time, or times, in your childhood when you felt very frightened and desperately alone. You were a very young, vulnerable child. You felt overwhelmed. That was when the child persona emerged in your psyche. It was the best thing your psyche could do to protect you from despair.

It does not have to mean that you had bad parents. Even with the best will in the world parents can't always protect their children from the 'ordinary catastrophes' of childhood. Those catastrophes include a young child being very frightened at a temporary separation from their mother or primary caregiver. But whatever it was, at the time you did not understand what was happening. You felt alone and unloved. And like all children who feel unloved, you felt it was your fault. You felt unlovable. Your Inner Child was wounded. And such childhood wounds stay with us. For some ABs, these wounds may not come from the ordinary catastrophes of childhood, but from abuse or neglect."

Rosalie Bent refers to the prospect of ABs recalling repressed trauma–

"Have you ever forgotten an important or traumatic incident that happened a long time ago and then suddenly, something triggered the memory and it came flooding back and was almost news to you? It happens to a lot of us at times and it happens to a Little One even more. The reason for this could be because Littles were often formed in their very young years and memories of that time seem to get filed in a dusty corner of the brain and forgotten as a matter of course.

Your Little One has as much access to all the adult's memories as the adult himself, right? Well, maybe not – it might be more. I don't want this to sound too overwhelming, but it is sometimes true that your regressed Little One might be better able to tell you about things in the past that were traumatic, than the adult. This might not always be a good thing, as some traumas are better left hidden, unless you are ready and able to deal with it. I bring this up though, because it may happen that your Little One dredges up an old memory from his distant past and it may or may not be related to how the regression began, or some other aspect to it."
['There's Still A Baby In My Bed: Learning To Live Happily With the Adult Baby in Your Relationship]

Validation

For ABs, the parallels with DID offer an important validation of their sense of self.

ABs are commonly mystified and confounded at the source and power of their compulsive demand for nappies. That is explained when we understand the power of alters within the psyches of people with DID. To describe alters as subjectively real doesn't adequately convey their power to affect a person's behaviour and bodily sensations. I have read references by mental health professionals to switches between DID alters where a person can go from displaying an allergy to having no allergic reaction; where medications will show greater or lesser or no effects; to presenting with convincing symptoms of physical maladies and then these quickly disappearing; or to experiencing pain or not from obvious physical wounds. These shifts are associated with switches between alters which do not share memories or even a knowledge of the other's existence. This does not apply to ABs, but it does indicate the power of the subjective experience of an alter to shape sensation and behaviour. If you doubt the power of subjectively real alters, read any autobiography of someone with DID (see Chapter 7).

As we have seen, subjectively real alternate identities are accepted as a valid phenomenon by authoritative diagnostic texts like the DSM. They are acknowledged as having real and significant effects on a person's sense of self.

Admittedly, the validation in the DSM is 'backhanded'. It's in the context of a catalogue of mental disorders. But it's a start. And it's based on work like that of Dr Marlene Steinberg which indicates identity alteration is only one of five components of dissociation. Identity alteration by itself is not debilitating (as we shall see in Chapter 11). As the DSM indicates, identity alteration alone, in the absence of distress or impairment, is not a mental disorder. In this sense, I think of AB's as the lucky kids on the dissociation 'block'.

ABs can also take validation from two other key perspectives from mental health professionals working in the field of dissociation. Firstly, alternate identities have their origin in childhood dissociation. That validates the obvious point that the AB's obsession with nappies and the other trappings of infancy points to origins in issues and unmet needs in childhood. Secondly, enlightened mental health professionals accept psychological health lies in accepting these alters and having a cooperative relationship with them – not denying them (for example Dr Yeung's approach to DID – see his books cited in the references).

A Note on the Book 'There's Still A Baby in My Bed'

Rosalie and Michael Bent's book *'There's Still A Baby in My Bed: Learning to Live Happily with the Adult Baby in Your Relationship'* was the first published work to consider being AB as a personal identity, not a sexual fetish. It is an evergreen book of groundbreaking courage. It helped me enormously in coming to terms with being AB.

The book describes a comprehensive list of AB traits and symptoms which are indicative of, or consistent with, ABs being an identity on dissociation spectrum. I refer to many of these citations in this book. Rosalie and Michael use the terms regression or regress where I use the term dissociation or dissociate. But I believe we are describing the same phenomena. The book has a firm grasp on the nature of co-conscious alters. It represents a remarkable feat of insight – to deduce a dissociative identity from observation and first principles.

Rosalie and Michael's book states being AB is not Multiple Personality Disorder (or DID as MPD was renamed). This is absolutely true. However, it also says being AB is *not* dissociative. I interpret this to mean being AB does not involve dissociative *amnesia*. This book affirms that view.

I believe the position in *'There's Still a Baby in My Bed'* can be readily understood. It was the first book to take issue with the offensive, harmful and empirically inaccurate categorization of being AB as a paraphilia (a sexual fetish) in the DSM. That categorization groups being AB with flashers, gropers, peeping toms and paedophiles. In seeking to rescue AB's from the harm of this error it would have been a doubtful gain to give the impression being AB was the same as MPD/DID.

Now, with the benefit of the cumulative understanding initiated by Rosalie and Michael, we can understand the breadth of the dissociation spectrum. And being AB and DID can be on that spectrum, and share much in common (alters), while also being very different (ie. ABs don't have amnesia or a fragmented psyche).

Summary

There is an important overlap between DID and being AB. DID is a combination of identity alteration and amnesia. Being AB is similar to DID, in that it is identity alteration without the amnesia. The identity alteration is common to both. Being AB fits the category of Other Specified Dissociative Disorder (OSDD). That puts it next door to DID on the dissociation spectrum.

5. Regression

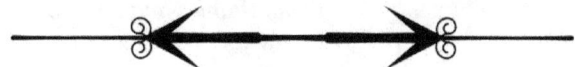

If being AB is a small subset of the much larger population with substantial dissociation symptoms, why does that manifest as a need, obsession and fetish for nappies? That isn't true for all the other people in the broader dissociative population.

I believe that's where regression comes in.

In regression, a person reverts to behaviours and a psychological state from their biological childhood. Those behaviours and states are not random. They represent points where the person's childhood development got stuck for a time, experienced difficulty or missed a step. This is referred to as a *fixation*. Most people have witnessed or read of situations where a young child, faced with an overwhelming crisis such as being hospitalized, separated from a parent, or the like, reverts to behaviours they had previously grown out of – bedwetting, thumb sucking, etc.

I suspect that ABs had issues, delays or setbacks in their continence and toilet training in childhood. I did. I posit the AB's regression to that point of fixation becomes the means by which a dissociated child alter breaks through from the unconscious and influences behaviour. The child alter is trying to signal both its existence and needs to our adult selves from behind high walls of repression, and later denial. The fixation with toilet training or bedwetting is the first hole in the wall.

There is no way of proving this hypothesis, but it fits with what we know about ABs. We know that the initial fetish for nappies typically blossoms eventually into a much larger repertoire of AB expressions and needs. That is consistent with the dissociated child alter eventually breaking through the hole in the wall of repression. Given the comparative rarity of ABs, it also makes sense there should be overlapping causal factors.

Okay, but why do we need to explain being AB in terms of dissociation at all? Why can't it be explained purely in terms of regression?

There are four key facets of being AB which regression alone cannot adequately explain (and dissociation does). These are –

1. Key traits and preferences of the AB's 'Little' or child alter were often not part of the AB's biological childhood.
2. An AB's Little typically manifests over time as a multi-layered persona consistent with 'identity alteration', one of the five elements of dissociation, rather than a set of disparate regressive behaviours.
3. Conflicted ABs commonly experience 'identity confusion', one of the five elements of dissociation, typically a conscious duality and conflict between an adult and child self.
4. For ABs who have accepted their identity, the positive experience of self-nurturing their Little is not adequately represented by the concept of regression.

Each of these aspects is discussed below.

Not Reversion to Biological Childhood

An AB's 'Little' commonly has important traits or preferences which were not part of their biological childhood. These are better explained as belonging to a dissociated alter which is a sub-conscious, and later conscious, construct of the AB's psyche.

A good example is that many ABs identify with having a Little with a different gender from their biological childhood. Rosalie Bent indicates -

> *'... around half of physically male Adult Babies and Little Ones identity as female infant/toddler, indeterminate or sissy. ... 'Sissy' and 'girl' are quite similar and when determining your Little One's gender, keep in mind the sissy option. It is a subset of the female gender, but for simplicity, I have used it as a separate one.'*

Some of these ABs did identify as female at an early age and hence regression might encompass baby girl clothing and behaviours. I suspect most did not identify as female at an early enough age for those characteristics to be caused by regression to their biological infant or toddler state. In my case I have a baby girl alter but my biological childhood was exclusively male, and in a family with an absolute demarcation between gender identities. For me, a female child self could not be the result of regression to any part of my biological childhood.

It is likely many of the traits and preferences of AB's child selves do not faithfully replicate those of the AB's biological childhood. This does not deny that some of the constructs of the baby/child self are influenced by the AB's biological childhood. But this influence is mixed with others, at least as strong, which come from elsewhere in the psyche. That is more consistent with a dissociated alter, rather than regression.

Identity Alteration

An AB's Little typically manifests over time as a multi-layered persona. It's not just wearing nappies. It's also a wardrobe of baby clothes, pacifiers, stuffed toys, perhaps bottles, and activities such as watching children's TV, colouring books or playing with dolls. And the physical manifestation of the Little is only the tip of the iceberg, on top of a large repertoire of fantasy involving an imagined life as a baby. This goes well beyond a limited number of disparate childish behaviours such as might be linked to regression.

The manifestation of such a multi-layered persona is more consistent with a dissociated alter. That represents 'identity alteration', one of the five components of dissociation. The AB's Little is sufficiently elaborated as an alternative personality they are often named by the AB. Again, that is consistent with a state experienced by the AB, not as a set of disparate behaviours but as an alternative personality.

Identity Confusion

Before AB's accept themselves, they typically experience an intermittent sense of turmoil and doubt about their identity. That experience is commonly one of living with dual and conflicting selves – the adult and the child. Even when the Little is denied by the AB, it is still experienced as a disruptive force which could unexpectedly manifest in the 'binge' part of the 'binge and purge' cycle, or in involuntary triggering of the need to put on a nappy. This is consistent with 'identity confusion', one of the five components of dissociation. This pervasive experience of uncertainty about identity is consistent with dissociation, rather than regression.

Self-Nurturing

When an AB accepts their identity, their episodes of 'baby time' (wearing a nappy, dressing in baby clothes, and the rest) represent self-nurturing of the AB's Little by the AB's adult self. That nurturing heals the AB's childhood wounds and supports a stable and healthy identity. The positive character of the AB's ongoing self-nurturing is more consistent with shared consciousness between an adult self, and a baby/child alter. It is less consistent with regressing alone to a past wounded biological childhood. Regression can be understood as a temporary psychological refuge when normal coping mechanisms have failed. The adult state is supplanted by a child state, and the former is not 'present' to comfort and protect the latter. Given the extent of Little related behaviours and traits in the lives and characters of ABs, that would suggest that ABs were neurotic failed adults.

This is not consistent with the fact ABs are both sane, functional adults *and* experience themselves as subjectively real children.

On the basis of the above, I believe regression alone is insufficient to explain being AB. The conjunction of dissociation and regression is a good fit with what we know about ABs, and the breadth of AB traits and behaviours.

5. Dax and Dylan

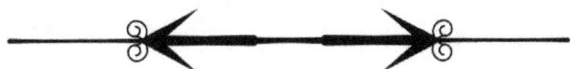

It is time to introduce Dax and myself.

Dax has DID and I am an AB. Dax is my wife's nephew by marriage, from a previous marriage. Our chance acquaintance offered the opportunity to compare our experience of ourselves with a depth and honesty that would otherwise not be possible.

Dax

Dax is one-of-a-kind, a larger-than-life personality. This is reflected in both his character and sometimes tumultuous life course. He is a gifted teacher. He has taught children with learning difficulties with an empathy derived from the challenges he faced through his life. He has held senior positions in schools around the world and has a successful online consultancy business.

Dax describes himself as 'a fully functioning cognitive adult who embraced his DID. He chose a profession and way of life that allowed for periods of hospitalization, therapy and isolation without it impacting his attempts to lead a normal life.'

Into his forties, he was a devotee of extreme sports and visiting remote exotic places. He has climbed mountains in most continents, and run marathons in the arctic and on the Great Wall of China. Dax has 'a thing' for islands. It led him to spend three weeks alone on a remote uninhabited island off the south coast of Australia and to make his current home on a beautiful small island in the Caribbean.

He grew up in the United Kingdom, where, as a child, he was subject to severe and repeated physical, sexual and psychological abuse. He found love and understanding with an adoptive family and was diagnosed with DID at age 16. In therapy, he began the process of getting to know his alters. Tragically, his beloved first wife died in a car accident and his adoptive parents died shortly afterwards. His birth personality contracted another marriage without the knowledge and agreement of other alters. The marriage was unhappy and ended in separation. It produced two daughters whom Dax has supported financially into independent adulthood.

In the latter half of his life, Dax moved jobs and locations around the world every couple of years as his DID fractured relationships. Now aged in his early fifties, he has married his partner and has a baby. He believes he will settle on his beloved island home.

Dax has nine alters. There are others but these are shadowy non-verbal 'presences', felt, rather than known. The nine are represented in a distinctive tattoo on the back of his hand – a spiral in circles and dots. It is a touchstone to remind all his alters, in the midst of amnesia, of his identity. Though Dax had an early diagnosis and therapy, the deep childhood trauma means debilitating amnesia is always present in his life.

All Dax's alters are male. He has one child alter, little Dan, aged 7. The others are adults or teenagers. Dax is the host, but not the birth personality (more on that topic in Chapter 11). The capabilities Dax needs to successfully navigate the external adult world are spread between several key alters – Dax, Jonah, Jinx and Ollie. Dax is the facilitator and lead; Jinx handles money and logistics; Jonah handles strategy and planning, and Ollie is the athlete and enabler.

Dax's life is the story of a unique journey and of unique courage. We are now working on his autobiography.

Dax on DID

The most compelling perspective on DID comes from Dax's verbatim descriptions. Dax speaks in the plural, speaking for his 'system' of multiple alters.

"DID for us is not having more than one personality, it is one personality that is divided into parts. It is inaccurate to conceptualise us as having 'multiple personalities'. A more helpful conceptualisation is that we have access to less than one personality (at any one time). Living with DID means our parts are separated from each other by dissociative barriers. As a result, we have developed separately and have very different skills, opinions, memories, friends, history, preferences from each other. For example, we have different ages, sexual preferences, skills, interests and beliefs.

I will always remember having this explained to me like a delicate vase being dropped onto the floor. It can be repaired, but the pieces never fit properly back together.

Living with DID is both a pleasure and a curse. We celebrate our individuality but the cost lies in our relationships with others being fragmented.

Diagnosis was a relief, but definitely not a badge to wear with honour. It has hindered our life at every stage and should never be used as an excuse. It is what it is, DID is a condition that provides a unique perspective on life but at the same time one that limits achievements. We had to accept the conflict that DID brought into our life, failure to do so would have resulted in suicide or institutionalization.

However, as DID took a greater hold on our life, the degree of self-doubt diminished as we learnt to become self-reliant as the roles of the alters evolved. Through embracing DID and not letting it rule our life, we became more self-sufficient.

Many years ago we got described as high functioning and able to hide in plain sight. So now we are invisible, alive but suffering in silence, in full view but alone."

I suspect many ABs will relate to Dax's observation about hiding in plain sight.

Dylan

By contrast, except for being AB, I (Dylan) am boringly conventional. I am in my late fifties and happily retired from a senior position in government service. I have been married for over thirty years to my wife, the love of my life. Through marriage, I have grandchildren and great-grandchildren. I was born, bred and have lived my whole life in a State capital in Australia. I had an insecure attachment with my parents as a child but this was not the result of abuse or neglect.

I first experienced behaviours linked to being AB - a compelling need to wear nappies and fantasise about being babied - around age ten. Being AB caused intermittent turmoil in my life but never became a clinical issue. For the greater part of my life, I experienced being AB as a sexual fetish with compulsive behaviours that tyrannized my life. It was completely and inexplicably at odds with my inhibited, responsible adult self. Early on I thought marriage would 'cure' me. Later, I tried many times to give it up, with willpower and therapy. It always came back, ultimately stronger than before. I was in my forties before I reluctantly accepted it would never go away. I was in my fifties before I accepted being AB was a personal identity with a subjectively real child alter originating in childhood trauma.

My principal alter is a baby girl, Chrissie. She originated from a traumatic temporary separation from my mother when I was aged three or four. This is described in my book *"Living With Chrissie: My Life as an Adult Baby"*
-

The Adult Baby – An Identity on the Dissociation Spectrum

My mother went to a sporting club, presumably for some much-needed respite from caring alone for two small children. While she was playing I was left with my sister in the care of other adults. My sister became inconsolably distressed at the separation. I felt responsible, either for caring for her or at least for showing a good example. But in the face of her distress, I couldn't contain my own and ended up bursting into tears and wetting my pants. I couldn't see my mother and she seemed to have gone beyond hope of return. I felt terrified, overwhelmed and abandoned. I had failed to be the 'big boy' I was expected to be. My sister was picked up and comforted by the other adults but I don't remember being so comforted.

I have two other child alters, boys, shy Joey and tough Robbie. Both are aged about nine or ten, my age when they split from my psyche. Joey originated from a traumatic fear of drowning, as described in my book -

> *My parents placed great importance on me learning to swim ... I had a fear of water, especially of putting my head under the surface. I had not been successful at government-run holiday swimming lessons that were a rite of passage for kids of my generation. My parents enrolled me for private lessons with a brusque, intimidating male instructor [I was physically afraid of men] ... It was the middle of winter. We were forced to jump into the deep end of a cold unheated pool. I desperately wanted to be brave but I was terrified. I thought I was going to die. My parents persisted. I would wait with mounting terror for the time for the next lesson to roll by. I remember being driven crying and distressed to early morning swimming lessons in the winter rain. Eventually, they relented and I was sent to a psychologist. Evidently, on his advice, I was allowed to give up swimming lessons until I was ready for them several years later.*

Robbie is the clearest example of a 'split' in my psyche. He originated from a traumatic bullying incident at primary school. It occurred on an oval out of sight of the main school complex. At breaks, it was only frequented by the older boys, unsupervised by teachers. It was 'Lord of the Flies' territory and you never 'dobbed'. I recall being alone and being circled by a large group of my taunting classmates. I blanked out, completely. When I recovered my senses I was sitting on top of a smaller classmate on the ground with my hands around his neck. My recollection is if I hadn't been pulled off by some older boys I would have strangled him. I was deeply shocked at my loss of control and what I was capable of. In the next several years I refused to fight again, even when I was hit by boys who were smaller than I was.

I have described these incidents to illustrate the 'ordinary catastrophes' of childhood can be sufficiently traumatic to lead to 'splitting'. In each incident, there were circumstances in my life at the time which may have increased my psychological vulnerability to trauma. Notwithstanding these childhood incidents, I grew up to become a strong-minded adult, capable of showing both physical and moral courage and leading others. I cite that to show I was not traumatized as a child because of an intrinsic weakness in my character. Trauma can briefly overwhelm a younger child's capacity to cope, no matter what that child's character.

Why didn't I understand as an adult, the impact of these traumatic incidents? In the case of the first incident, when I was aged three or four, it was part of family history and I had a visual recollection of the event. I always recalled the other incidents but buried the feelings associated with them. It was only after I talked to a skilled therapist in later life I recalled my emotional memory and joined it with the visual memory. Only then did I understand how traumatized I had been in each case. Therapy started the process of healing the trauma carried by my alters. Self-acceptance and the acceptance of my wife carried that healing through.

Accepting Chrissie as a real, fundamental and healthy part of my psyche has transformed my life. I feel whole, contented and safe in a way I never did before. That extends beyond my AB side to my life in general. Chrissie is a delight to me.

> *"Sure she can be a real 'little miss', at her worst a selfish brat. But she's also a shy, easily scared, innocent, loving, affectionate, warm-hearted, fun-loving little girl who melts my heart. My adult-self feels very good about comforting and protecting her."*

I now embrace being AB as a liberating and redeeming personal identity. My wife does not act as Chrissie's mother or caregiver, but she accepts Chrissie as subjectively real and can laugh with and about Chrissie, in ways that are deeply affirming and healing to me. Now, in retirement, there is a kind of 50:50 balance between my adult self and Chrissie. I sleep each night and spend each morning dressed as Chrissie in a nappy and baby clothes.

Stage of Life When We Accepted Our Identities

Dax and I consciously accepted our identities at different stages in our lives. For Dax, that was in young adulthood, and for me, it was in late adulthood. In this, neither of us is necessarily representative of our identities.

Both people with DID and ABs can accept their identities either early or late in their lives. Dax is representative of people of either identity or any minority identity, who do so early in life. I am representative of people with any minority identity who reach acceptance only later in life.

For Dax, the extent and effects of childhood abuse resulted in medical intervention early in his life. He was clinically diagnosed with DID aged 16 by mental health professionals and experienced that diagnosis as a relief from uncertainty. Conversely, there are many people with DID who do not accept their identity until mid-life, and some who never accept themselves.

I did not accept being AB as a minority personality until I was aged in my mid-fifties. This is despite showing the first behaviours linked to my identity (craving nappies) as early as age 10 and seeing therapists in relation to these behaviours several times as an adult. Conversely, there are many ABs who accept their identity as adolescents or young adults. This pattern has become much more prevalent with the advent of the internet and social media age.

The balance of this book explores what it feels like to live with DID and being AB, based on the experiences of Dax and myself. It points to when it feels similar, and when it feels different.

7. DID Autobiographies

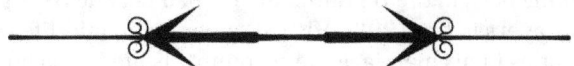

No individual is representative of an entire identity – whether DID or AB. I had an awareness of where my circumstances and traits fitted within the broader ABDL population. I didn't have the same awareness of where Dax fitted within the DID population. To seek that awareness, I read case histories and five autobiographies of people with DID that covered a breadth of different circumstances.

The five autobiographies are summarized below -

Robert Oxnam was a prominent US and international academic leader whose career in Asian studies brought him into contact with the US President and business leaders like Bill Gates and Warren Buffett. His DID emerged in mid-life as he recovered from alcoholism and bulimia. His DID was caused by childhood physical, psychological and sexual abuse by men and women within his extended family. His first marriage ended before or during the early stages of treatment of his DID. His second wife, another prominent academic, accepted his DID and lovingly embraced his alters. He was 'outed' with DID and seems to have had to start a new career as an artist.

Before and after accepting his DID, he seems to be a self-important, grandiose and self-absorbed personality. Robert describes a dramatically gothic, compelling interior landscape peopled by his alters. His psychiatrist promoted fusion of his alters. Robert's account focuses on his treatment journey which led to eleven original alters integrating into three. He describes how his host personality switched from an alter back to his birth personality. He embraced his alters. One of the remaining triumvirates of healed alters was a child, and another a woman. His autobiography is '*A Fractured Mind: My Life With Multiple Personality Diso*rder'.

Christine Pattillo is an everyday woman from the northwestern US who earned her livelihood in the retail and financial services sectors. Alone of the five autobiographies cited here, she was consciously a multiple from childhood. She was not diagnosed with DID until crises in mid-life caused her to seek treatment. Her DID originated with physical and psychological childhood abuse from her father and childhood sexual abuse from a person outside her family.

Before her DID, she seems to have been a warm but deeply conflicted personality, suffering from sometimes debilitating bouts of anxiety, self-harm and bulimia. After accepting her DID, she is a warm, vibrant, optimistic personality. Her loving husband was at her side throughout her therapy. Her altruistic therapist emphasized cooperation between alters rather than fusion. She warmly embraced her alters who include children and a male teenager. Her remarkable account has the voice of the host/birth personality, each alter, and the host's husband and mother. It vividly describes her alters' characters and their relationships with each other. She lives openly as a 'multiple' and her husband embraces her vibrant, healed alters as his family. Her autobiography is '*I Am We: Living With Multiple Personalities*'.

Olga Trujillo was a high powered lawyer in the US Justice Department and later became an influential advocate for survivors of child abuse. Her DID emerged in mid-life. Both it and the memories of childhood abuse came as a complete and shocking revelation. Her DID was caused by a childhood of depraved, sexual, physical and psychological abuse by all members of her family. Her psychiatrist seems to have pursued treatment which emphasized abreaction – re-experiencing the trauma. She was re-traumatised over an extended period and her marriage to her loving husband did not survive. She later married a gay partner who accepts her DID. Before and after accepting the DID, she seems to be a highly controlled person focused on her work. She seems to have a functional, impersonal relationship with her alters. Her final relationship with her alters is unclear. Her autobiography is '*The Sum of My Parts: A Survivor's Story of Dissociative Identity Disorder*'.

Herschel Walker is the most highly visible person I know who has come out as having DID. He had a highly successful career as a running back in the US National Football League (NFL) and as an Olympic athlete. He was one of the highest-paid NFL players in the 1990s. His DID emerged in mid-life as he grappled with the end of his NFL playing career and difficulties in his marriage. He recounts his life from childhood, describing how his at-the-time unrecognized alters helped him overcome being an overweight, stuttering child to become a superstar athlete. After his career finished, without an outlet for his competitiveness and aggression, his alters became dysfunctional. He entered therapy, but his marriage ended in divorce.

Alone of the five autobiographies cited here, his DID was not caused by sexual abuse or abuse within the family. He attributes it to a temporary separation from his mother after birth, but mostly to prolonged bullying and ostracism in primary school (he also witnessed a terrifying assault by hooded KKK thugs as a six-year-old). Before and after accepting his DID, he was a highly controlled, emotionally-avoidant person. He seems to have a functional, impersonal relationship with his alters. He doesn't refer to any child alters or alters of a different gender. His psychiatrist seems to have aimed for fusion of his alters. His autobiography is '*Breaking Free: My Life with Dissociative Identity Disorder.*'

Cameron West is an everyday person from the US who was a prosperous small businessman before his DID. It emerged in mid-life after a debilitating crisis with his physical health. His DID was caused by childhood sexual abuse by his mother and grandmother. His loving wife had a background in working with special needs children and supported him through his diagnosis and recovery. Alone of the five, he had a young child when he was diagnosed with DID. His account focuses on his therapeutic journey and shows his struggle with denial. His therapists did not purse the fusion of his alters. His alters were co-conscious from the outset but switched uncontrollably.

Before and after accepting the DID, he seems to be a warm empathic person. Both he and his wife warmly embraced his alters, especially his child alters. His alters included an adolescent girl. He lives as a multiple with a remaining core group of healed, mainly child alters. After his DID was diagnosed he reinvented his working life. His autobiography is '*First Person Plural: My Life As a Multiple*'. It was publicized by Oprah Winfrey.

I hope these brief sketches show people with DID come in many guises and walks of life. Each of them showed inspirational courage in facing repressed memories of abuse, and coming to terms with a new and challenging identity that their hidden pasts had foisted on them. They represent people you might work with or meet every day. I refer to their experiences throughout the rest of the book.

There is an implicit bias in these five accounts. All the people survived torment, found therapists who understood dissociation, and in varying degrees, healed themselves, to be able to publish their stories. Psychiatrist David Yeung's 14 case histories provide a more representative range of outcomes for people with severe DID (see his book '*Engaging Multiple Personalities Volume 1: Contextual Case Histories*' cited in the references). For those with severe dissociation, it can be an unkind world, with unaccepting partners, relatives, and mental health professionals. Of those 14 who eventually found an empathic and skilled therapist in Dr Yeung, two committed suicide and three others remained at high risk with uncontrolled fragmentation. However, for the greater majority, an accurate diagnosis and effective therapy was a route to healing and psychological health.

8. Living With Alters

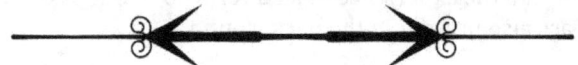

For Dax and I there is a compelling similarity in our sense of self. We both live with alters which are real to us, and which influence our perceptions, thoughts, feelings and actions on a daily basis.

The next three chapters discuss this common experience. The effects of amnesia shape living with alters in ways which are unique to DID. These differences will be discussed in Chapter 11.

The experience of living with alters which are common to both of us include-

1. how it feels to live with alters;
2. triggering;
3. alters' fundamental place in our psyche;
4. alters' effect on relationships with loved ones.

Each of these topics is discussed below.

How It Feels

Our alters feel completely real. They never go away, they are part of our psyche 24/7. People are familiar with this perspective on DID. It is also true for ABs. Rosalie Bent recognized these two fundamentals for ABs in her book *'There's Still A Baby in My Bed'*. Addressing the partners of ABs she says –

> *"The startling news for you is that the child is always there. ... In the case of your Little One, however, there is a very real Inner Child that is well-formed and accessible via deep regression."*

When an alter is 'out' – at the forefront of our consciousness – we experience the world in real-time through the lens of that alter's perceptions, feelings and thoughts.

When an alter is not 'out' they are always sitting in the background, each processing the same events and sense impressions according to their age and character (and in my case, gender). A sense-impression may have a different meaning for one alter than another. It is common for at least one alter to have the function of 'watcher'. Thus multiples always have more than one pair of eyes 'in the room' (or rather they process the same sensory stimuli from multiple viewpoints). This can be positive or negative. In the positive, it can mean multiples don't miss much when they focus. In an earlier quote, Dr Yeung referred to how teachers or therapists with DID can be exceptionally perceptive and sensitive to their students or clients. In the negative, when a situation triggers unconscious memories of past trauma, it can result in hypervigilance – being on high alert that can shade into high anxiety or a panic attack.

My principal alter, Chrissie, is deeply comforted by wearing nappies, and the familiarity of a wet nappy. Ditto for soft-to-the-touch, pastel pink, pyjama-style baby clothes. She loves an afternoon nap and calmly drifts into sleep on her back, comforted by her pacifier and with her beloved soft toys, Bunny and Dolly, cuddled on either side. Each night she sleeps soundly between child-patterned flannelette sheets and feels deeply protected by the presence of Bunny and Dolly. She has an instinctual comfort from the constant presence of an array of stuffed toys in her bedroom looking out at her when she wakes or goes to sleep. Her dolls set inspires a deep desire to play, cuddling and feeding her dolls. She has a spontaneous delight at seeing a pretty baby girl's dress or outfit, or an appealing soft toy.

This repertoire of feelings and reactions are completely at odds with my inhibited adult self. Yet I have slowly learned to trust their instinctual nature, consistency, and spontaneity as being real and honest. They are not an act or even my conscious imagination. They really do belong to a little girl in my psyche. My other alters, Joey and Robbie, are less prominent, but just as real.

It is the same for Dax. For him the experience of an alter who is 'out' is even more compelling because that alter is less aware all the others are also present in the background.

Whether an alter is 'out' depends on conscious choice, or whether the alter is 'triggered' by a sense impression (sight, sound, smell – a familiar or confronting situation). *Choice* is the optimal situation. For Dax, that means the adult alter with the capabilities most appropriate to a situation is 'out'. For Dax and myself, it means a child alter can come out to 'be' or play when it's safe and congenial. In this benign sense, it's not much different than a 'singleton' who shifts between different roles and contexts in their daily life.

A common experience is a person can have alters of a different gender from the host personality. This is prevalent in both identities. I earlier quoted Rosalie Bent saying about half of male ABs have a female/sissy Little. That's me. Colin Ross indicated in a sample of 236 people with DID, 62% had an alter of a different gender (cited in *'Dissociative Identity Disorder'* p151). In three of the five DID autobiographies, the author cited having an alter of a different gender. That can be true for hosts of any gender. Christine Pattillo gives a humorous account of being a middle-aged woman with an alter who is a hormone-driven male teenager. Some other people with DID, or ABs, only have alters with the same gender as their host personality. That is true of Dax.

Sensationalist accounts of DID often emphasize the high number of alters. ABs commonly identify as having one 'Little'. That can make it seem ABs must be completely different from people with DID. It is not so. If you have one alter besides your host personality you are a multiple. An experience of self, based on a subjectively real alternative personality, is still very different from an experience of self-based on a unitary psyche.

But sometimes ABs can also have multiple 'Littles' or alters. Rosalie Bent recognized this -

> *"Your Little One may be more than one! … For example, a Little might have behaviours ranging from ages twelve months up to eight years old. In this case, they may separate into one, three, five and eight-year-old identities and have different names for each. They may have separate clothing preferences, toys and other objects. Their behaviours may range from a non-walking, baby-talking one year old, to an eight-year-old with all the abilities and more of a typical child of that age."*

For people with DID, a large number of alters belongs to a highly fragmented state before healing. This can happen where a person is exposed to repeated trauma over an extended period. Dissociation and splitting become an established pattern to protect the psyche. The DSM IV-TR indicates males diagnosed with DID have an average of around eight alters, while females average fifteen or more. Some of the large number of alters may be what Dr Steinberg refers to as personality 'fragments' which are feeling states without a developed personality. Healing seems to result in some alters becoming inactive, fusing with others or disappearing. After the process of healing people with DID commonly seem to have a core group of alters numbered in the single figures – Robert Oxnam has 3, Christine Pattillo has 6, Cameron West has 9, and Dax has 6.

Triggering

Triggering is an involuntary process. People are used to talking about triggering for people with DID or Post Traumatic Stress Disorder (PTSD). It also applies to ABs. Rosalie Bent describes it as follows -

> *"A stressor or trigger occurs to begin the process. This may be an event, a sight, a memory or a sudden emotion. It can also be a smell or the presence of a specific object …"*

> *"You need to become aware of triggers which can start a deep regression, rather than just a shallow one. Sometimes, there are triggers to avoid, such as baby shops, children's books or sights and smells that push regression into higher levels."*

Any alter can potentially be triggered any time, 24/7. It can be nice, such as when a child alter sees a friendly dog or an enticing toy, and spontaneously comes out to enjoy the experience. It can be confronting, such as when a situation prompts a feeling of threat, discomfort or distress, and suddenly you are experiencing your body and the world through a personality that may be agitated, angry or frightened. Other times it can be a strong feeling of unease and tension.

My triggering is now manageable. I accept the existence of my alters and understand their personalities and triggers. All are co-conscious, so while a single event and sense-impression can produce different reactions, all know what the others are experiencing. Mostly my host and alters are co-present, sharing the sensations and control of my body (more on this later). Outside of that, changes are more a case of 'shifting', a smoother and less abrupt experience than 'switching'.

It was far more confronting when I didn't accept and understand the nature of my identity. My alters held unrecognized and unhealed trauma from my childhood. At times that was like an emotional tinderbox waiting for a spark. Then the influences on my feelings, thoughts and actions, sometimes seemed capricious and unpredictable. I sometimes experienced abrupt switching. I can remember occasions in my adult life when I had to flee from social situations, desperately trying to disguise the incomprehensible panic of my unrecognized alters.

For Dax, the situation is far more difficult. His triggering is abrupt -

> *"When we switch it's fast, it's a blink, the click of the fingers and that's ...it my lights go out, although I have got to understand a lot more about the triggers that cause the switching..one second I'm conscious the next I'm unconscious. My next conscious thought maybe 4 hrs later or the next day or longer."*

Some of his alters are co-conscious with others, but others are not. Some of the alters live with childhood pain so deep it will never fully heal. As Dr Yeung indicates, they have PTSD. At its worst it's like 'flashbacks' for combat veterans – Dax's system can go from zero to full fight-or-flight mode in a heartbeat. He can be confronted by the reactions of others to words or actions by an alter that is no longer 'out', and have no recollection of their words and actions. That is living with present-amnesia and makes triggering a sometimes-confronting experience.

Both of us can be plagued by symptoms another might take as chronic or acute anxiety. It might be construed as social anxiety, linked to apprehensions about interacting with others. But it's not anxiety in the way most would understand it. If you have alters who can be triggered involuntarily at any time, walking into a crowded bustling room of strangers can be the equivalent of trying to take a gaggle of skittish or boisterous dogs across a busy four-lane highway. That experience can be nerve-wracking. The 'anxiety' is a realistic apprehension of risk and potential difficulty.

Alters Are Fundamental

For Dax and myself, our alters hold indispensable pieces of our psyches. Dax uses an analogy of a broken vase to describe his psyche – each alter is a fragment of the whole. They have different, complementary roles. The alters also give Dax access to a different sexual orientation than his birth personality and represents that fulfilment of his psyche. For me, as an AB my child alters, kept the capacity for tenderness and innocent joy, alive within my psyche. It also allowed me to express an important female part of my psyche.

For Dax and myself, the character of our alters is not random. It follows an unconscious logic. For example, for both of us, the gender of key alter(s) is the one that is psychologically safest. All Dax's alters are male. Dax, the host, is gay. He experienced the most wounding psychological abuse in childhood from his biological mother, making males a safer gender. It is the reverse for me. There was no abuse or violence in my childhood but there were no safe, embracing male role models. As a child, I was emotionally estranged from my father and afraid of him.

Our alters are permanent. Some therapists believe the outcome of successful therapy is that alters are fused into the undifferentiated Self. Some people with DID follow that route. Conversely, many seem to retain their alters, but build cooperative relationships with them. That's the way it is for Dax and myself. What peace I have with myself is the product of a long process to accept my subjective reality. Each alter represents an indispensable part of me. Dax and I both experience a suggestion or expectation our alters will, or should, disappear, as negating our identity. (See the discussion on the different expert views of alters in Chapter 14).

Relationships With Loved Ones

Alters have a big impact on our relationships with those closest to us, and in turn, those relationships have a big impact on our alters. It's a two-way street.

For people with DID, and ABs, there are two important factors which are not present in most other peoples' relationship with their partners.

Firstly, alters are fundamental to how a person experiences themselves and life, and there is a vast difference between having to conceal that fact and being able to share it. A partner's acceptance of the subjective reality of alters is a big issue. The process of reaching that acceptance is just as confronting, complicated and lengthy as it is for the person with the identity.

Secondly, with the presence of alters, the partnership is not just a one to one relationship, it is one to two or more. The relationship dynamics can get complicated. This aspect is succinctly highlighted in the comment by Dr Yeung –

"For DID patients, marriage is very complicated. It is often the case that some alters are very fond of the spouse while others are not."

There is an overlap between these two issues. For a partner who hasn't yet, or doesn't ever, accept alters are subjectively real, they are left with seeing their partner as 'bad' – moody, irritable, angry – or 'mad' – unstable, delusional etc. Even for an accepting partner, there can be a sense of loss for the person they thought they knew, bewilderment, and fear of where this is all leading.

For some people, either with DID, or ABs, it doesn't work out well. In three of the five DID autobiographies, the author's marriage did not survive the diagnosis and early treatment of DID. Dax's partner loves and accepts Dax but prefers to think of Dax's identity as autism rather than DID. For Dax, that leaves a space and a yearning.

Dax's marriage to his beloved first wife is an example of where a loving partner accepts the subjective reality of alters. Of the five autobiographies of people with DID, two had loving partners who supported them through diagnosis and treatment, and two others had second partnerships with people who accepted their DID. Three of the autobiographies show the giant leap of empathy and imagination an accepting partner makes – they have a relationship, not only with their partner's host personality but also with each of their alters. My wife accepts and relates to each of my alters. For every accepting partner, this represents a gift of the deepest and most healing love.

The issues and relationships between a partner and child alters is a related - but distinct - issue. That is discussed in the next chapter.

Summary

Both people with DID, and ABs, are multiples. Our sense of self is intertwined with our compelling experience of our subjectively real alters. Those alters process our sensory impressions according to their own unique characters, traits and histories. Each of our alters influence, and are influenced by, our relationships with others, especially loved ones.

9. Child Alters – The Key Similarity

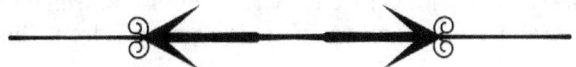

The most compelling similarities between people with DID, and ABs, can be seen in their child alters, and in the relationship between their child alters and their partners. These two aspects are discussed separately below.

DID Young Child Alters

<u>Child</u> alters are the defining characteristic of ABs.

But people with DID usually also have child alters. Dr Yeung says of the latter –

> *"Because the traumatic experiences occur primarily in childhood, child alters are almost always present. There are usually several of them. Each has his or her distinct characteristics and performs a specific function. … Most child alters are locked in their ages and never grow up."*

The public view of DID commonly focuses on the number of alters, and does not grasp that child alters are often central to the psyche of functional people with DID. Their experience of their child alters echoes that of ABs.

Dax says of his child alter -

> *"Dan is a child, I think around around 7, he loves the color red and dinosaurs. He likes to paint and role play, has lots of different voices. I know he plays with Aaron [Dax's baby son with his partner] a lot."*

We have already met Christine Pattillio's six-year-old alter, Chrissy, in the second chapter. Christine also has a delightful two year alter, Cyndi. Her autobiography provides the following accounts of Cyndi by her mother, Christine herself, and another of Christine's alters-

> *[Christine's mother says of a two-year-old child alter] "Cyndi could not walk, barely spoke, and on occasions wet her pants – ie. Christine's pants. This was not good. My daughter is a grown woman who could at any provocation turn into an infant sucking her thumb. That was a hard adjustment, but the more time I spent with Cyndi, the more I was amazed at all her little nonsense songs, her funny little sounds, and how she breathes while sleeping, so clearly a young child. It's been extraordinary watching her."*

> *[Christine says of Cyndi] "… Christopher, family and friends would try to let me know the minute I shifted back out after a visit from [by] Cyndi. Christopher would even videotape her and I would see myself singing and acting like a baby. I was mortified. I had visions of being out in public as this self-conscious, overweight, middle-aged woman sucking a thumb and peeing my pants. (Yes, Cyndi wasn't potty trained and we guess she was about two years old.)"*

> *['Q' one of Christine's alters, a young woman with a speech impediment describes an incident with Cyndi] "One day I at a craft store getting supplies for my business. Cyndi need go poop. Cyndi hates going big potty and cries and cries. I walk us to the restroom and shift Cyndi out. While Cyndi crying, 'No Poo Poo Koo', someone else enters the bathroom. Nothing can do so just let Cyndi stay out and fuss. I can't potty for her. After a few minutes, I hear woman asking if Cyndi OK. Cyndi keep crying. Woman ask if Cyndi want her to go get her Mommy. I think fast and shift back out saying, 'No I right here. She just not like go poop.' The woman laugh and tell me*

her grandson same. Now Cyndi done, but sit and wait for woman to leave. Was not sure what she might think if only me walk out of stall and no physical child."

The child alters of people with DID are subjectively real young children with similar capacities for wonder and fun, and similar needs for love and protection, as young biological children. This is understood by empathic mental health professionals and in DID self-help books.

Dr Yeung says –

> *"Child alters think, feel, speak, and sometimes write, as young children. This is how they see themselves, regardless of their chronological age. The therapist must refrain from judging or treating them as adults."*

The DID self-help book 'Got Parts: An Insider's Guide to Managing Life Successfully With Dissociative Identity Disorder', says of child alters -

> *"Remember to love, to cherish, to value these young parts. ... It can take great patience, finesse and wisdom to deal with wounded 'littles' ... Yet, as they realise the 'bigs' in the System [psyche] will keep them safe, the rewards are well worth the investment of time and effort as they shed layers of fear and distrust and to learn to be open and loving and inquisitive and playful as they do their own healing work."*

'Got Parts' goes on to discuss the need for an internal sanctuary within the mind, in terms which emphasize the needs of child alters –

> *"Within these guidelines, your 'dome' can contain within it anything that brings you all comfort, pleasure, peace and security. Do you want a reading area with a fireplace, an area to play or listen to music, a playground for the littles? Would you like to have a perpetual rainbow, or lots of soft, warm blankets and cuddly pillows, or a lake or pool to swim in? Would you like to have unicorns, hummingbirds, butterflies, or a gentle-to-the-System [psyche] but fiercely protective dinosaur? You may have it in your Dome."*

There is a striking similarity in the character and needs of the child alters of people with DID, to the child alters of ABs is striking.

The autobiographies of Christine Pattillo and Cameron West are exceptional in the warmth and openness with which they embrace and describe young child alters – in Christine's case, a baby alter. I wonder if their experiences might be less exceptional amongst people with DID than they seem. To publish an autobiography about DID in the face of deep misunderstanding takes great courage. I wonder if others have self-censored accounts of the character and needs of their young child alters for fear of exacerbating the stigma and ridicule amongst the uninformed.

This supposition is supported by the following comment in a recent (2016) text for therapists on dissociation -

> *"It is not uncommon for patients to report they have infant dissociative parts. Often, very young behaviours are associated with the activity of these parts, such as thumb sucking, rocking and bedwetting." [Treating Trauma Related Dissociation: A Practical Integrative Approach]*

DID Child Alters and Partners

Subjectively real child alters are similar to biological children. Typically they seek love and acceptance from the host's partner. Dax's description of the relationship between his loving wife and his 7-year-old child alter affirms this -

The Adult Baby – An Identity on the Dissociation Spectrum

"Amelia treated Dan like a loving protective big sister, with compassion and empathy. Dan's needs are simple, he needed to be shown kindness - being hugged, having a story read to him or just listening to music. Dan wanted someone to listen and help him understand why certain things happened."

A partner's acceptance of the existence and needs of child alters was central to the happiness of three of the five authors of DID autobiographies.

For Cameron West, the turning point in his journey with DID was his wife Rikki's loving embrace of his child alters. She had understandably held them at a distance to protect the couple's nine-year-old son, Kyle. The breakthrough came in a conversation between Cameron, Rikki and Cameron's psychiatrist Steve, cited below -.

[Steve asked Rikki] "What if you agreed to spend time with Cam's alters, say in the evening after Kyle's gone to bed. Give them some time out in the house. Help them feel accepted … not just by saying that they are, but by being with them. In exchange, we could ask them to wait until Kyle gets a little older before they meet him.

"What I'd like to do, Rikki," Steve continued, "is talk with Cam's alters, in particular with Clay [8 yo alter] and the other young ones, and see if they'd be willing to kind of watch out for Kyle and be his protectors, and know that you'll be their friend and protector after Kyle goes to bed and he's not around."

"Steve, that's an excellent idea," Rikki said excitedly. "I'd be happy to spend time with Cam's guys. I'd do it every night. …"

[Cameron] Suddenly the world was in color again. Inside Clay was telling Per yes, he'd do that, he'd be Kyle's protector, and Switch [8 yo] was saying the same thing, and Wyatt [10 yo] too, they were puffing their chests out like they were the new sheriffs in town. And Dusty [12 yo girl alter] was even saying she'd like to be able to talk to Rikki. …

She said, "I promise to talk to everyone at night after Kyle's gone to bed."
"Oh God, Rik", I [Cameron] said, tears forming in my eyes. "That'd be wonderful."

She said, "I want everyone inside to know that I'd appreciate it tremendously if they'll kind of watch out for Kyle and go in when he's around, at least until he's old enough to understand a little better. And I'll be their friend and talk to them when he's not around, even if it's during the day. Okay?"

Then Clay switched out and said in his little voice, "Okay. L-like a sheriff, right Rikki? To watch out for Kyle."

Rikki laughed. "Yup, Clay. Just like a sheriff." ['First Person Plural: My Life As a Multiple']

After being tormented by her DID Christine Pattillo arrived at a place of happiness and contentment based on the warm acceptance of her alters, especially her child alters, by herself and her loving husband Christopher. This is described below -

[One of Christine's other alters, says] "Most nights, it's Cita [Christine Pattillo] who is physically shifted out and sleeping in bed next to her husband. The rest of us snuggle down in our own beds [in the sanctuary in Christine's mind]. It is common for the two youngest, Cyndi the [2 yo] baby and [6 yo] Chrissy, to shift out and say their goodnights to Christopher."

"… it's as harmonious as it gets for us. That is, until Cyndi, the youngest alter, all of about two years old, wakes and shouts, "Pee Pee Poppi, Pee Pee!" ("Poppi" is Christopher.) Then

of course, one of us is shifting out and taking us to the restroom before Cyndi takes a leak in Cita's pyjamas. Yes, that has happened a time or two. ..."

Christopher says of Chrissy – "If I gently touch her arm she'll continue to sleep, but then she quietly says, "That's My Christopher." If I tickle her, she busts a gut laughing. She won't wake up and I'm warmed by her own special giggle. I feel as close to her then as if I'm sitting right next to her in her internal bedroom. Chrissy has an extraordinary ability to touch my heartstrings, the high pitches and low tones that no one else can play.

But he also had to work extremely hard on his patience:

Christopher: I was now a first-time father and I had to learn to reach her on her own level. Chrissy's feelings were easily hurt and there were times when I would accidently squish them. I was learning how to be around a small child. I became aware of how frightened she became when I sounded too harsh or used profanity." ['I Am We: My Life With Multiple Personalities']

Robert Oxnam, a more controlled and status focused person, also cites his second wife's loving embrace of his alters, especially his child alter, as a turning point in his life.

AB Child Alters and Partners

We can compare the above accounts with several from the partners of regressive ABs.

The first is by 'Kayley' and refers to her AB husband's 'Little', a toddler named Jenny –

"It took me a long time to connect with my husband's toddler inner child especially since she is a girl inside! At first it seemed like I would never find her and he would never find me, but eventually, we connected, and things just started to happen. ... Jenny bubbled out all this stuff about his own mother who was distant and uninvolved and how he felt cheated out of a mother. ... He cried for hours as he just dumped all this raw emotion onto me about never feeling properly loved. ... it was pretty clear that he wanted me to pretty much assume a genuine step-mother/adoptive mother with him. ... I decided to informally adopt Baby Jenny as my daughter and then set about working out how to do it. ... Since then the relationship has just blossomed. I think by adopting her I now feel free to be her mommy in every aspect when she is a Little. And when she is my husband again I still feel this special bond that extends beyond the norm. ... as far as we are concerned, Jenny is my REAL daughter and we wouldn't have it any other way. A new complication arrived a year later in the form of twins. But even though I have real children, I still have a child who is every bit as real to me, and while the twins will grow up and out, Jenny will not. My daughter is mine for good. ['There's Still A Baby in My Bed' – Case Studies]

The second is by the wife of an AB named 'Joe', and refers to her husband's Little, 'Joey' –

"... He also very slowly and carefully let me know he has a thing for diapers. ... I did understand where it was coming from as I know the extremely long history of abuse that started when he was 2 years old. The other tell tale sign that this had a much deeper cause was the frustration fits that were thrown. Joe would get so mad and worked up when he was stressed that he would basically throw a temper tantrum. If I managed to get to hold him he would calm down and snuggle into me. He would put his thumb in his mouth and curl up with me and stay that way for up to an hour sometimes. This was the start of me understanding his deep need to regress especially after a wet lap a few times.

The Adult Baby – An Identity on the Dissociation Spectrum

Some people may not believe in regression, but Joe is two different personalities. It isn't as far as a multiple personality, but a toddler version of him. Knowing it has had more than its challenges, but also benefits to both of us. His two big conflicts where admitting he had a need to regress and dealing with how deep his need for diapers is. It became much more obvious to me how much happier and relaxed the adult Joe was when he had a diaper on. It made a huge difference in our relationship and his stress levels. The diapers seemed to tie both worlds together. Joe accepts that there is a little inside and Joey feels that he is accepted and has a place in our lives and a tie to the outside world." ['There's Still A Baby in My Bed' – Case Studies]

In the above account, Joe's wife rejects the idea his Little represents multiple personalities. I suspect this echoes the views of many other ABs and their partners. It reflects a misunderstanding that only people with DID / MPD have alters. As we have seen, this is not the case. It is notable the account includes key features of a dissociated identity – childhood abuse and trauma; and a personality distinct from Joe's adult self which manifests beyond conscious control, with its own infantile needs.

In her groundbreaking self-help book for the partners of ABs, Rosalie Bent says -

"There is a very special kind of relationship that can exist between a loving couple, where one of them is a regressive adult baby, or what I call a 'little one'. … It is what I call the Parent/Child relationship and it is where you have a deep, meaningful and substantive relationship, not just with your adult partner, but also with their Inner Child (or Baby) as well. … The Parent/Child relationship operates at two basic levels. In the primary level, you will relate to your partner as adult to adult, just as you do right now. The secondary level is where you relate to your Little One as a child or infant, with you as their parent.

If there is one aspect of the Parent/Child relationship that is truly unique, it is the depth of interaction that can eventuate from it. Within a functioning Parent/Child relationship, there can be a level of communication between two souls which can be truly unique and exquisite. … Rather than treat regression as a curse, it should be treated as an opportunity to have a relationship that combines the very best of both worlds [ie adult to adult; adult to child] …
['There's Still A Baby in My Bed']

My wife and I now accept my alters. She is not a mother or caregiver to my alters, but more like a kind and fun-loving aunt. I don't have to hide my alters and she is no longer afraid of my identity. That is wonderful - liberating, healing and life-changing. I have greater contentment and happiness than at any previous time in my life.

Similarities In Relations With Partners

There are compelling similarities between people with DID and ABs, in terms of relations between partners and child alters.

In the negative, child alters desperately want love and kindness, but can be vulnerable, fearful and skittish. They will commonly quickly withdraw in the face of any sign of rejection by partners. (In the early days, those signs are typically of the behaviours of the child alter, rather than of their explicit existence.) The hurt and anger that comes from such interactions can be disruptive to a relationship and typically misunderstood by a partner as immaturity, petulance or moodiness. It can be awful for all concerned.

In the positive, a partner's acceptance of a person's child alters is transformative. There is a striking similarity between the two identities in the descriptions of a partner's acceptance. All these partners discerned their loving acceptance of their spouse's subjective reality was make-or-break for both their spouse's psychological health, and their marriage/relationship. In each case, the partner's acceptance was an act of courage, empathy and love.

The Adult Baby – An Identity on the Dissociation Spectrum

The renown psychotherapist Donald Winnicott lets us understand how a partner's acceptance works psychologically. It fits with Winnicott's widely accepted concept of transitional phenomena. Things as diverse as a baby's security blanket, child's play, and all culture such as sports, politics and religion, belong to the category of transitional phenomena. Such phenomena are neither wholly subjective (solely inside the mind) nor wholly objective (physically tangible) – but somewhere in between. We can tacitly agree with others to invest shared activities with common meanings which are not inherent in objective forms. Winnicott says of transitional phenomena (here called 'intermediate' phenomena) -

> *"Should an adult make claims on us for our acceptance of the objectivity of his subjective phenomena we discern or diagnose madness. If, however, the adult can manage to enjoy the personal intermediate area without making claims, then we can acknowledge our own corresponding intermediate areas, and are pleased to find a degree of overlapping, that is to say common experience between members of a group in art or religion or philosophy."* [Playing and Reality]

For people with DID, or ABs, alters are subjectively real – to them. But if they insist that anyone else take that alter as objective reality ie. the same as a biological child or person, then people will perceive them as mentally ill (this is discussed in Chapter 15). However, a person with DID, or an AB, who is happier, more vital, because they have accepted their own subjective reality, invites a partner to share an intermediate or transitional space – where the person and their partner accept the alters are subjectively real to the former. That can be a healthy, happy space as per the above.

A Difference

There are many similarities between people with DID, and ABs, in terms of the relationship between their partners and their child alters. One difference is I did not come across any reference to power exchange in the relations between people with DID and their partners. Power exchange refers to dominance/submission practices where one adult sometimes exercises authority over a consenting partner in a manner outside normal, equal relations between adult peers eg. one person taking the parent role and treating the other like a child. Dominant Daddy/Little Girl (DDLG) is an example of a power exchange relationship. On-line many ABs seem to have or seek DDLG relationships – or the gender converse, variously identified as Dominant Mummy or Caregiver / Little Boy, or similar. These relationship patterns are found within and beyond the ABDL community.

I suspect the presence or absence of doubt is responsible for this difference between the two populations. People with DID have less cause to doubt the subjective reality of being a multiple with child alters. They will often have a diagnosis by a mental health professional. Prior to diagnosis and treatment, they and their partners will often have lived through the trauma of amnesiac alters with uncontrolled triggering and switching. After that DID is all too real. They have tangible indications they are dealing with a subjectively real child.

By comparison, being AB is regarded as a fetish or a kink. Those are labels which explain nothing. Both are pretty flimsy hooks on which to hang the challenging subjective reality of child alters who need regular nurturing for the AB to avoid becoming neurotic. So for both the AB and their partner, there is doubt about what being AB *really* is, and no model for the place of child alters in a partnership. I suspect some people fill in the gap with power exchange relationship models. Those are borrowed from sexual fetishism and bondage and discipline (B&D). Power exchange relationships become a vehicle for the acceptance and nurturing of dissociated child alters within a partnership.

The downside of power exchange relationship models is they further fetishize being AB through dominance and submission practices borrowed from B&D. Secondly, it can foster the perspective the AB's partner is the primary source of nurturing and parenting for the AB's child alter. In a psychologically healthy multiple that role belongs to the multiple's adult host (see the discussion in Chapter 15.) This is why it is important to understand being AB is an identity on the dissociation spectrum. It gives ABs and their partners greater capacity to choose relationship models which do not borrow inappropriately from fetishism.

Summary

The overlap between people with DID and ABs is strikingly clear in their experience of child alters. Some of the accounts of child alters I have read could be transposed from people with DID to ABs, or vice versa, and people of the other identity would not readily pick the difference. For both identities, a loving partner's acceptance of child alters is affirming and healing. It is often a turning point in people's lives.

10. Alters Don't Stand Still

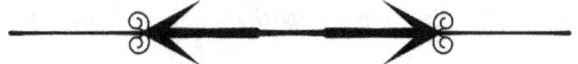

Alters are subjectively real.

They are not metaphorical in the same way as the 'inner child' of a singleton. They have their own personality, their own perspective on life, their own needs, their own virtues and vices. Alters are an 'engine room' of the psyche of multiples. They drive change in our sense of self, and in what we want and get from life.

It starts with our alters breaking through the repression that kept them hidden in our sub-conscious. That forces us to come to terms with their existence and their needs. The dynamism continues after we have accepted ourselves as multiples. These processes of change are discussed below.

Coming to Terms with Alters

Coming to terms with our alters was a long and complex process for Dax and myself.

I believe people with DID, and ABs, go through the same stages of accepting their identity as other people with a minority identity. That process moves through stages of initial discovery and confusion, denial, ambivalence, reluctant acceptance, to full acceptance and pride, and hopefully, finally to a transcendent view which sees the commonalities across different identities. These follow the six stages of identity formation described by Dr Viv Cass in her widely accepted *'Theory of Lesbian and Gay Identity Formation'*. (See my book *'The Adult Baby Identity – Coming Out As An AB'* for a discussion of Dr Cass' theory and its application to ABs.)

For people with DID, and ABs, the different stages of identity formation can best be seen in their acceptance of their alters. Some, like Christine Patillo and Cameron West, end up warmly accepting their alters. They explore and celebrate their individual character, give them personal names, schedule 'out' time to enjoy activities, and share them with partners and close family. In short, they proudly celebrate their alters.

Others like Herschel Walker and Olga Trujillo seem more ambivalent. They appear to hold their alters at a distance. The alters' character remains an outline, defined only by their behaviours, or function or dysfunction in the psyche. The alters are given only functional labels like 'the consoler,' rather than personal names, or they are identified only by their age. This seems to apply even for child alters.

The difference between tolerating and warmly embracing alters seems to be reflected in the person's experience of life. Christine Pattillo and Cameron West's books show personal destinations lit by warmth, optimism and openness. This is despite overcoming earlier torment with their identities and childhood trauma. There is a kind of equality between their adult host personality and their alters.

The other autobiographies of people with DID are different. Their personal destinations don't seem as warm and buoyant. They seem to place greater emphasis on the outward control and success of the adult host personality, and hold the child alters at arm's length. Dr Ross refers to this phenomena as 'host resistance', and describes it as follows -

> *"The problem of host resistance is a frequent theme in the treatment of DID. … the host personality often believes that she is 'the person' and the alters are second class citizens with no rights. This is a form of resistance. All the parts are parts of the whole – the host is just the part who has the job of being the host. There is only one person, but she is fragmented into parts who think they are separate from each other. …*

The Adult Baby – An Identity on the Dissociation Spectrum

*The host commonly thinks that the alters are the problem, when actually they are
holding intolerable feelings, conflict and memories so the host can function in the outside world.
Also, often, they are reacting to rejection and devaluation by the host.*

*"It is important to remind yourself that DID work is the same as work with a non-DID
person, just broken into parts. Developing empathy for the self, treating the self more kindly,
accepting rather than avoiding difficult feelings, taking responsibility for one's actions, learning
self-soothing, and so on, are basic recovery tasks for anyone. The same is true for people with
DID."*

ABs seem to span a similar spectrum in terms of their relationship with their child alters. That ranges from embracing to just tolerance.

Some alters can have dysfunctional behaviours. This is particularly so before self-acceptance and healing. There can be a fierce conflict between alters and some can be abusive and damaging to others. Christine Pattillo and Robert Oxnam describe how some of their alters would terrorise others. The abusive alters represented the internalized negative feelings from abuse or trauma. Often the child alters are on the wrong end of those conflicts. All of that is tormenting for the whole psyche. In my case there was a horrible three-cornered conflict between a punitive parent alter, my child alters and my adult host personality. (This is described in my book *'The Adult Baby Identity – A Self Help Guide'*.)   Dax had similar experiences with his alters.

For Dax and myself, our alters held the trauma from the original events which led to their splitting from our psyches. For Dax, those are deep wounds from childhood abuse. Those wounds never fully heal. Dax has learned to live with them. Likely that is why amnesia continues to have such a large part in his psyche. Dax does not dwell on these matters, I believe because he does not wish to be defined by them. Instead, he focuses on living with his DID the best way he can.

For Dax and myself, psychological health came from accepting our alters as real, and building a cooperative relationship with them. Our alters influence our feelings, thoughts, actions, our sense of self, and our experience of the world on an hourly and daily basis. Not accepting something that powerful and pervasive within our own psyche would cause us psychological harm.

For Dax, with DID, that acceptance is literally a matter of life and death. He explains -

*"Most, if not all, of the other DID sufferers we encountered over 30 years ago have died,
some through old age, most through suicide. Many people fail to understand and integrate their
alters. Most develop a psychosis that drives them mad. So their DID in a collective sense,
consumed them."*

For both of us, getting to know our alters was a lengthy process. Alters don't jump out and announce themselves like the genie-in-a-bottle in Aladdin. Alters are a product of our sub-conscious. Before we accepted our identities, we experienced our alters only as disruptive, incomprehensible behaviours, at odds with our adolescent or adult personality. We didn't connect those behaviours with our alters. It was only after we accepted our alters as real that we could really start to get to know them. Each is as unique as our host personality. They are multi-dimensional with their own likes, dislikes, fears, 'hot buttons', virtues and vices.

Starting when Dax was diagnosed with DID as a teenager, with therapy and the support of his adoptive parents, he developed a cooperative relationship between his alters. He explains -

*"There are 9 alters. Through a lot of therapy, support and hard work their roles have
become very clear over the past 30 years. Each has a particular skill, trait or characteristic and is
signified by the tattoo on my hand. The tattoo is a reminder that we are more than one..we are
the sum of each of us. When the "Power of Nine" was built over many years, we were each asked
to describe who we felt we were, each of us had therapy time explaining how important our roles
where. I feel that it gave us a sense of responsibility that we respected because we were*

recognized. It took a huge amount of time and money to map through...lots of dead ends, negativity from the alters and silence.

Enlightened medical professionals who accept the subjective reality of alters, recommend people with DID seek this kind of cooperative relationship with their alters. (For example, see psychiatrist David Yeung's books cited in the reading list.) Rosalie Bent urges the same approach for ABs, to accept and come to terms with their child personas.

For me, as an AB, accepting my alters wasn't a matter of death, but it was a matter of life - the difference between a happy fulfilled life, and neurosis. In the latter, doubt, self-loathing and anger intermittently but persistently tormented my mind, spirit, and marriage. Accepting my baby alter, Chrissie, as real, lead to positive and powerful cognitive and behavioural changes. I would never have anticipated the strength of those changes and the power of self-acceptance. The compulsive behaviours that formerly tyrannized my life disappeared. That includes compulsive masturbation, involuntary 'triggering', the 'binge and purge' cycle, a shopping addiction (for baby clothes), and psychologically unsafe fantasies. All gone! Try changing that with just will power (not happening)! In its place there is a comfort and safety with myself, that has extended to my marriage.

Having accepted my alters, I have looked back over my life with different eyes. I am beginning to see how, even when they were unrecognized, they played a big part in my experience of self and life. It's a bit like the way a person who discovers in mid-life they were adopted, looks back and re-interprets their life. Herschel Walker's autobiography is a good example of the retrospective application of this new perspective.

Alters Are Dynamic

For Dax and I, the presence of alters within our psyches changes and grows stronger through life. My reading suggests that is often true of people with DID, and ABs.

These changes are driven by three things –

1. the erosion of the repression that concealed the full presence and character of our alters;
2. changes in external circumstances, especially less necessity for concealment; and
3. self-acceptance.

Each of these is discussed below.

The presence and character of our alters are progressively revealed by the erosion of repression within our psyches. Childhood dissociation has a deep and pervasive effect on the psyche. The repression of dissociation in the unconscious breaks down very slowly, often over many years and decades, well into later life. The erosion of the repression does not proceed at a uniform pace. Crises in life, especially in mid-life, can suddenly release chunks of repressed memory and the expression of alters. But in my experience, rarely all of it at once. The rest, especially the full character of alters, continues to slowly come to the surface in an intermittent series of quietly surprising insights and subtle changes. Four years after the therapy where I first fully accepted my alters, this is still happening for me. Herschel Walker indicated it was still happening for him ten years after his DID was diagnosed. It was similar in Christine Pattillo's account.

Rosalie Bent, addressing the partners of ABs, discusses this dynamic in a manner I find consistent with the progressive emergence of a repressed alter -

"The truth of the matter is that the extent of the regression for a Little One does progress over time. ... The real question however is: does it expand regardless of what you do? And the answer is a qualified yes. The needs and behaviours of the Little are constantly evolving, even if sometimes quite slowly. Different circumstances develop different needs and wants. New experiences alter their feelings and perceptions. In short, like any biological child, your partner is changing. The difference is, that while a biological child matures, the Little One generally

remains the same basic age. What does change, however, is the expression of that age. He will add new behaviours, modify others, and remove some altogether."

Change is also driven by our external circumstances. Our alters have been held back by fear and necessity. When those inhibiting factors abate, the presence of our alters grows stronger. Rosalie Bent recognized the extent and character of an AB's child self grows and develops over time, and it is often held back by circumstance rather than choice.

Felix Conrad in his book '*How to Jedi Mind Trick Your Gender Dsyphoria*' describes a parallel in the way external circumstances influence the expression of transgender people. He says the conformity involved in full-time, out-of-home work, conflicts with the expression of self for transgender people. That was also true of me as an AB. It is not just the constraint to present as 'normal' while at work. Mostly it was how that lifestyle suppressed, 24/7, the space in my psyche I could afford to give my alters. It was only after I retired from my job a few years ago that changed. My principal child alter, Chrissie, now takes a large space in my daily life in a way that would have been impossible before I retired. Only arriving at that point has created a feeling of a stable, safe and cooperative co-existence. Dax is currently on the cusp of shifting to working from home. The prospect of greater freedom for those of his alters that have had to stay more in the background, is both welcome and a source of concern.

The authors of four of the five DID autobiographies describe making changes to their careers after the diagnosis and acceptance of themselves as multiples. In part or whole that was to allow greater space and freedom for their alters.

Self-acceptance also drives change. In my case, I got tired of being hostage to fear about others finding out about my identity. I set much of that fear aside. I don't mean to court harm by 'outing' my identity in an unsafe way. But in the safety of my private life, I find happiness and contentment in giving space for my alters to be themselves – for me to be me. I am well into the second half of my life. I have a sense of '*if not now, when?*' I suspect that is true for many people with any form of non-conforming sense of self.

Living in an accepting household lets alters feel safe and express their personalities more. This is not just a conscious process. I can provide an example. When I was writing this book my wife spontaneously pointed out one of my latest mannerisms. Sometimes when I am standing, I find myself absentmindedly taking the sides of the hem of my T-shirt in each hand. With kind laughter my wife observed it was the sort of thing a little girl would do with her dress. It was initially completely unconscious on my part. Now I am aware, it feels very Chrissie (my baby girl alter).

Nature of Changes

The shifts described above, are in turn, reflected in changes within, and between alters. The changes can include -

1. some alters heal and transform positively;
2. some alters can disappear or fuse with another;
3. at the most extreme, the function of host personality can shift from the birth personality to an alter, or from one alter to another;
4. alters, singly and as a community, can 'relapse' to previous dysfunctional behaviours in the face of neglect, or denial by ourselves; and
5. alters can get out of balance, just like any biological personality.

Each of these is discussed below.

The most positive change is the way alters can heal with self-acceptance, the acceptance of partners or therapy. This leads to a transformation of alters from angry or frightened with dysfunctional behaviours, to being happy and settled. Christine Pattillo, Cameron West and Robert Oxnam describe such transformations and how that powerfully changed their lives for the better. Some had formerly harsh or angry adolescent or adult alters who transformed into protectors and nurturers of their child alters. They each had child alters who became sources of innocent joy. Christine Pattillo provides a vivid account of how those transformations were experienced by the alters themselves. I believe this trajectory can be seen for each AB who's life has been transformed by self-acceptance. When I didn't recognize or accept her, my baby girl alter, Chrissie, was alternately frightened and needy, or a tantrum-throwing brat. Now she is happy and content, secure in the knowledge she is loved and protected by myself and my wife. The change in Chrissie has transformed my life.

In the process of change, some alters can disappear or fuse with another. This is linked to the process of healing. How it plays out seems to be different for each person. Robert Oxnam describes how most of his original alters fused with the one's that remained, the positive capabilities of the former now accessed by the latter. Christine Pattillo describes how a beloved female alter passed away when her protecting and nurturing role was taken over by Christine as she grew stronger. Cameron West indicates now he has healed, some of his most wounded alters are rarely seen anymore. I suspect that after I accepted myself as a multiple and retired, an unnamed punitive alter that was focused on duty in my vocation has integrated or fused with my birth-host personality.

The extreme form of change is when the host personality changes. It can move to or from the birth personality to an alter, or from one alter to another. This is the case with Dax. It is not applicable to the vast majority of ABs. Yet it may be relevant in some rare examples. This issue is discussed in Chapter 11.

When there is a life crisis or a reversal of progress in self-acceptance alters can revert to former dysfunctional feeling states, behaviours and conflicts with each other. Alters are subjectively real. When they are neglected and disregarded they react badly. Robert Oxnam gives an example of how such a relapse undid much of the healing he had accomplished and threatened his marriage and his life.

Alters are also like any other biological personalilty, they go through ups and down, times when they are happy and content and times where they are selfish and 'off beam'. Remember our alters are present 24/7 processing the same sensory impressions and life experiences as our adult host. Life is a moving picture and our alters move with it.

For ABs, this dynamic is even more true of our child alters. Their senses, experiences and reactions can be more vivid than those of adult personalities. Self-accepting ABs love their Littles as the apple-of-their-eye. In the positive, they bring the joy and contentment of well-loved children. But sometimes, an AB's adult host can be overindulgent and over permissive, spoiling our child alters. And like biological children that can sometimes make them spoilt brats - greedy, selfish and demanding.

Summary

Alters are dynamic – they drive change in the psyches of multiples. That is clear in the process of coming to terms with being a multiple. But it continues after self-acceptance. As a multiple, we experience life through the kaleidoscope view of each of our alters. And each can bring change to our life as a multiple.

11. DID and Being AB Are <u>Not</u> The Same

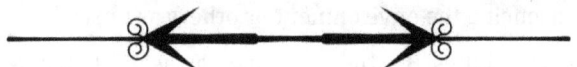

We have seen powerful similarities between the two identities, but DID and being AB are NOT the same.

This chapter focuses on the key differences between the two identities. For Dax and myself, these include -

1.   the origins of our identities;
2.   the nature of the division in our psyches;
3.   the complexity of relationships within our psyches; and
4.   the psychological function served by our identities.

Let's look at each of these in turn.

Origins

There is a difference in the origin of Dax's DID and my identity as an AB. For Dax, DID had its source in severe and repeated physical, sexual and psychological abuse in childhood. Dax's experience is representative. The ISSTD's 2010 Guidelines states -

> *"DID develops during the course of childhood, and clinicians have rarely encountered cases of DID that derive from adult-onset trauma (unless it is superimposed on preexisting childhood trauma and preexisting latent or dormant fragmentation)."*

The DSM-5 indicates childhood abuse is present in 90% of people with DID (cited in the Wikipedia article on DID). Dax has learned to live with those wounds, but they may be too deep to fully heal. They leave a legacy that forever contests with hope and joy. The idea of suicide never completely goes away (for one or more of his alters).

DID can have other childhood origins. For example, Herschel Walker cites a temporary separation from his mother after birth, and severe and prolonged bullying and ostracism in primary school, as the origin of his DID. (He also witnessed a terrifying assault by hooded Klu Klux Klan thugs as a six-year-old which may have contributed). Dr Yeung states –

> *"Deprivation of emotional support in a child's early years can constitute a passive type of severe abuse powerful enough to result in pathological dissociation."*

For me, the child alters that are my AB identity, came from being traumatized by the 'ordinary catastrophes' of childhood (as detailed in chapter 6). There was no abuse or neglect. Based on posts in on-line ABDL forums, I believe these ordinary catastrophes of childhood are a more typical origin for ABs than child abuse.

The Nature of Division Within the Psyche

Dax experiences DID as a pervasive fragmentation of his psyche. By contrast, before self-acceptance, I experienced being an AB as a conflicted Jekyll-and-Hyde duality. Fragmentation is a lot more damaging and difficult to heal than duality.

When I was conflicted, I experienced being AB as a competing dual nature – adult versus child. Was I an adult or a child? How could I be both? Did the baby side of me mean I was a failed adult? (For a full discussion of the symptoms of this conflict see my book *'The Adult Baby Identity – A Self Help Guide'*.) Although the duality could be tormenting at times, it was not fragmentation. The bugbear for me was identity confusion, not amnesia.

My only amnesia was the repression of the original childhood trauma and the existence of my alters. In the present, my alters are all co-conscious. I suspect it is the same for most ABs. Even when I was conflicted, I had the benefit of a consoling faith and a distinct sense of a higher self. I had only moderate levels of depersonalization and no significant derealization (experiencing the environment or others as unreal).

My alters have distinct personalities. But there is some permeability between their character and my host personality. That's because memory is shared and the original trauma is largely healed. That permeability is shown in several ways.

Firstly, communication within my psyche is non-verbal - 'sensed' rather than heard. My alters are not so distinct from my host personality that I hear a concrete dialogue with them.

Secondly, my child alters influence traits in my adult host (and presumably vice versa). For example, my principal child alter is a baby girl, and my adult host now identifies much more with the perspective of women in politics. I have also come to prefer girls as the leading protagonists in the young adult fiction I like to read, and to write.

Thirdly, my adult host personality is *co-present* with my alters. That is a term used by psychiatrist Colin Ross to indicate both sharing the sensations and control of the body. For example, now I am retired I don't always shave every day. My adult male host self is untroubled by short bristly stubble but my baby girl alter doesn't like the feel or appearance of it.

This permeability is characteristic of sub-DID dissociation – OSDD (Other Specified Dissociative Disorder). Rosalie Bent identified this permeability (described as behavioural leakage or crossover) as a characteristic of ABs. For me, this permeability means the experience of living with alters doesn't feel fragmented. After accepting my identity, I experience being AB and a multiple as a loving internal family lead by my adult host.

Co-presence produces a different experience of alters in ABs than for many people with DID. Let me explain. In both identities, alters are present 24/7 and potentially can trigger and come 'out' at any time. For people with DID with amnesia, if an alter is 'out' it controls the thoughts, feelings, perceptions and actions of the person to the exclusion of the other personalities.

It's different for self-accepting ABs. Amnesia is not an issue. So once an AB accepts their 'Little', that alter is commonly co-present with the host. Co-presence also happens for people with DID who heal their trauma. But the special character of ABs is their child alters are commonly very young – infants or toddlers. So the unique character of a self-accepting AB is co-habiting your body with an incontinent small child almost 24/7. The longer an AB has accepted their Little the stronger than sense of co-habitation grows.

I believe that explains why self-accepting ABs progress to wearing nappies for longer periods each day. Some ABs need to wear nappies 24/7. The co-presence of an incontinent toddler may have an adverse effect on continence (as with Christine Pattillo and her alter Cyndi) – although for many ABs the co-present adult self maintains continence. But whether continent or incontinent, wearing nappies for an extended period meets an emotional need. It is the need of the co-present child alter for a physical sensation which is familiar and comforting. This is true for me. I sleep every night and spend most mornings in a nappy. The co-presence of my baby alter also explains why the constant presence of a comforting array of stuffed toys in my bedroom, and the nappy bucket in the laundry, have such a soothing effect.

Because their psyches aren't fragmented, ABs are also less likely to experience an alter unilaterally taking executive control of their body from their host. That is generally uncommon for ABs, but it does happen. It happens in periods of high stress or triggering, probably related to the original trauma. The example of Joanne, the baby girl alter traumatized by a nighttime storm cited in Chapter 2 fits the latter circumstance. Before I understood and accepted myself as a multiple, I experienced these changes in executive control in the 'binge and purge' cycle or in confronting social situations (as discussed in Chapter 4). Curiously, I believe that the circumstance where ABs generally experience changes in executive control is sex (as discussed in Chapter 16).

In contrast, for Dax, every day is a struggle to pull the pieces of his fragmented psyche together. That fragmentation is driven by–

- amnesia which divides the real-time memories of some of the alters, and limits the cooperation between them; and
- derealisation and depersonalization, the sense the world and the self, respectively, are not real, caused by the amnesia.

This fragmentation is driven by the extent of his childhood trauma. Dax says of his amnesia-

> *"compartmentalised memory was our bodies response to memories that couldn't be processed. they are not forgotten, not resolved and will be forever with us. they hang over us like a hangman's noose!"*

For Dax, that trauma is an insurmountable obstacle to faith in a divinity. He has a diffuse sense of his higher self. There is limited co-consciousness and no co-presence between alters. Dax experiences his alters as highly distinct from the host, and 'hears' concrete dialogues between alters. He says -

> *"... there is often noise, voices in my head. I tended to regard these as the alters talking but it could be my conscious, subconscious and co-conscious thoughts are fighting to be heard. Filtering them out is not easy and when it gets too invasive we tend to switch."*

Dax's verbatim descriptions provide a compelling understanding of what it is like to live with a fragmented psyche.

> *"We switch about 4/5 times a day. This occurs when a situation becomes unbearable for the conscious alter, or there is a trigger that causes the switching or a change of environment, or the one most common to us on a daily basis, is the changing of roles due to the time of day. We have no idea, who will be conscious when. The concept of time means nothing. I refer to time as being 'present' and 'lost' time. I guess I'm [Dax] present maybe a few hours a day or not at all, depends on triggers.*
>
> *I have a fractured perspective of any given day, week, month; memories are broken, incomplete or not there at all (amnesia). As many of us are conscious over any given period of time, no one has the complete picture, emotional reactions are often missing or inappropriate decisions are made when only some of the facts are known to the conscious alter.*
>
> *How do you stand in front of someone and tell them you have no idea what they are talking about yet they are adamant you had a conversation not 3 hours ago... trying to explain that it was with another alter, seems farcical, comedy to the extreme !!*
>
> *So we are spectators in our own lives. Because nothing is real, we try to fill in the gaps by reading body language, guessing some responses or just passing over certain things or people as irrelevant.*
>
> *Daily life is chaotic, disjointed and often it's hard to decide what was thought, what was a recalled memory and what is an action. So when I stress and worry, I was always taught to rehearse what you want to say but after lots of repetition and if the stress remains or the day ends for me, I never know whether that thought became an action and then a memory. Hence, this fugue state of existence means that most things seem unreal because you're never 100% sure that the action happened.*

The Adult Baby – An Identity on the Dissociation Spectrum

We are constantly detached from environments we should know and the people we interact with. Think of this as Groundhog Day occurring over several days/weeks. We don't relive the same day over and over but we do continue to make the same mistakes because we are disconnected, no one and nothing is familiar. It causes us to become distressed and in its severest form causes trauma.

Dissociation unplugs us from our own senses, dulling or even removing altogether our sight (I am often blind, unable to read or focus). De-realisation occurs often, where we feel totally disconnected from the world around us, it feels like being in a dream. Nothing feels 'real'. This may not sound so bad but it is very distressing.

Throw 500 jigsaw pieces in the air many times, each time they land you are left with a completely different pattern. That's what fragmentation is like for us. I'm trying to make sense of everything ..with a constantly changing set of data.

We are probably awake on average 16-18+ hours a day, consume massive amounts of information, are constantly trying to find ways to be safe."

Dax uses 'Post-It' notes to communicate between alters that are barely co-conscious. One alter will write a 'stickie' to another. Dax explains –

"these are simple messages, a few words, a song title, a keyword, a number, a cash figure....but rarely a sentence. Unfortunately, too often we ignore a message meant for us, so during the time of high volume interactions and at certain times of the year..it can fail as we simply forget.

We do not have any link or awareness of the actions of each other. These events are compartmentalized within each of us. If we have been respectful and followed protocol then someone will leave a " stickie" to prompt/ remind one of us to follow up on something. Let me explain – I [Dax] can make a conscious decision to drive to the shops, but I will not make the decision to go to the ATM and withdraw cash. Jinx is responsible and retains knowledge of codes, pins, passwords, internet access addresses..etc although I'm aware of the banking Apps on our iPad.

The experience of time loss due to amnesia and switching is characteristic of DID. Dr Yeung says -

"Most of us have experienced situations in which time seems to disappear, such as when we are driving long distances or deeply absorbed in something we enjoy. … Qualities of time-loss characteristic of DID are different, and returning to the ordinary experience of time is a terrifying jolt. After conventional experiences of time loss, we do not find ourselves with cigarettes in our pocket when we are confirmed non-smokers, nor are we greeted by people we do not know who obviously know us by a different name."

Dax's perspective lets us see how disorientating and painful this experience can be –

"We have no idea, who will be conscious when. The concept of time means nothing. I refer to time as being " Present" and " Lost" time. I guess I'm present maybe a few hours a day or not at all, depends on triggers. We never wear a watch or have any clocks visible on the walls. Clocks represent pain, isolation and loneliness."

Dax's experience shows it is the traumatizing effect of living with amnesia on a daily basis which drives de-personalisation and de-realisation. It is unhealed childhood trauma and the amnesia it produces, which is the debilitating component of DID, rather than identity alteration or alters, per se.

The Complexity of Relationships Within the Psyche

The relationships between alters within Dax's psyche are more complex than they are for me. In this, we are representative of our respective identities.

The relationships within my psyche are straight forward. I have three alters. They all 'split' from my host-birth personality. All are co-conscious, that is they share memories. While my principal alter, the youngest, a baby girl, is the most prominent in my psyche, there is no hierarchy or sub-systems within my psyche.

In DID terms, Dylan is both my birth and host personality. I have never felt the need or inclination for my birth personality to relinquish being my host personality. All my alters are pre-adolescent children who cannot negotiate the adult world unaided. Any suggestion of relinquishing my host personality to a child alter would feel psychologically unhealthy. I believe this is similar for most ABs. As Michael Bent explains, for ABs the adult self is the primary personality (the host in DID terms) and the baby or child persona is a sub-personality (alter in DID terms) (see *'The Identity Conflicts of the Adult Baby'* in the book *'Being an Adult Baby'* or in the article tab on the AB Discovery website).

Dax has a more complex set of relationships within his psyche. He has 9 alters. Starting with abuse at age seven there were successive waves of 'splits' as dissociation became the pattern for coping with trauma. The initial alters split directly from the host-birth personality. However, later, alters split from other alters. Christine Pattillo is another example of such a pattern. This has a bearing on which alters are co-conscious (although it is not the only factor). The fact that Dax's capacity to function in the external world is spread across alters also results in more complexity.

Dax is also not his system's 'birth' personality. Dax became the host personality by necessity and circumstance. His system's birth personality, bearing the burden of childhood wounds, grew tired and less able to act as host. The course of Dax's life and his relocations around the world have separated the birth personality from familiar places. In turn, after hectic years of travel and relocation, Dax has grown tired and is relinquishing more space to other, more energetic alters.

For people with DID, sometimes the host personality and the birth personality will be the same, other times not (as with Dax). Robert Oxnam discovered the host personality who had fronted his life and career for decades had taken over from his birth personality after high school. His healing involved his birth personality taking back the host role. Christine Pattillo gives a compelling account of grappling with the terrifying prospect her birth personality would relinquish the host role in her psyche to one of her alters.

For people without DID, like myself, it is confronting to hear of the birth personality withdrawing from being the host personality. It can seem like the death of identity. DID is a challenge to expand our conception of what the 'self' can mean for different people. Dr Ross explains -

> *"Most people with DID have had the same host personality since childhood. Sometimes, though, a previous host got overwhelmed or tired and went away inside. Another alter personality then took over and became the host. The main point is that the host personality is not 'the person' – or the 'real person' – the host is just one of the alter personalities, whose job is to be out front most of the time."*

This separation of the host personality and the birth personality is fortunately not applicable to the vast majority of ABs. It may be relevant in some rare examples. There are several published accounts written by the partners of ABs which describe a lifestyle where the AB's child self appears to be equal to, or more salient, than their adult self. The parallel with DID shows the birth personality relinquishing being the host is a serious psychological threshold. That is increased where an adult personality is potentially relinquishing being the host to a child alter. This is discussed in Chapter 11.

I believe DID and being AB serve different psychological functions. Let me explain.

The term 'psychological function' sounds very rational. That's misleading. We are referring to the deepest parts of our identities which are formed in the unconscious. The unconscious logic can only be discovered many years after the initial trauma.

I have read a few on-line posts indicating there are some ABs who are also DID. There is no indication this overlapping population is a significant proportion of either identity. This suggests that dissociation and alters serve a different psychological function for people with DID, compared to ABs.

For Dax, DID is about survival at its most fundamental level – both physical and psychological. It was about surviving childhood abuse that threatened both his will to live, and his capacity to develop a functional self that could navigate the external world. Dax's adult alters provide essential capabilities that complement those of his host personality. For Dax DID was, and remains, a functional alternative to suicide. This is not being dramatic. The ISSTD's 2010 Guidelines state -

> *"Suicidal and/or self-injurious behaviors are exceptionally common among DID patients; studies have shown that 67% of dissociative disorders patients report a history of repeated suicide attempts and 42% report a history of self-harm ... "*

For me, being AB is about overcoming an inner emotional deadness. Compared to the life-and-death issues of DID that might sound unimportant. It isn't to me. The legacy of an emotionally austere childhood threatened to suck much of the joy, tenderness, and hope out of my life. All my alters are children, and my principal alter is a baby toddler girl. Those alters give my psyche access to the life-giving and life-affirming qualities cited above.

For me, being AB is a functional alternative to neurosis.

We can see this difference between the two identities in terms of their childhood attachment with their mother/primary caregiver. I suspect for people with DID, the depth of their childhood trauma, and the sense of betrayal by those who should have protected them, shattered their attachment with their mother/primary caregiver in their unconscious. In contrast, for ABs the lesser level of trauma, has broken rather than shattered their trust and attachment with their mother/primary caregiver. In turn, that leaves the AB with a compelling unconscious desire to revisit and repair that attachment.

To understand this we need to look at childhood attachments. We understand them based on the widely accepted and empirically-based Attachment Theory developed by the psychiatrist and psychotherapist John Bowlby. (For a discussion of Attachment Theory see my book *'The Adult Baby Identity – Healing Childhood Wounds'*.) A positive bond between a child and their mother/primary caregiver is called a secure attachment. It allows a child to grow up feeling secure, confident to explore their world and express themselves, and to trust themselves and others. A broken bond is called an insecure attachment. It has a reverse, negative effect on a child's self-esteem and trust. Children with insecure attachments are more at risk of being traumatized by the 'ordinary catastrophes' of childhood. People with insecure attachments have lifetime issues with loneliness, a hunger for love, and distrust either of others or themselves.

Insecure childhood attachments are very common. Studies replicated across advanced western countries indicate around one-third of all children have an insecure attachment. An insecure attachment arises because a mother/primary caregiver is not sufficiently attuned to the needs of their baby or young child. That can happen for any number of common reasons – fatigue, anxiety, depression, lack of family modelling. An insecure attachment can also be caused by abuse or neglect.

Both people with DID and ABs have insecure childhood attachments. No surprise there. But I believe they have different types of those insecure attachments. ABs have either one of the two most common types – either

- minimizing their own emotional needs, reflecting a lack of trust in others (called an avoidant insecure attachment) or

- becoming clingy and demanding, reflecting a lack of trust in themselves (called an ambivalent insecure attachment).

However, people with DID have a third, much more damaged type of insecure attachment, labelled a disorganized attachment. They flip between the two other attachment types, alternating between a phobia for attachment (avoidant) and a phobia for detachment (ambivalent). A disorganized attachment is essentially a label for the seemingly capricious, alter-driven shifts in behaviours which derive from severe amnesiac dissociation.

Unlike people with DID, ABs revisit infancy and early childhood for emotional comfort and psychological safety. We are unconsciously revisiting the broken childhood attachment with our mother/primary caregiver (the psychological mechanism we use is discussed in Chapter 13). AB's child alters are an unconscious attempt to get or regain our caregiver's love. This is described in my book '*The Adult Baby Identity – Healing Childhood Wounds*' -

"The character of the child persona of each AB is unique, just as the adult selves of ABs are unique. Yet I suspect that there is important common ground in the characters of AB's child personas. They emerge in response to the brokenness of an insecure childhood attachment and childhood trauma. They are a response to the fact that ABs, as children, often felt unloved. And like all children who feel unloved, ABs felt it must have been their fault. They felt themselves to be unlovable.

Our child persona is the antidote to feeling unlovable. Our subconscious created the most lovable child it could. I can best illustrate this from my own life. Chrissie emerged from a temporary traumatic separation from my mother when I was aged three or four. My baby sister and I were left in the care of strangers. My sister was picked up and comforted by but I don't remember being so comforted. Is it any wonder that my child persona is a baby toddler girl? In my eyes it was my baby toddler sister who got the love. As the elder male child, instead, I got expectations to be grown up beyond my years and felt ashamed for not meeting them. In my eyes, I wasn't picked up and comforted because I was an unlovable failure.

Our child personas are a way of affirming to our wounded Inner Child that they are lovable. ..."

"Dressing to feel authentic is very important. The more I dress in baby clothes that look, and more importantly, feel right for Chrissie the more I feel like a real baby girl. I sometimes say to my sceptical wife that an outfit or piece of Chrissie's clothing is 'cute' – more accurately Chrissie feels 'cute' wearing it. There's a world of meaning in that word. It means more than just nice or pretty. It means feeling like a loveable, adorable baby girl – a little princess. That is central to the 'primal drama' in my psyche – I can go back to a time when there should be a secure attachment between baby and mother. Being cute means (this time), I'll be loved and comforted and protected."

An essential difference between DID and AB is the former is an unconscious flight from catastrophic childhood trauma (typically abuse), while the latter is an unconscious attempt to revisit childhood trauma (probably not abuse) to change the outcome.

A Final Word on Differences

A key purpose of this book is to show the hitherto unrecognized similarity between DID and being AB. Both are on the dissociation spectrum. However, DID and being AB are not the same. Amnesia fragments the psyche of people with DID in a way that is not true for ABs. That fragmentation creates a deeper wound and is far more difficult to heal than the Jekyll and Hyde duality of ABs. An analogy would be to say there is a 'family relationship' between the two identities, but the differences make us first cousins rather than siblings.

DID represents an unconscious flight from catastrophic childhood trauma while being AB represents an unconscious attempt to revisit childhood trauma to change the outcome.

12. Alienation and Self Absorption

We have discussed alters, the key similarity between DID and AB, and we have looked at the major differences between Dax and myself.

Now we can return to look at other similarities between Dax and myself. They include alienation from self and others and self-absorption. Each of these is discussed below.

Alienation

For Dax and myself, alienation from both ourselves and others is a powerful part of our experience of life. It is a legacy of an insecure child attachment and childhood trauma. It is reinforced by having to live in the closet with a stigmatized personal identity. It can be overcome by healing and conscious effort, but it remains a stress point in our psyches which comes to the fore in adverse circumstances.

The alienation comes from childhood trauma. It is particularly the experience of 'aloneness' identified by psychiatrist Jeffrey Smith and discussed in Chapter 3. Childhood abuse is commonly perpetrated by a family member or someone known to the family. The abused child sometimes tells someone and is disbelieved. Or they don't tell because they are afraid they will not be believed, or because the abuser has threatened them or others. Abused children feel alone and often betrayed by adults who should have protected them from harm.

Dax captures how the sense of childhood betrayal lives on-

> *"This is true for us even today, although we are adults ourselves ... We may appear to be physically mature but ... our growth has been stunted and fragmented because of trauma and our intense loathing of all adults is very prevalent in the way we perceive the world. We start from the perspective of don't tell, don't trust anyone, and maybe with time gradually learn to trust and open up, although this has not got easier with age. ... We crave kindness, love and stability, simple things but often far outside our reach or the capabilities of the adults around us to provide."*

The trauma I experienced had these same elements of aloneness and broken trust, even though it was not abuse. For example, in my generation, you didn't complain to anyone about schoolyard bullying because you would be thought of as weak. A traumatized child's experience of aloneness and betrayal is the deepest wound and it is the hardest to heal. It leads to lifelong issues of alienation and mistrust of others.

But not all the wounds belong to the past. Our identities are stigmatized by the world at large. Of necessity, we have lived the great majority of our lives 'in the closet'. Public understanding of both DID and being AB is growing, but it is off a very low base. We know disclosure of the true nature of our identities to the great majority of our acquaintances, colleagues, friends or family would commonly result in shock, fear and rejection.

Those are issues faced by people with many different minority identities. Because of the hard-won victories of gay and lesbian liberation, much of society has come to accept many LGBTQ identities. Difference on the basis of sexual orientation has become accepted by many. We have learned to understand being gay or lesbian or bisexual is not a contradiction with, for example, being a truck driver, a nurse, a mother, a father, a sibling, a friend. But difference on the basis of multiple consciousness is still not accepted. And it will not be accepted for some time to come. And when people don't accept multiple consciousness they must adopt other pathological views of our identity – we are 'bad or mad'. People still experience our identities as an irreconcilable and unacceptable contradiction of our visible personas.

As with any closeted and stigmatized minority identity, Dax and myself internalized much of those negative views. We did not trust ourselves, we pathologised our non-conforming sense of self, blamed ourselves for it and felt ashamed. We have both moved on, but you can't completely let go of the baggage when you need to remain closeted because of a genuine fear of detriment. We are both committed to changing the public misunderstanding of our identities. We share that goal with many others.

Alienation does not just apply to your sense of self. It applies to your relationships with others. The aloneness and betrayal that comes with an insecure childhood attachment and childhood trauma creates a deep mistrust of others. We are too quick to believe we are on our own in a dangerous and uncaring world. We doubt we can ever truly connect with anyone but our most loved partners. Dax sums up this alienation from others -

> *"we see alienation as a response to survival. As much as we want acceptance and support we also want to be left alone because trying to function in an adult world ignorant of our mental health issues is unfathomable."*

The cruel irony is alienation from others is a self-fulfilling perspective – the more alienated we feel, the more we cut ourselves off from others. I am conscious of the potential for a downward spiral. That can make me discount my resilience and feel more fragile than I really am. The alienation overlays and exacerbates the difficulties of coming to terms with living with alters.

But people with DID, and ABs, are not alone in facing alienation. And like everyone else, there is an onus on us to find our way beyond it, to seek and affirm a healthy relationship with ourselves and with others. Most of the alienation belongs to experiences in the distant past. We don't need to carry that baggage into our future. Therapy can help if it's needed.

Self Absorption

I believe people with alters have a propensity for self-absorption, and for self-centeredness and selfishness in their relations with partners. Anybody in distress or crisis is necessarily self-absorbed and self-centred. I am talking about people with DID, and ABs, in our everyday lives.

The self-absorption is understandable. Our alters are as real to us as our host personalities. We are living with an internal community or family which can demand, and also entertain, our attention. That is particularly true of child alters. Their delights and play are a source of fun and entertainment. Their tantrums can preoccupy us. Christine Pattillo's autobiography provides a vivid picture of a mesmerizing, warm, vibrant and boisterous family life amongst her alters. Cameron West's alters include a gaggle of engaging children. The interior landscape inhabited by Robert Oxnam's alters is dramatically gothic and entertaining. In both positive and negative states our alters constantly pull our attention inwards to ourselves. As necessary or satisfying as that can be for us, it can be experienced very differently by those closest to us. At worst we can be moody and withdrawn, and even in better times, we can simply be self-absorbed and oblivious to the needs and feelings of our loved ones.

For those of us who are more emotionally inhibited and mistrusting of others, our alters can be celebrated as a source of self-sufficiency. Dax says -

> *"My alters are a comfort to me, they are my brothers, they have my back and they share the same goal of survival as me. Because we are many, there is little or no time/space to have others in our lives. It doesn't negate the desire for acceptance or having friends but the reality is that self-absorption is all-consuming."*

This can become a way of pushing others away. Herschel Walker attributes the breakdown of his marriage to this mistaken self-sufficiency.

The Adult Baby – An Identity on the Dissociation Spectrum

I suspect people with identities based on alters can be self-centred and selfish in their close relationships. Our loving partners carry a burden of sensitivity, care and protection of a multiple that is not wholly reciprocated. We often fail to understand what being on the 'wrong' end of one to many relationships means. We take relating to one personality for granted. Our partner is relating to multiple personalities. That was still true even before we recognized we were multiples. Our partners dealt with the moodiness, irritability, withdrawal and outright tantrums by our unrecognized alters. Being on the 'one' end of a one-to-many relationship can be hard work.

The extra mile that loving partners go is clear in Christine Pattillo's description of her marriage to her loving husband Christopher, of Cameron West's description of his wife Rikki, Robert Oxnam's portrayal of his wife Vishakha, and Olga Trujillo's description of her first husband David.

That asymmetry is exacerbated by the natural self-centredness of child alters. Like any biological children, they can be demanding, selfish and greedy. Rosalie Bent says *"little Ones can be vain, selfish and arrogant."* Like biological children, they have to be taught to build reciprocal relationships with others.

Wounded, unhealed alters can also have a survival mentality. One of Dax's alters describes it so –

> *"Our DID is all-consuming, you have to be selfish, and focused on self-preservation at all cost."*

Unless we consciously seek to balance it out, we can take more of our partner's lives and energy than we give. Every human being has a capacity for self-centredness and selfishness. Our conscience is the measure of our honesty about this capacity. Those of us who have alters have a stronger propensity to be self-absorbed than most, and all too often that becomes a stronger propensity for selfishness. We need to be careful that consciousness of our unique identities does not become emotional entitlement. Everybody is unique. Everybody has hidden pain. We need to strive that bit harder to overcome our negative traits and ensure we give at least as much as we ask of those closest to us.

Summary

Alienation from self and from others, and a capacity for self-absorption and asymmetry in close relationships are traits common to both people with DID and ABs. We need to recognize those traits and respond to them positively or we risk making living with alters more difficult than it needs to be.

13. Are AB's Child Alters Real Children?

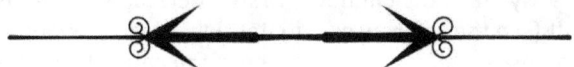

I t is obvious AB's child alters are not real in a physical sense. But what about psychologically?

Many ABs experience their Little or child alter, as a psychological refuge from the stresses and strains of adulthood. When they become their Little, they see and experience themselves as inhabiting the headspace of a baby or young child which is soothing and tranquil.

So, via their child alter, do ABs have the psyches of biological babies or young children?

To answer these questions we need to look at both subjective reality, and objective reality. We'll start with subjective reality.

Subjective Reality

Alters are subjectively real.

That statement can seem condescending or pejorative – like the way you might characterise a child's imaginary friend. For adults, it can sound like an alter is an indulgence – perhaps of a weak mind.

That is not so.

Although our alters are later elaborated by our conscious minds, they originated in our sub-conscious when we were biological children. AB's involuntary triggering of the need for nappies, or the conflicts of the binge and purge cycle, are testament to that. Trauma rewired our psyches. We have lived all our adult life with that rewiring. Initially, with repression, our conscious mind may not even know we have alters. And when repression breaks down, our conscious minds can spend years or decades denying what our unconscious wants to foist on us. For example, I was horrified to realize my principal child alter, might be a girl. I fought accepting that for years.

We know how powerful the mind, especially the sub-conscious mind, can be in relation to the body. I refer in Chapter 4 to the way for some people with amnesic DID, switches between alters can manifest in changes in the physical body – shifts between being allergic and non-allergic, to medicines working and not working, to feeling pain and not feeling pain etc. Our psyche genuinely experiences our alters as real. They are more than metaphorical in the way singletons have an 'inner child'. This is not imagination or 'creative visualisation'.

Because they originate deep in the subconscious we know from DID dissociated alters cannot be wished or reasoned away. Removing alters as separate personalities, takes years of intensive psychotherapy to rewire the psyche (more on this in Chapter 14). Medication has little or no effect on dissociated trauma and alters (although it is sometimes used for associated symptoms like depression or anxiety).

Validation

There is a compelling validation that AB's child alters do replicate part of the psyche of a biological baby or very young child. The replication is in the way AB's gain a deep level of grounding and comfort from their nappies and other baby items. It is not an affectation. But how? Why is a soft or wet nappy so comforting? Why is a favourite soft toy so calming? Or favourite baby clothes? Or a pacifier? Or a bottle? After all a wet nappy or any of these things are not intrinsically comforting for most adults – most would find them annoying, if not downright discomforting. They ARE deeply comforting and calming for adult babies.

The answer is these objects provide comfort to the AB's child alter through exactly the same psychological mechanism as they do for biological babies and young children. It is commonly understood these objects serve as a substitute for the continuous presence of the mother/caregiver. That's why they help the child go to sleep or tolerate the temporary absence of the caregiver. They are called transitional objects.

The way they work in the psyche of the child was first understood by the renowned paediatrician and psychotherapist Donald Winnicott (see the references for citations). It is not just a case of a child deriving comfort from a familiar, but physically inanimate object. In the psyche of the child, it represents and embodies the caregiver – the object *is* the caregiver. It is called a transitional object because it exists between subjective and objective reality. The child's psyche endows an inanimate object with a subjective meaning which is not intrinsic in its objective, physical form. As transitional phenomena, the object's meaning goes beyond the confines of the child's mind, and is apparent to, and can be shared with, others. So a caregiver might ask a crying or fussing child, 'want your teddy,' knowing it has a special meaning for the child.

This psychological mechanism works at the deepest, earliest levels of a child's psyche. Biological children first create transitional objects when they are between 4 and 12 months old. That is before they have language or abstract thought. For ABs to gain such a deep level of comfort from childhood transitional objects means they must be replicating part of the psyche of a baby or young child. That is not something normal adults can access. I find that a compelling argument.

So now we understand why nappies are such a powerful part of being AB. The familiarity of nappies is a source of comfort for our child alters. But it's a lot more than that. Because the nappy is a transitional object, when we wear them, ABs are unconsciously recreating the presence of a loving caregiver. We are doing that because our child alter replicates *some* of the deepest parts of the psyche of a biological child. A wet nappy increases its efficacy as a transitional object. Presumably, that harkens back to the time when a wet nappy made the presence and attention of a caregiver more likely. That's why ABs find nappies so comforting.

Similarly when my baby alter Chrissie, hugs her favourite stuffed toys in bed they are not just cuddly but inanimate objects. She really feels like they are friends protecting her – just like any small child feels.

When AB's accept their child alters, through the psychological power of transitional objects, we have access to this deep level of self-nurturing. That can comfort and heal our the insecure childhood attachment with our caregiver - if we pursue a psychologically healthy path (more on the latter in Chapter 15). It is important to remember that transitional objects are a means by which a child comforts *themselves*. They represent the child's first step towards psychological independence.

Objective Reality

So, from the above discussion, we might think ABs have the psyche of a biological child.

It is not so.

That's for two reasons. Firstly, our child alter exists in the same psyche as our adult host. Secondly, the Little or child headspace we visualize is an artificial construct of our adult psyche. Each of these points is discussed below.

Because ABs do not have amnesia, our child alter is co-conscious with our adult host. Each knows of the existence and capabilities of the other. Thus our child alter co-exists with our adult mind. We cannot unlearn what we know as adults about the trials and tribulations of human existence. Thus we are not truly innocent as children are. We cannot jettison our responsibility to do for ourselves and for those who need us, as best we can, without being self-indulgent and incurring realistic guilt. Thus we are not truly carefree as children are. A securely attached young biological child can feel completely safe in the arms of a protector they sincerely believe to be infallible, selfless, omnipotent and immortal. But we cannot truly re-experience that safety because as adults we know no protector is endowed with all these qualities.

The Adult Baby – An Identity on the Dissociation Spectrum

Even if we had amnesia as do people with DID, replicating our biological infancy or early childhood would not be a safe refuge from our adult lives and selves. In reality, biological infancy and early childhood is not the tranquil psychological refuge AB's imagine it to be. Such a view is the artificial construct of our *adult* minds.

Arguably, the human psyche never faces more daunting challenges, including powerful fears and conflicts, than between the age of six months and three or four years old. Look at the dramatic changes in the physical and psychological capabilities in a child over these years. The psyche has to work incredibly hard to accommodate and drive those changes. These stages are beyond conscious recall, but we understand them through the work of child development experts like the psychotherapist Donald Winnicott (see my book *'The Adult Baby Identity – Healing Childhood Wounds'* for a description of the development of a child's psyche in the first year of life.) These stages of life are not the ones you would really want to go back to for a soothing calm respite.

So, the way we see or experience our child alters is not an objectively accurate facsimile of the psyche of a biological baby or child. Our child alters are a construct of our sub-conscious, later consciously elaborated. Rosalie Bent understands this. As well as being the partner of an AB she is the mother of four biological children and a grandmother. Writing for the partners of ABs she says -

> *"What is actually happening is that your partner has deep un-met needs and therefore constructs a pseudo-personality that can help meet these needs. The power of an intelligent and creative mind takes a set of behaviours and thinking patterns that are deeply separated from the usual adult patterns and then builds an age, name and pseudo-personality around these needs and behaviours. Thus a 'little one' is born."*

The 'artificial' nature of this construct is also evident in Rosalie's observation that ABs typically dress or behave as Littles in ways which combine elements from different developmental stages that would be unlikely to coexist at the same time in a real child. This applies to me and my baby girl alter, Chrissie. I have jackets and knitted bonnets that belong to a very young baby's layette, onesies and babysuits such as a crawling baby might wear, and two-piece pyjamas and dungarees you could see on a toddler. I visualize Chrissie being breast and bottle-fed, sleeping in a cot and playing in a playpen – behaviours which are probably most consistent with the 'crawler' stage. But I also visualize her feeding herself (messily), running around (unsteadily), playing with dolls and watching kids' TV shows, attributes which belong to an older age, toddler or beyond.

Psychiatrist Colin Ross puts the case that child alters do not replicate the psyches of biological children -

> *"Many child alters do not actually function at their alleged age level cognitively. They often understand long words, abstract concepts, and moral dilemmas in a way that would be rare for a normal child of that age. Others do seem to have a childish way of thinking. ...*
>
> *A scientific demonstration that child alters do not function cognitively at their alleged age would not invalidate DID. It would only prove that they are not real children. Such evidence, however, would challenge the overliteral view, according to which alters represent a concrete fixation in cognitive development. In my view, child alters are not packets of childness retained in a surrounding sea of adult psyche. They are stylized packets of adult psyche. ...*
>
> *The therapist shouldn't believe that child alters are really children, any more than he believes that demon alters are really demons, or that the patient is really possessed by her dead mother when an alter claims to be the mother. On the other hand, clinicians work within the patient's beliefs and worldview to a varying extent. The child alter personalities are always key components of the personality system in terms of the planning of therapy."* [*Dissociative Identity Disorder: Diagnosis, Clinical Features, and Treatment of Multiple Personality p147]*

As Dr Ross indicates, there are many examples of alters in DID which we could never confuse with objective reality, even at a psychological level. Many people with DID who had been sexually abused as children by people in overtly religious contexts had alters who were demonic or satanic. Two of Robert Oxnam's original alters were a witch and a pair of disembodied eyes (reminiscent of Sauron in the fantasy Lord of the Rings). The uninformed might think of this as crazy. But we understand these alters as the psyche's response to childhood trauma; the child's psyche way of making sense of their experience. An AB's child alters belong to this broad phenomena of dissociated alters. We should not expect they replicate objectively real psychological states.

But I disagree with a key point made by Dr Ross. As per the previous discussion, I believe the child alters of ABs do replicate part of the psyche of biological babies and very young children. They do that through the mechanism of transitional objects. It is one of the deepest and earliest psychological mechanisms developed by biological children. We can see this most in the comfort ABs derive from their nappies and those other transitional objects (stuffed toys, pacifiers, bottles or whatever) which are most instinctual to them.

But beyond this deep subconscious mechanism, the rest of how AB's see and experience their child alters, is a construct of their adult psyches. That doesn't make it false or make-believe, but we should not confuse it with the psyche of biological children.

Summary

Because alters are not objectively real doesn't mean they are imaginary, an affectation, or the indulgence of a weak mind. They are deeply rooted in the subconscious and are compelling real to the person who has them. They cannot be willed, reasoned or medicated away.

ABs do not have the psyche of a biological child. Because we don't have amnesia, our child alter and our adult host are aware of each other's existence and capabilities. That means we cannot be truly innocent, or truly carefree, or feel as protected, as a biological baby or child. The way we visualize and experience our child alter is a construct of our adult psyches. But our child alter does replicate part of the psyche of a biological baby, specifically through the comfort we gain through transitional objects.

14. Are Alters Psychologically Healthy?

O kay, so we understand people with DID and ABs both have subjectively real alters.

But is having alters psychologically healthy?

Amongst the experts on dissociation and DID there are a range of views. The prevailing expert view is alters are a risk to psychological health. Other experts believe people can live safe and happy lives with alters. Both views emerged early in the development of the contemporary understanding of DID, and have persisted ever since. Each of these is discussed below.

Alters Are a Psychological Risk

The prevailing expert view is living with alters will always be a risk to psychological health. The strongly preferred outcome of the treatment of DID or OSDD is to fuse the alters back into a unitary psyche. I refer to this as the 'fusionist' view.

Psychiatrists Richard P Kluft and Colin A Ross are pioneers in the treatment of DID. From the 1980s and 1990s, they have been proponents of this adverse view of alters. It is reflected in the current (2010) version of the ISSTD's Guidelines. They state -

> *"R. P. Kluft (1993a) has argued that the most stable treatment outcome is final fusion—complete integration, merger, and loss of separateness—of all identity states. However, even after undergoing considerable treatment, a considerable number of DID patients will not be able to achieve final fusion and/or will not see fusion as desirable. Many factors can contribute to patients being unable to achieve final fusion: chronic and serious situational stress; avoidance of unresolved, extremely painful life issues, including traumatic memories; lack of financial resources for treatment; comorbid medical disorders; advanced age; significant unremitting DSM Axis I and/or Axis II comorbidities; and/or significant narcissistic investment in the alternate identities and/or DID itself; among others. Accordingly, a more realistic long-term outcome for some patients may be a cooperative arrangement sometimes called a "resolution"—that is, sufficiently integrated and coordinated functioning among alternate identities to promote optimal functioning. However, patients who achieve a cooperative arrangement rather than final fusion may be more vulnerable to later decompensation (into florid DID and/or PTSD) when sufficiently stressed."*

For its' proponents, the idea of fusion is a positive one. The alters merge with the host and the positive capabilities and traits of the alters are not lost but become available to the whole psyche. Colin Ross in his book *'Dissociative Identity Disorder: Diagnosis, Clinical Features, and Treatment of Multiple Personality'* describes a 'fusion ritual' – mental imagery intended to reassure clients nothing positive is lost from their life as a 'multiple'. The damage and the pain held by the alters from the original trauma(s) is resolved in therapy before fusion, and is not carried forward. The person now has a unitary psyche. There are no 'fault lines' remaining in the psyche which might again fracture in the face of future stresses or crises. To effect fusion requires years of intensive weekly therapy to rewire the psyche.

The problem with this view of alters is not the idea of fusion. For some people with DID, moving to a unitary psyche may be a Godsend which relieves them of symptoms that have blighted their lives. There is nothing wrong with giving 'multiples' the option of fusion in therapy. The problem is the proponents of fusion stigmatise the other pathway to psychological health, cooperation between alters, in terms which are biased and harmful.

Opposition or reluctance by a person with alters, to see them disappear, is stigmatized as psychological weakness or ill-health. The return of alters after their fusion into a unitary psyche is stigmatized and referred to as a 'relapse'.

This can be seen in several points in the description of Dr Kluft's views above. There is scant regard for a 'multiple' not choosing fusion. It is largely stigmatized as an inability or failure. In particular, attachment to alters is referred to as a possible example of a 'narcissistic investment in alternate identities'.

In a later passage, the ISSTD's 2010 Guidelines focus on 'narcissistic investment' as the sole reason why a multiple may not choose fusion –

> *"Fusion rituals are useful when, as a result of psychotherapeutic work, separateness no longer serves any meaningful function for the patient's intrapsychic and environmental adaptation. At this point, if the patient is no longer narcissistically invested in maintaining the particular separateness, fusion is ready to occur."*

In his recent (2018) book Dr Ross says –

> *"The goal of treatment for DID is stable integration – according to me. But that may not be the client's goal. Some people want to stop at the stage where all the parts are co-conscious and working together – this is their choice and it may be the right choice for them, and that's fine.*
>
> *Why do I think that integration is the best goal? For several reasons: (1) Why would you want to live with a little bit of mental disorder rather than none? (2) It takes less time and energy to be one person compared to managing a whole group inside. (3) Who knows how long the 'everybody in harmony' status will last? It seems that if you stop at the cooperating system stage, then life deals you severe trauma in the future, you are more likely to lapse back into conflicted, symptomatic DID – if you are integrated, this is less likely.*
>
> *There is no research literature comparing the long-term outcomes for fully integrated versus partially integrated DID. All opinions on the subject are opinions, not scientific facts – some opinions are educated, some are not.*
>
> *Reasons people give for not wanting to be fully integrated include: (1) I'll be lonely. (2) I'll miss them. (3) I don't want to get rid of them. (4) I'm functioning fine as I am. (5) I can't handle it on my own. Each of these reasons can be legitimate or just a form of denial and avoidance. It varies from case to case. The main thing is not to be dogmatic about integration, either pro or con."* [Treatment of Dissociative Identity Disorder: Techniques and Strategies for Stabilisation]

Dr Ross's terms 'stable or full integration' is synonymous with Dr Kluft's term 'fusion'. Dr Ross makes clear he sees the continuing presence of alters as a risk. I characterise this as tolerating rather than accepting alters. However, he pays greater regard to the self-determination of people with alters, and 'owns' his views as (educated) personal opinion in the absence of clear research evidence backing either position.

This adverse view is reflected in the fusionist approach to alters in therapy. Even though fusionists recognize it is necessary to work with alters, the latter is still regarded as a risk to be contained. We can gain an idea of the nature of that risk from the following reference in the ISSTD's 2010 Guidelines -

> *"It is countertherapeutic to suggest that the patient create additional alternate identities, to name identities when they have no names (although the patient may choose names if he or she wishes), or to suggest that identities function in a more elaborated and autonomous way than they already are functioning."*

The Adult Baby – An Identity on the Dissociation Spectrum

This passage reflects an understandable concern to avoid either (a) the accusation the therapist is 'seeding' alters in the mind of a suggestable client or (b) exacerbating fragmentation in the psyches of distressed multiples. However, it refers pejoratively to the alters functioning in an 'elaborated' way. Presumably, this will then be an obstacle to a person agreeing to fuse their alters with the host – the 'narcissistic investment' referred to above.

The problem is this stigmatizes the cooperation option where multiples warmly embrace their alters. I suspect Olga Trujillo and Herschel Walker's distant and impersonal relationship with their alters reflects their psychiatrists' adverse, fusionist view. This runs counter to the usual trajectory discussed in Chapter 10 whereby the expression of alters grows and expands. Presumably, mental health professionals with this perspective would regard most ABs elaboration of the personality of their Little or child alter as psychologically unhealthy.

A recent (2016) text on dissociation for therapists, *'Treating Trauma Related Dissociation: A Practical Integrative Approach'*, refers to the re-emergence of alters after fusion as a 'relapse'. It discusses strategies for 'relapse prevention'. This makes it clear alters are seen as pathological.

This adverse view also extends to the interaction between a person's alters and their partner. The above text cites the following instruction -

> *"It is important for the partner not to call out parts other than the adult self of the patient, but to learn simple ground techniques that help the adult part of the patient to stay present and to return should there be a switch. Partners should not interact regularly with child or other parts of the patient, except to help the patient return to an adult and grounded place. This is essential because the more parts are active in daily life, the more autonomous they become, and significant relationship issues may be avoided by both parties by only dealing with more functional adult parts."* [Treating Trauma Related Dissociation: A Practical Integrative Approach]

From the perspective of the cooperative approach to alters, the above instruction is cruel and inhumane. It would preclude or stigmatise the warm accepting relationships between a person's alters and their partner described in earlier chapters. We have seen in several of the autobiographies these relationships were a positive turning point in the lives of people with DID. That was the case for Dax and myself. All of that healing would be prevented or undone by a therapist following the above text.

Presumably, this adverse view would also extend to any concrete recognition of Littles by partners. The ISSTD's Guidelines state –

> *"Reparenting" techniques such as sustained holding, simulated bottle or breastfeeding, and so on are clinically inappropriate and unduly regressive behaviours that fall below the current standard of care for any patient."*

Colin Ross explains in his book *'Dissociative Identity Disorder: Diagnosis, Clinical Features, and Treatment of Multiple Personality'* the simulated breastfeeding refers to that action by a therapist, rather than a partner. However it still clear that actions by either an AB or their partner which physically meet the needs of their Little or child alter (like wearing or changing nappies) would not be viewed positively.

This adverse view of alters places therapists in a difficult ethical position with their clients. Therapists are aware their view that alters should fuse back into a unitary psyche would not be well received by many of their clients. The ISSTD's Guidelines state -

> *"However, clinicians should not attempt to press for fusion before the patient is clinically ready for this. Premature attempts at fusion may cause significant distress for the DID patient or, alternatively, a superficial compliance wherein the alternate identities in question attempt to please the therapist by seeming to disappear."*

Therapists with an adverse view of alters seem to be placed in the difficult position of dissembling with their clients. They seem not to disclose their views about fusion in the first stages of therapy because that would be an obstacle to the trust and safety their clients need to feel for an effective therapeutic relationship.

Dr Smith says –

> *"When therapists are too enthusiastic about integration, patients tend to become suspicious of their motives. The decision of whether to integrate is best left to the patient."*

Dr Smith's injunction to respect the choice of the patient is an ethically sound resolution of this difficult position. Dr Smith did exactly as he enjoins – his client, Robert Oxnam, chose to live happily with his three remaining alters.

Unfortunately, some therapists are so certain of their view about what is best for their clients, that dissembling shades into ethically doubtful intransigence. The 2016 text referred to above, coaches therapists on how to manipulate clients towards their hidden agenda of fusion -

> *"Once therapy has progressed to the point where the parts are working well together for the most part and at least some traumatic memories have been integrated, the therapist can begin to pique the patient's curiosity about fusion in an indirect way. **The therapist should regularly ask in a curious way,** I wonder what keeps those parts of you separate from you? Or, Have you ever thought about why those parts still need to be separate from each other? Have you ever thought about why that part of you has never grown up? I'm curious about what it might be like for you if those parts were closer together?"*

The three authors of this text are respected experts on dissociation. One, Kathy Steele, is the past (2008-9) President of the International Society for the Study of Trauma and Dissociation. Their certitude is reflected in the explicit endorsement of manipulative intransigence. There is scant space in this certitude to acknowledge there is no clear research evidence favouring fusion as an outcome, or to respect a client's choice there is a different way to psychological health (as per Colin Ross above).

Amongst therapists, there may be an association between this intransigent certitude about alters and an adherence to the more mechanistic therapist-driven schools of psychology. Those are schools such as Freudian psychoanalysis, or B.F. Skinner's Behaviourism and its derivatives; Learning Theory, Cognitive Behaviour Therapy (CBT) and Dialectical Behaviour Theory (DBT). The 2016 text cited above seems to be strongly influenced by DBT. These mechanistic theories can be contrasted with the greater respect for the client's self-determination in humanistic theories of psychology.

In fairness to the mental health professionals who hold an adverse view of alters, we need to understand many have spent decades working with clients for whom dissociative conditions are distressing, debilitating and life-threatening. These mental health professionals have in the last four decades contributed to a vast improvement in public and professional understanding of debilitating dissociation and its treatment. That being said, in my view, manipulative intransigence is therapeutically and ethically doubtful.

A Positive View of Alters

Fortunately, there are other experts and mental health professionals who have a positive view of alters. They believe it is psychologically healthy for alters to continue to exist as separate personalities, provided they work together as a team or a family. I refer to this as the 'cooperation' view.

One of the other pioneers in understanding dissociation, psychiatrist and paediatrician Frank W. Putnam, propounded this view in his 1989 text the *'Diagnosis and Treatment of Multiple Personality Disorders'*. This perspective has been recently restated by Psychiatrist David Yeung in his 2018 book -

"Although much of the writing on DID suggests that the goal of therapy is to integrate the alters into a unitary personality, that was never my goal. My approach is to help them become, as Putnam recommends, a fully functioning unit. If the alters are fused into one personality, there is a risk that without their main defence – dissociation – integrated patients may lack sufficient protection against the ordinary stresses of life, and thus be subject to splitting again in the future." [Engaging Multiple Personalities Volume 1: Contextual Case Histories]

The cooperation option means the alters work as a team with the host. The extent of cooperation can vary. At one end of the scale, it can be sufficient for daily functioning although dysfunctions remain. Dax has this level of cooperation. Some of his alters are co-conscious, although most are not. There is little or no conflict between alters. Amnesia is still an issue and so is switching.

At the other end of the scale, full cooperation means the alters are like a family, each loving and respecting the others. There is no amnesia and all the alters are co-conscious. Shifting is more common than switching. The alters may be co-present. I fit this pattern. I suspect non-conflicted ABs would also fit this level of cooperation. Christine Pattillo, Cameron West and Robert Oxnam are examples of people with DID who have completed therapy and chosen to live with healed alters as an essential part of their personal identity.

This is the view in the self-help book 'Got Parts: An Insiders Guide to Managing Life Successfully with Dissociative Identity Disorder' which says –

"Parts are never going to disappear or go away; they will always be there, and part of you. Individual parts will always remain separately individual, but the goal of re-integration is to become aware of each other and working so seamlessly and cooperatively together, with shared information and regarding switches, that you can live and function in the outside world with a minimum of distress, without others, even knowing about your multiplicity unless you choose to disclose it."

Dr Yeung's position has the ethical and therapeutic advantage that it does not require him to dissemble with his patients. He is not pursuing a hidden agenda which he knows is contrary to their wishes. As can be seen in his published case studies his position also allowed him to welcome an accepting relationship between a client's partner and the client's alters. This is a humane and therapeutic position, compared to the prohibition on such acceptance by proponents of fusion.

Dr Yeung's comment that people who formerly had alters may be less resilient after fusion, is important to understand. People with alters have been living with multiple consciousness since they were young children, albeit this may have gone unrecognized until much later in life. Typically, their alters split within their psyche in childhood, before adolescence. Often they are in mid-life before they are correctly diagnosed. They have never lived with a unitary psyche as a teenager or an adult. Requiring a person who has lived with alters to transition to a unitary psyche is effectively a bold experiment. It is analogous to hitting the command 'restore factory settings' on a vintage laptop computer or PC which has decades of patches and upgrades, while hoping (with your fingers crossed) you can successfully load new, better software.

The 2016 text '*Treating Trauma Related Dissociation: A Practical Integrative Approach*' recognizes the significance of the change from multiple consciousness to a unitary psyche. It cites a range of difficulties the person may encounter. None of these are debilitating but they do suggest a decreased level of resilience, hopefully just for the short term. This underscores that pushing a 'multiple' to fusion is an experiment with that person's psyche. In this context the intransigent certitude and lack of humility of some of the therapists quoted above is disturbing.

Stigmatizing opposition by a multiple to fusion as a 'narcissistic investment in their alters' is the clearest example of this lack of humility. It disparages the psychologically healthy reasons for multiples to prefer accepting their alters as a team or family, over fusion into a unitary psyche.

Take me. My psyche split off alters between the ages of four and ten. I have been living with the behaviours driven by a child alter since I was ten. I am in my late fifties. I have never lived with a unitary psyche as an adult. Discovering I am a multiple helped me make sense of myself and my life in a deeper way. Making friends with my child alters has given me a sense of 'coming home' to myself. My whole psyche has access to their positive qualities. My girl child alter has helped me move beyond seeing things from a purely male perspective. My alters are a healing response to an insecure childhood attachment and its legacy; a life course shaped by the resulting emotionally inhibited, avoidant and anxious host personality. You cannot 'cure' an insecure childhood attachment, nor overthrow an entire life course. But you can find an internal source of warmth, safety and inspiration that enables you to better love yourself and others. My alters are a loving internal family. They overturn a lifetime fear of emptiness and loneliness. I am better, happier and more resilient for accepting them. I have fulfilled my obligations to society. I don't have anything to prove. I can be me. I am human, imperfect, but labelling all of that a narcissistic investment is inaccurate, arrogant and offensive.

AB's sexual fetish for nappies is also likely to be an obstacle to fusion. After adolescence the means by which we derive sexual pleasure is pretty hard-wired into our psyches, it's been reinforced many times by a powerful reward and isn't amenable to change. So even after fusion, our sexual fetish is going to keep pulling AB's back to the nappies which powerfully evokes our child alter.

I suspect many multiples will have their own sound reasons for choosing to continue to live with their alters. There are indications a significant proportion, probably the majority of people with DID in therapy do not want or effect fusion. The ISSTD's Guidelines state -

> *"Systematically collected outcome data from case series and treatment studies indicated that 16.7% to 33% of those DID patients achieved full integration (i.e., final fusion; Coons & Bowman, 2001; Coons & Sterne, 1986; Ellason & Ross, 1997)."*

Remember that fusion takes years of intensive weekly psychotherapy. That is accessed by a tiny minority of the much larger population who have substantial dissociative symptoms. So stigmatizing the option for psychological health which is available to, and chosen by, most people with significant dissociation symptoms is harmful and counterproductive.

The cooperation approach is supported by a school of psychology named Internal Family Systems (IFS) therapy which has emerged since the 1980s. It is premised on the cooperative team approach. IFS is applicable to multiples with dissociated alters, and to singletons with metaphorical inner parts. It was developed by psychotherapist Richard Schwartz based on his work with bulimic clients. This may not be coincidental. I have read eating disorders may sometimes have their origin in dissociated trauma. For a discussion of IFS see my book *'The Adult Baby Identity – A Self Help Guide'* or search Amazon for books by Richard Schwartz or Jay Earley.

Dax, from the vantage point of reconciling DID with a functional and full life, says -

> *"There are risks attached to both perspectives [fusionist and cooperation]. The various approaches to therapy are constantly evolving and we learn more about the complexities of DID. The category of DDNOS didn't exist when I was diagnosed, it has evolved as more and more individuals are identified as having DID. As professionals continue to map and share the facts of cases we hope that patterns will emerge that can be supported by corrective therapy. Failure to understand the causes of trauma will ultimately result in more fragmentation and mental health suffering. A professional with a balanced approach, an open mind and a non-judgemental attitude will have a positive impact on the individuals they work with."*

> *"Treatment protocols only have merit when you truly understand the footprint of the individual. Trying to cookie cut a solution is not productive, and in the long term can cause more fragmentation. Positive support, guidance and clear communication are key factors inhaling someone with DID to understand their condition and its complexities."*

I believe these sentiments are valid for any multiple.

The Adult Baby – An Identity on the Dissociation Spectrum

What the adverse, fusionist view of alters does not take into account is the issue of personal identity. Let me explain.

Remember, for a person to be diagnosed with DID they have to satisfy four criteria. The fourth criteria was –

> *The symptoms [listed in the other three criteria] cause clinically significant distress or impairment in social, occupational, or other important areas of functioning.*

There is a similar criteria for Other Specified Dissociative Disorder (OSDD).

We have seen multiples who live with their alters as a cooperative team or a loving family can be free of distress or impairment. If there is no distress or impairment, the fourth diagnostic criteria above is not satisfied. The person satisfies the other criteria for DID or OSDD but there is no mental disorder. So what do you call it?

If a psychologically functional multiple chooses to live with alters it is a minority personal identity. They have a non-conforming sense of self. That makes it similar to, but not the same as LGBTQ identities. Transgender people are LGBTQ by virtue of having a compelling, non-conforming sense of self – they experience themselves as being of a different gender from the one they were born with. Having subjectively real alters is a non-conforming sense of self. That deserves the same respect and freedom from prejudice as LGBTQ identities.

It is not the place of the mental health professions to be the arbiter of minority personal identity. There is already a long dismal history of those professions causing harm to stigmatized minorities while being certain they were doing good. This includes stigmatizing gay and lesbian people as having a mental disorder, and stigmatizing transgender people as being fetishists or covert homosexuals. This harm is associated with unwavering certitude on the part of mental health professionals they knew what was good for their clients, disregarding and stigmatizing any contrary views by those same clients. The need of multiples in acute distress for guidance from mental health professionals does not validate a disregard for the personal experience and choices of the large population of people with significant dissociation.

The Nature of Identity

If we accept DID and being AB as identities on the dissociation spectrum, it prompts the question, how can a positive identity be borne from trauma?

The answer lies in understanding the nature of identity. For all of us, I believe the foundation of our identity is formed in the sub-conscious. That is different from the 'superstructure' of our identity, which we build in both our conscious and sub-conscious mind. We can come to understand why our identity has the foundation it does. We can make something positive of that foundation. But it is beyond our conscious mind to change those basic building blocks. I believe this is true for all, LGBTQ people and non-LGBTQ people.

The sub-conscious foundation of our identity, no matter how strange it may seem, represents our psyche's best solution to what our biology and our early environment bequeathed us. That foundation was our psyche's way of optimizing our chances for 'life, liberty and the pursuit of happiness', even in the face of factors which threatened to diminish or even destroy those chances. When we think about identities born from trauma, like being AB or DID, we need to remember they are the *responses* to difficult or pathogenic circumstances.

We should not judge such identities by the difficulties or trauma from which they arose, but rather by their success in creating a capacity for happiness and self-determination.

I owe this perspective to the psychotherapist Dr Michael Bader. In his book *'Arousal: the Secret Logic of Sexual Fantasies'* he takes the approach our sexual fantasies are our psyche's sub-conscious solution to finding sexual arousal and pleasure in the face of pathogenic beliefs formed from our upbringing. Those pathogenic beliefs would otherwise destroy any capacity for sexual pleasure. No matter how strange our sexual fantasies they are perfectly comprehensible and serve a healthy function. I have extended this compelling and liberating logic to identity and happiness more generally.

Summary

There are conflicting expert views about whether living with alters is psychologically healthy. The 'fusionist' view is living with alters, even after therapy and self-acceptance, remains a psychological risk. Proponents of this view hold the definitive outcome is to fuse alters back into a unitary psyche. The positive traits and capabilities of alters become available to the whole psyche. The alternative, 'cooperation' view is multiples will be more resilient by living with their alters as a mutually supporting team or loving family. Both fusion and cooperation are valid options. It should be the choice of the multiple, not their therapist. Neither option should be stigmatized. I believe many ABs will favour the cooperation option. If a psychologically functional multiple chooses to live with alters it is a minority personal identity. That deserves the same respect and freedom from prejudice as LGBTQ identities.

15. The Challenges for ABs Living With Alters

ABs cannot be blind to the psychological challenges of living with our alters.

I disagree with the fusionist view of alters discussed in the last chapter. Even where a multiple can access and afford years of intensive psychotherapy, I believe many will be more resilient by choosing cooperation; to live with their alters as a team or family. But it would be unwise to dismiss the concerns of the experts about the risks of living with alters.

We have complex psyches. That brings both unique gifts and unique risks. Dax describes his alters as a 'two-edged sword'. We have seen that alters are dynamic. They are a source of change within our psyche. So it is not a case of reaching some endpoint and saying 'it's all okay now'. We need to periodically check if our path is taking us in the right direction.

As a multiple, I have learned to think of my psychological health in terms of my alters. If I'm out of balance, getting stressed, compulsive or obsessive, I ask myself 'what's up with my alters?' My wife will ask the same question. Often (not always) the source will one of my alters getting 'off beam'. Unfortunately, as multiples, sometimes we are only as 'together' as our most 'off' alter.

For multiples, psychological health means your alter(s) and your host are working well together. Each has a role to fulfil. Each respects the feelings, needs and role of the others. It's like a happy, psychologically healthy family. As a multiple, our psychological health reflects the state of our whole psyche, not just one personality. If one personality (either alter or host) is having everything their way, to the detriment of the other(s), then we are heading into trouble.

The Middle Road

I believe for ABs, living with alters in a psychologically healthy way, involves walking a middle road between pitfalls on either side.

The **first** pitfall is not accepting the subjective reality of our child alter(s).

The **second** pitfall is not accepting the objective reality that we are not biological children, either physically or psychologically.

Failure to accept either reality is psychologically unhealthy. Rosalie Bent describes this as the "all-important goal of balancing the need to be Little, with the real world requirement to be an adult."

Our child alters are subjectively real. They are more than metaphorical in the way singletons have an 'inner child'. They are a compelling presence in our psyche. A part of us really does think, feel, perceive, and at times act, like a young child (or rather our version of a young child). That got hard-wired in by trauma when we were biological children. Denying that reality twists our minds like a pretzel. It can make us neurotic. Denying the needs of that subjectively real child for nurture and safety leaves us feeling depleted in a way that cannot be salved by anything else.

Despite our child alters, in objective reality, we are not biological children, either physically or psychologically. Although we replicate *some* aspects we do not have the psyche of a biological child. While we can feel comforted and protected by nurturing our child alter, our adult minds and responsibilities cannot be jettisoned.

And in reality, biological infancy and early childhood is not the tranquil psychological refuge AB's imagine it to be. Such a view is the artificial construct of our *adult* minds. Our alters are a construct of our sub-conscious, later consciously elaborated. That doesn't make them fake. They hold fundamental components of our psyche we need to live whole lives. They can be a healthy part of our psyche. But we should not make the mistake of thinking they are a complete or accurate facsimile of the psyche of a biological child.

Challenges to Our Psychological Balance

So it's keeping on the middle road. How difficult can that be?

Sometimes it can be very difficult. As a multiple, we need to accept a subjective reality which contradicts objective reality. As a result, we live with two unwelcome but constant adjuncts to our identity – doubt and cognitive dissonance.

'Got Parts: An Insider's Guide to Managing Life Successfully with Dissociative Identity Disorder' tells us -

> *"There may be times when you may begin to wonder, or doubt whether your traumatic experience ever happened, or if it was really 'that bad'. There may also be times when you may question, even go into denial about whether or not you really are DID [AB]. This is very normal. ... Don't get stuck here, or let this de-rail you. ... Sometimes it comes down to intuition, faith, trust and deciding that even though you don't have all the answers, or don't know everything you long to know ... you can still move on in reclaiming your life."*

The doubt is about our sense of self. How can our AB identity be real when it is such a contradiction of our adult and visible selves? Is it just an over-active imagination? Are we crazy? We are the only ones who directly experience the child inside. We know we can never convince someone who chooses not to believe our subjective experience. To them, we are 'bad or mad'. Even after we accept ourselves, our doubt still lurks in the shadows. One of the cruel ironies of being AB, is before we accept ourselves we are afraid our child alter is real, and after we accept ourselves we are afraid they aren't.

Another key reason that ABs wear nappies, and all the rest, is to reassure ourselves our child alter is real – to bridge the chasm between our subjective reality, and visible, objective reality. The nappies are a visible sign of a compelling sense of self which is otherwise invisible and unprovable.

Cognitive Dissonance

We also live with cognitive dissonance. The Wikipedia article of the same name defines that as –

> *"cognitive dissonance is the mental discomfort (psychological stress) experienced by a person who holds two or more contradictory beliefs, ideas, or values."*

For ABs, our cognitive dissonance comes from the contradiction between being functional adults who also experience ourselves as infants or young children. There is a stark disparity between how our child alter feels to us, and what we see when we look in the mirror. That is especially so for the estimated 50 per cent of male ABs who have a female Little. In my case, the hirsute older man dressed in 'baby drag' in the mirror can look grotesquely different from the cute adorable baby girl in my psyche. That difference is reinforced by most of our interactions with the world. Those interactions confirm only the existence of our adult host, to the exclusion of our child alter.

This cognitive dissonance can make us feel bad. Depending on what is going on for us, it can make us feel uncomfortable, or painful, or even tormented. If this seems overdramatic we need to consider several parallels that demonstrate the power of cognitive dissonance when it comes to personal identity. One is transgender people, another is people with anorexia.

The Adult Baby – An Identity on the Dissociation Spectrum

Felix Conrad in his book *'How to Jedi Mind Trick Your Gender Dysphoria'* describes the pain some male-to-female transgender people experience when they realize, even if they fully transitioned and had gender reassignment surgery, they will never pass for a woman in a way that fulfils the self-image in their psyche. It can be tormenting. Failure to accept the cruel constraints of biology can become an obsession that takes over and blights their lives. (Though both dysphoria and cognitive dissonance are describing the same experience, I prefer the latter. Dysphoria is associated exclusively with transgender people and cognitive dissonance better describes what creates the discomfort or distress.)

People with anorexia have a cognitive distortion; when they look in the mirror they see a fat person that contradicts the trim self-image they have in their psyche. The cognitive dissonance between those two images is tormenting and drives their self-destructive behaviour. In this context, it is not too much of a stretch to compare being AB and anorexia. Psychiatrist Colin Ross describes DID and identity alteration (alters) as a cognitive distortion. I think the description is unkind, but accurate. I am not suggesting ABs are transgender or anorexic, rather pointing out the power of cognitive dissonance when it comes to personal identity.

It doesn't seem people with DID have the same struggle with cognitive dissonance as ABs. I believe this is because of the different psychological functions dissociation serves for the two identities (as discussed in Chapter 11). People with DID are not driven by the same unconscious need to revisit childhood as ABs.

The only long term, psychologically healthy answer to doubt and cognitive dissonance is self-acceptance – to accept our child alter is subjectively real, *but not* objectively real. Self-acceptance is learning to trust our experience of our self - to trust it even when we are struggling with ourself, or with life. Self-acceptance really does work: to the extent that we trust our subjective experience, we are fortified against doubt and cognitive dissonance. Self-acceptance is continual, slow-yielding, self-disciplined effort.

Denial of Subjective Reality

So, sometimes painful doubt and cognitive dissonance will cause us to veer off the middle road.

In the first half of our life course as ABs, before we accept ourselves, the culprit is most likely doubt. With few or no signposts to guide us, we doubt our experience of ourselves. *I'm an adult. How can I sometimes feel like a baby or very young child?* That leads us to deny the subjective reality of having a child alter. The problem in this stage is what psychiatrist Colin Ross calls 'host resistance' (discussed in Chapter 10). Our adult host identifies itself as "us", our psyche, to the exclusion of our child alter(s). They reject the existence of our child alter because they want to disavow the alter's needs, and the alter's origin in trauma and insecure attachment. Our adult host struggles to accept our alters are a real and valid part of our psyche. The worst form of host resistance is the savage rejection of our child alter in the purge part of the 'binge and purge' cycle.

We have two choices. We can deny and reject our child alter, or we can accept them and make what we want of our identity. For people with DID, and ABs, denial of our subjective reality is our enemy. It *will* screw us up. The way to psychological health is to accept and nurture our child alter, and to build a loving and harmonious relationship between our child alter and our adult host. Speaking from personal experience, I can say this is healing and transformative. That's the same route as for people with DID. Other books cover accepting child alters extensively so I will provide just a summary here.

Nurturing

Child alters are subjectively real. They have real needs. Imagine having a neglected or ignored small child in your household. Sooner, rather than later, they are going to get distressed or angry, or both, and they are going to let you know about it. If you're a person with DID, or you're AB, your child alter is no different.

Like biological children, child alters need to be nurtured on a daily basis and to feel protected. Every AB, and every child alter is unique. You need to work out what best nurtures your child alter. See Rosalie Bent's book *'There's Still A Baby in My Bed'* or my book *'The Adult Baby Identity – A Self Help Guide'* for useful thoughts on

311

nurturing. Because child alters are subjectively real, they have access to the same deep sources of comfort as very young biological children. I'm talking about nappies, but also stuffed toys, a security blanket, or pacifiers or bottles.

Nurturing our child alters is self-love in the best sense of the term, and heals not just the child alter but the other alters as well. Providing nurturing turns angry, dysfunctional adult or adolescent alters from persecutors to protectors. They feel good about themselves and that removes the dysfunctions. This is true of both Dax and myself. The autobiographies of Christine Pattillo and Cameron West show how embracing and nurturing child alters can work for people with DID as well as it does for ABs.

Denial of Objective Reality

In the second half of our life course as ABs, the problem is usually cognitive dissonance. It goes like this: 'I have a compelling experience of sometimes feeling like a baby or very young child. But daily, my interactions with the world, keep telling me I'm 100% adult. It's painful having my feelings fight my mind'.

That leads us into toying with denying the objective reality that we are not biological children. I discuss this at greater length than the denial of subjective reality as it is not as widely covered elsewhere. It is the reverse of host resistance. It comes from our adult host growing tired and demoralized by cognitive dissonance and wanting to surrender that burden by giving way to our child alter.

It is an AB's adult host that struggles most with our identity of being a multiple with a child alter. Our child alter doesn't need to convince themselves they are real. They know they are. It is our adult host that bears the burden of cognitive dissonance. They are the alter who 'fronts' our psyche to the world. They are the alter that is most impacted by having to live with the fact that almost all of their daily interactions with others affirms only our adult side and denies the existence and need of our child alter(s). ABs alters are co-conscious and often co-present. So, our adult host is always aware of our child alter but they have to keep up the pretence to the rest of the world that the child alter doesn't exist. This can be cognitive dissonance at its worst. It can be exhausting and demoralizing.

From this place, it can seem like a solution for the adult host to step back, and cede more space in the psyche to the child alter.

Some ABs come to believe it is not their (adult host's) role to nurture and regulate the demands of their child alter, but their partner's. It's nice for our child alter(s) to have the love of the adult host's partner. A loving partner accepts the AB's child alter as subjectively real. The partner relates to the alter in some fashion as a caregiver. For some that will include changing nappies and bottle feeding or the like.

But our partner, no matter how accepting and loving, cannot supplant the role of the adult host in the psyche of the AB. Some ABs believe they can completely transfer this role as adult host to their partner. It represents trying to export the self-regulation and resilience of a healthy psyche to another person. That is incompatible with psychological health and stability.

Why? Because it denies the objective reality we do not have the psyche of a biological child. ABs do not have amnesia, our subjectively real child alter is co-conscious with our adult host. Each knows of the existence and capabilities of the other. Thus our child alter co-exists with our adult mind. A young child's psychological dependence on a parent is a necessary stage of their development. The same thing in an adult is unhealthy. That's for two reasons:

1. because a child's psyche is yet to gain adult capability, their dependence is not a denial of reality, indulgent or unhealthy; and
2. we do not share the child's sincere belief that our caregiver is infallible, selfless, omnipotent and immortal and thus can provide absolute safety for our psyche. As adults, we cannot unlearn the understanding that no caregiver can provide absolute safety, and we must be the first guarantor

of our own psychological safety and well being. Others can add immeasurably to our sense of safety and well being but they cannot substitute for the strength we must find within our psyche.

Remember too, that the deepest part of a child's psyche that is replicated by our child alters, transitional objects, represents a biological child comforting *themselves*. It is their first step beyond depending completely upon the nurturing of a primary caregiver. For an AB to read their child alter's need for transitional objects as consistent with their complete dependence on a partner's nurturing, is a misunderstanding of biological infancy.

The adult host ceding its space in our psyche to our child alter might seem like positive self-acceptance. It might seem like a kindness to our child alter. It is not so. For their child alter to feel safe and protected ABs need a strong adult host within their own psyche. In this, we are no different from other multiples. The DID self-help book *'Got Parts: An Insider's Guide to Managing Life Successfully With Dissociative Identity Disorder'*, describes this -

> *"Remember to love, to cherish, to value these young parts. … It can take great patience, finesse and wisdom to deal with wounded 'littles' … Yet, as they realise **the 'bigs' in the System [psyche] will keep them safe**, the rewards are well worth the investment of time and effort as they shed layers of fear and distrust and to learn to be open and loving and inquisitive and playful as they do their own healing work."*

The key point (bolded) in the quotation is that child alters need to be cared and protected, primarily, by the adult alters within the person's *own* psyche.

Only finding the strength within our psyche to care for our child alter is consistent with both our subjective *and* our objective reality. There is no sustainable safety for our child alter if our whole psyche renounces adult strength and resilience and is weak and vulnerable. It is impossible to remake ourselves into a biological child and trying to do so will cause us psychological harm. You can't be genuinely psychologically safe when you know you are consciously denying objective reality.

That is a fraught road for anyone with an identity which originated in childhood dissociation. In the original childhood trauma, we lacked adult coping skills. Denying objective reality was a survival mechanism which detached us from adverse circumstances that threatened to overwhelm our psyche. It was a source of resilience. But unhealthy DID shows us continuing to rely on dissociation, into adulthood when we do have adult coping skills, becomes dysfunctional. The reality we don't want to acknowledge doesn't go away. Continued reliance on dissociation makes people less resilient and more vulnerable.

How do you know if you are veering off the middle road into denying objective reality? I believe this commonly manifests in two ways –

1. an unhealthy infatuation with fantasies of permanent regression; and
2. seeking to replicate the physical lifestyle of a biological child for the greater part of the day or even 24/7, and an unhealthy infatuation with the child alter supplanting the adult host.

Each of these is discussed below.

Fantasies of Permanent Regression

There is a vast stock of AB fiction on-line. One of the most common themes is permanent regression to infancy, whether voluntary or involuntary. The reach of this theme indicates this is a powerful idea for ABs.

Sometimes indulging fantasies of permanent regression is positive or harmless – a temporary respite from the lesser discomforts of cognitive dissonance, and the self-discipline involved in accepting our complex dual identity. But when we are in a bad place and stray off the middle road these fantasies are both a symptom and a cause of psychological malaise. I stress the difference between these fantasies being harmless or negative is the state of mind of the AB.

When we are in a bad place, cognitive dissonance grows more burdensome. The temptation is to set aside the hard work of self-acceptance for a quick or easy fix. Then our use of AB fiction can become unhealthy. Fantasies of permanent regression can express and feed a desire to deny the objective reality that we are not biological children. It can get into our heads in a bad way.

ABs are a sub-DID group with a subjective identity derived from dissociation. For us, fantasy can be a particularly psycho-active ingredient. Let me explain. The ISSTD Guidelines describe people with DID as being 'highly hypnotizable'. This does not only refer to trances induced by a therapist. It also refers to the use of imagery and fantasy by multiples themselves. The ISSTD Guidelines state -

> *"... dissociative patients, usually unwittingly, use a variety of self-hypnotic strategies in an unbidden, uncontrolled, and disorganized way, and teaching them to exert some control over spontaneous hypnosis and self-hypnosis may allow them to contain certain distressing symptoms and to use their hypnotic talents to facilitate constructive self-care strategies."*

An example of the positive form of this self-hypnosis is using creative visualization to make a safe internal sanctuary for our alters, or nurture our child alter.

In the negative, it includes how off-balance ABs can become infatuated with fantasies of permanent regression. ABs can resort to these fantasies and the related on-line material frequently and compulsively. This is a powerful form of self-hypnosis as described in the Guidelines. That can lead to a negative trajectory. It can fetishize our identity as a multiple through an infatuation with B&D / power exchange themes. It can be reinforced by compulsive masturbation driven by painful cognitive dissonance (see the discussion in Chapter 16 about the relationship between cognitive dissonance and sexual climax). Eventually, that makes the cognitive dissonance and the doubt worse. In turn that feeds the need for more quick or easy fixes and a preoccupation with a 24/7 AB lifestyle.

Sometimes, when doubt and cognitive dissonance are weighing us down and drawing us into fetish depictions of our identity or power exchange relationship models, we need a reality check. Conduct a thought experiment. Take any given circumstance or depiction, either from fantasy or from real life. Take the nappies and the AB themes out of the equation. Is that situation psychologically healthy or unhealthy? Nappies and AB themes are not a magic ingredient. If the situation would be unhealthy without them, adding them, doesn't make it healthy. There are no quick or easy alternatives to self-acceptance of our dual identity.

Given that ABs are susceptible to triggering, it would be helpful for AB fiction or true-life books to carry trigger warnings. The warning would list the key themes in the book ie. permanent regression, power exchange or B&D relationships etc. The warning would alert potential readers who had recently experienced shame, compulsive behaviours or obsessive thoughts in relation to being AB, to look after their self-care and delay reading the book until they were in a better place with their identity.

Replicating the Physical Lifestyle of a Biological Child

For some psychologically vulnerable ABs, the denial of our objective reality can lead to wanting to replicate more and more of the physical lifestyle of a biological infant or small child in a way that is detrimental to the healthy role of their adult host.

By this, I mean going beyond providing physical comfort for our child alter in a way that allows our adult host to have an equal share of our daily life. It's fine to wear nappies openly in private, wear nappies discretely in public, have a private room which is a child's bedroom or nursery or sleep at night as an infant or toddler. None of these stops our adult host being able to live an adult life (and be accepted by others as an adult).

But some ABs want to go beyond this. On-line there are hypnosis tapes that purport to assist an AB to become incontinent, or to adopt on a full-time basis, other infantile traits such as a need for pacifiers or bottles. In social media, it is not uncommon to read posts by an AB seeking to become incontinent 24/7. Others advocate for the public permission to live openly as a child and go out in public dressed and acting as a biological child.

These ABs are seeking to physically replicate the lifestyle of a biological child. It represents an attempt to validate a reality that is subjective, to avoid painful doubt and cognitive dissonance. For psychologically vulnerable ABs this is a dangerous road to take. This is emphasized in the ISSTD Guidelines -

> *"In addition to being highly hypnotizable, some DID patients have been thought to be highly fantasy prone .... A minority may be so, although several studies suggest that most DID patients are only moderately fantasy prone ... Nonetheless, there is concern that at least some DID patients are vulnerable to confusing fantasy with authentic memory and/or mistaking experiences within the inner worlds of the personalities for events in external reality whether or not hypnosis is induced ..."*

I suspect the Guidelines are concerned with avoiding 'false' memories of childhood abuse. But for ABs the concern about multiples being fantasy-prone includes an obsession with the 24/7 AB lifestyle (which is based on an artificial 'fantasy' view of childhood).

Remember, being AB is an unconscious attempt to revisit childhood trauma and effect a different outcome – a secure attachment with a caregiver. We can make our peace with that. But when that becomes a flight from adulthood it becomes unhealthy.

It represents the adult host wanting to cede its proper place in the psyche to the child alter, and perhaps to cede the healthy self-regulation of their own psyche to a partner. We know from the above discussion, it is because the adult host has grown exhausted and demoralized by the constant burden of cognitive dissonance. In the extreme, this parallels situations where someone with DID changes their host personality. That is a major psychological threshold. For someone with DID, a child alter supplanting an adult personality as the host would be a grave indication of psychological deterioration. It is no different for ABs. It is a denial of the objective reality ABs are not biological children, either physically or psychologically.

This is akin to the obsession Felix Conrad indicates can blight the lives of some transgender people. It is akin to the self-destructiveness of anorexia. For ABs, it represents the renunciation of adult resilience and surrender to self-absorption. One of the problems in going down this road is that an AB or their partner may believe they are in conscious control of the trajectory when they are not. They are using dissociation as a coping strategy. We know from DID, the real driver of that trajectory is repressed or denied childhood trauma. Good things don't drive trajectories that undermine our adult resilience and make us more psychologically vulnerable. Denying objective reality hits a fault line in our psyche as a multiple. Pursue that denial too hard, for too long and there is an escalating risk to psychological health. In a previous chapter, I quoted Dax saying he knew of people who failed to come to terms with being a multiple and it consumed them.

Understanding that ABs are multiples with a child alter which originated in childhood trauma means there is help for AB's struggling with this situation. Psychotherapy with a skilled psychotherapist, based on an accurate diagnosis of dissociation, offers the prospect of healthy relief and healing for a struggling AB and their demoralized and exhausted adult host. See appendix 2 for thoughts on finding the right therapist and psychotherapy.

What's Real?

Sometimes living with our dual identity can feel like living in a no-man's land betwixt subjective and objective reality. Sometimes we can lose track of what's real.

So what is real?

Our dual identity is real.

The need to balance the needs of both our adult and child alters is real.

Our broken childhood attachment is real. If it wasn't, you wouldn't need nappies.

The childhood trauma is real. If it wasn't, you wouldn't have a Little/child alter.

I believe, like DID, being AB is a childhood-onset post-traumatic developmental disorder.

You didn't ask for any of it. It's not your fault. But you got it. You need to make your own peace with it.

The broken attachment and the trauma can be healed. You can't 'cure' either of them away, but you can make your peace with them.

Summary

For ABs, our child alters can be a gift. They give us access to innocent happiness and contentment which approaches that of a securely attached biological child. But as multiples, our psyches are complex and there are risks if we do not find a way to live safely with that complexity. We have to walk a middle road between denying the subjective reality of having child alters with their own needs, and denying the objective reality we are not biological children, either physically or psychologically.

As a result of our complex psyches, we cannot completely escape living with doubt and cognitive dissonance. They are sometimes painful. We are not the only minority identity with that challenge – for example, people who identify as transgender but chose not to transition, are in a similar boat. The only psychologically safe sustainable antidote to doubt and cognitive dissonance is acceptance of our dual subjective child/objective adult reality. Self-acceptance is a long, slow, self-disciplined effort. But it works. It does fortify you against doubt and cognitive dissonance. You can love and enjoy your child alter without having to prove they are objectively real.

16. Alters and AB Sexuality

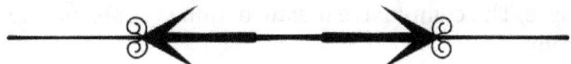

I am an unlikely person to be writing about sexuality. I am inhibited and strongly introverted. These are not the best qualifications for writing about this topic. But it's important and it's a big part of being AB. It contributes a great deal to the confusion and shame that conflicted ABs feel about their identity. And I believe that I have found insights that might help others to better understand themselves.

Most of what I understand about AB sexuality is based on my own experience. In the introduction, I said take what is helpful from this book, and leave the rest behind. That applies doubly to this chapter.

From what I have read in online forums and AB non-fiction books, I believe that my experience conforms with many other male ABs. However, there is comparatively little written from the perspective of female ABs, particularly when it comes to sexuality. So I don't know how similar or different this issue is for female ABs. For example, do they suffer, in the conflicted stage of our identity, from the same compulsive masturbation as male ABs? I don't know. There is a clear need for more writing from the perspective of female ABs.

For ABs, sex can be complicated. That's for three reasons –

1. we have a sexual fetish;
2. sex can involve a lot of involuntary switching between alters; and
3. the erotic 'target' of an AB's sexual fantasies may not be sex with a partner, but their own fantasised transformation into an adorable dependent baby.

Each of these is discussed below.

Fetish

Many mental health professionals and laypeople consider that being AB is a sexual fetish. That is how it is defined in the DSM. That's wrong in as much as the fetish for nappies/diapers is a *symptom* of being AB, not the cause. We are ABs because we have a subjectively real child alter, which dissociated in childhood trauma. But we still have a sexual fetish for nappies. Why? How?

The key is understanding the sequence of developments. I believe what came first was the broken (insecure) attachment with our mothers/primary caregivers. Remember, attachment patterns are established very early in life. They are well developed by the time a child is 12 months old. The insecure attachment made us more vulnerable to being traumatized by the 'ordinary catastrophes' of childhood, such as temporary separations from mother. The traumatic event or events came next. It was probably when we were still very young. In my case, the first traumatic event was when I was three or four years old. That's when our psyche first split off a child alter.

It seems for many ABs, the first experimentation and compulsion to wear nappies didn't manifest until some years later. Around the age of ten seems to be a common experience. For some it was much younger, even going back to age five or six. Whatever the exact age, it was before puberty. The nappies started off being a source of emotional comfort-driven from our subconscious by the needs of our unrecognized child alter.

Then along comes puberty and our adolescent host develops sexual needs and the beginnings of their sexual identity. This is grafted onto the existing most powerful dynamic in our psyche – our child alter. Voila! Nappy/diaper fetish. Nappies now serve two needs – our child alter's need for comfort and nurturing, and our adolescent host's sexual needs. Nappies are both a transitional object and a fetish object. And as we don't know we are multiples, these different needs are experienced as a tormenting conflict within ourselves.

How we derive sexual pleasure gets hard-wired pretty early in adolescence. Thereafter, the constant reinforcement of pleasure means those preferences aren't amenable to change. So even after we have accepted our identities as ABs, and as multiples, we will still have a nappy fetish. For me, nappies and fantasies of being babied are indispensable to sexual pleasure. The compulsive masturbation is gone, but the nappy fetish remains. I believe that would be true for ABs generally.

Switching and Sex

Sex is the circumstance most associated with involuntary and unrecognized switching between my alters. Switching commonly occurred in sexual arousal, and again immediately after sexual climax. That means in a short space of time three different alters were in executive control of my body. There was the alter before sexual arousal, a different one during sexual arousal and climax, and a third one after climax. When I was conflicted about being AB the switching was abrupt and brought confronting changes in my emotions and thoughts.

Take the example of the involuntary triggering of the need to put on a nappy. My experience is described below -

> *"I wanted nappies because they met a deep need within me. I wanted to enjoy the wonderful feeling of freedom, of coming home to myself, that wearing a nappy represented. I was often stressed, tense and anxious. The prospect of wearing a nappy promised at least a brief respite of being able to lose my adult worries and feel comforted and safe. But that goal always got hijacked with me becoming sexually aroused, and masturbating while wearing the nappy. A powerful climax was pretty much always guaranteed. But immediately after I would be filled with feelings of shame and remorse. I would hurriedly fling the nappy aside, put on my adult clothes and quickly tidy everything out of sight. The goal of being comforted in a really deep and satisfying way always seemed to be just out of reach." ['The Adult Baby Identity - A Self Help Guide']*

My reading suggests this is a fairly typical experience of male ABs. We can look again at this situation with our understanding of ABs being multiples. It was my child alter coming 'out' and desperate for nurturing and the comforting familiarity of a nappy that triggered my need to put on a nappy. But that purely emotional need didn't hold sway for long because nappies are a sexual fetish for my adult host. They needed the release of masturbation as an antidote to stress, anxiety and also to the conflicts about being AB in the first place. So, as the fetishized nappy caused sexual arousal, my adult host switched 'out' replacing my child alter in executive control.

Then, immediately after climax, my punitive parent alter switched out. They were angry and scared at the loss of control caused by the needs of my child alter and adult host. It was the revulsion of my punitive parent alter that caused me to immediately throw off the nappy and rush to 'tidy away' all the evidence of my AB side. No wonder masturbation was so compulsive and emotionally convulsive! Of course, before I accepted I was a multiple I didn't recognize this switching for what it was – I just lived with the abrupt and confronting shifts between emotional states.

Rosalie Bent describes the switching which occurs after sexual climax –

> *"One problem that may occur is known as the 'crash'. Orgasm usually causes the Little One to temporarily disappear and for the adult to re-emerge. In masturbation, this is expected and understood and is normally, relatively gentle. During sexual intercourse, however, the feelings and emotions are far more intense and can cause the re-emergence to be powerful, fast and at times, overwhelming. Be aware of it and comfort your adult if this happens. It is also a good reminder for both of you to realise that sex was actually between two adults, but the 'crash' can also sometimes be disturbing. Be prepared for tears at times. It is all worth it, however. The recovery from the crash is usually quick and becomes easier if the Little One is permitted to crash and then recover with you there, as his primary support."*

Now that I have fully accepted myself as an AB and a multiple, it works a bit differently. Thankfully! My child alter gets to wear nappies at regular times each day. Most days that doesn't result in any inclination for my adult host to masturbate. On the occasions that I do masturbate, when I start to think about sexual fantasies that precede sexual arousal, my child alter switches inside. It is my adult host which enjoys the fetishized fantasies and reaches sexual climax. Afterwards, it is my child alter which switches back out to resume the comforting feelings of being in a nappy and have a nap. My punitive parent alter plays no part (I think with self-acceptance and retirement, they have either become dormant or fused with my adult host). The switching is not abrupt, more like shifting, without the conflicting emotions and needs.

Understanding all this has let me see that sex and specifically, fetishized sex, is driven by the needs of my adult host, not my child alter. As a result, I believe that AB's child alters seek only emotional comfort from wearing nappies.

The Erotic Target

That brings us to the third point above, the erotic target of an AB's sexual fantasies. What do I mean by erotic target? It is what fulfils your sexual fantasy, the endpoint that brings you to sexual climax. In researching this book it was a revelation to me to realise that the erotic target of my sexual fantasies was not sex with a partner. It was imagining myself to be an adorable, helpless and dependent baby. A desirable adult woman was always part of my sexual fantasies. But I realized that they are there as caregivers, not sexual partners. In my fantasies, they are treating me as a baby, not as a sexual object.

I owe this understanding to Felix Conrad's insight into transgender erotic fantasies. In his book *'Transgender: Fact or Fetish'* he indicated that the erotic target of at least some male to female transgender people was not sex with a partner, but imagining themselves with the body of the woman that met the idealized self-image in their psyche. I realized this applied to me, except as an AB, I wasn't imagining myself as a woman, but as an adorable baby girl.

Sexual fantasies are notoriously individual and diverse. Perhaps this was just my 'thing' and had no relevance to other ABs? But then I looked at the erotic AB fiction I liked to read. All of it was based on stories where the protagonist was psychologically or physically turned into a helpless dependent baby. Depending on the story, the women characters may have played a sexual role, but that was ancillary. Their main role was to 'baby' the protagonist, not to relate to him as a sexual adult. Most of the detail elaborated in these stories is not about sex, but about how the male protagonist's adulthood is stripped away and how that makes him feel, willingly or unwillingly, like a baby. That's where the author's and the reader's attention lies. That was the erotic target, not sex with a partner.

There are a lot of these stories on-line which meant there was a market for them. It wasn't just me! I'm not saying this is the only game in town when it comes to AB sexual fantasies and AB fiction. But it does look like it's a sizeable part of the market, and hence a sizeable part of the AB population.

But how does this erotic target fit with an AB's alters? As we have seen, it is the adult host who is 'out' in an AB's sexual arousal and climax, not their child alter. Why does our adult host need sexual fantasies where they are transformed into an adorable baby? Because as we saw in the previous chapter, it is an AB's adult host that bears the burden of the sometimes painful cognitive dissonance about being AB. The fantasy and the erotic target salves that burden. At the point of climax, our adult host's identification with the child alter is complete and the painful cognitive dissonance is momentarily dispelled. For that brief moment, we are not a multiple. We are just our child alter. And we are adored – loved and protected – so that the broken childhood attachment is also repaired. That's why the need for masturbation is so compulsive and powerful for conflicted ABs. All this logic happens in our sub-conscious so most aren't aware of it.

I found corroboration of my experience in an account by Maggie Joyce. She is the partner of an AB, and the mother of her husband's Little, a baby girl named Melissa who identifies as a nine-month-old. Maggie provides the following account of her AB partner's sexual climax -

"The truly fascinating and possibly freaky aspect of this is that at the point of orgasm, she is as young as ever I see her. I can only imagine the psychological processes at work, but as she approaches orgasm, I can see in her face a lowering of her age until at that point, she is perhaps as close to a new-born as she gets. It only takes a few moments for her to return to her nine-month-old age again, but for a moment, she is new-born." ['The Full Time Permanent Adult Infant']

I believe Maggie is describing the point where the adult host is completely identified with the child alter. The rapid transition back to reality after sexual climax also helps us better understand the 'crash' earlier described by Rosalie Bent.

But what about all the fetish bondage and discipline (B&D) and power exchange themes in AB fiction? Doesn't that contradict the idea that our erotic target is not about sex? No. Those themes are what our adult host needs to bridge the chasm between what they believe sex should be about (sex with a partner), and the real erotic target of seeing ourselves an adorable helpless baby. Remember the phenomena of host resistance identified by psychiatrist Colin Ross and discussed in Chapter 10. Our adult host struggles to accept that our child alter is an equally real and valid part of our psyche. This is especially true of sex. A healthy child alter does not have an interest in sex. Sex is the province and need of our adult host or alters. But the deepest need of our adult host is to dispel the pain of cognitive dissonance. And that leaves a chasm between what our adult host believes sex should be about and what it's really about when you're an AB. That's where the fetish, B&D and power exchange themes come in.

In an earlier chapter, I mentioned psychotherapist Michael Bader's insightful understanding of the role of sexual fantasies. No matter how strange they may seem, our sexual fantasies allow us to find sexual pleasure in the face of pathogenic beliefs that we derived from our upbringing – beliefs that would otherwise prevent us from reaching sexual arousal and climax. For example, for someone who enjoys the submissive role in B&D, the fantasies are an antidote to our childhood fears that we are unimportant to our loved ones. If we could not counter this unconscious belief it would be impossible to gain sexual pleasure. Who could get sexually aroused either with a real partner or in fantasy, if we really believed that we are insignificant and undeserving of attention? The intense attention and focus of a 'dominant' in B&D fantasies is a reassurance that we do matter to them, we are important – loved. Again, this logic happens in our subconscious and most are unaware of it.

ABs have a broken childhood bond with our primary caregiver. A young child unconsciously takes responsibility for the broken bond because it is too terrifying to see a deficit in the caregiver upon whom they are completely dependent. So, unconsciously, the child believes the broken bond must be their fault. They are unloveable.

So an AB faces two major obstacles within their own psyche to sexual pleasure. Firstly, sex is an adult need and means sex with an adult partner, but the deepest need is release from the painful cognitive dissonance of the contradiction of simultaneously being both adult and child. Secondly, we have an unconscious belief that we are unloveable – we were unloveable as children, we are still unloveable as adults.

As Michael Bader says, fetish and B&D fantasies are the solutions to these obstacles. Typically the fantasies start with the protagonist being an adult. That's the starting point our adult host needs to feel okay about sex as an adult activity. Typically, (but not always) the fantasies involve the protagonist with someone who is, or has the prospect of being, a desirable sexual partner. Another tick for our adult host. The fantasy involves the 'partner' progressively transforming the protagonist into a submissive, dependent, infantilized figure. The protagonist may be willing, but is typically unwilling, with some ineffectual show of resistance. Unwilling submission is a sop to our punitive parent alter that we do not want what we really want, to surrender being an adult and the cognitive dissonance that goes with it.

As the fantasy progresses, the partner figure asserts their dominance. They effectively transform into a parent/caregiver substitute for the emerging unified adult-child figure. In some fantasies, the parent/caregiver may have had this character from the outset. In this situation, the unconscious mind converts B&D themes of dominance to signals the emerging baby of the fantasy is adored and safe. This works for both the adult host and the child alter. The eventual submission of the infantilized protagonist to the 'partner'/substitute parent-caregiver represents the adult host surrendering the burden of cognitive dissonance, of maintaining the pretence that the psyche is wholly adult. That goes to our adult host's deepest but unacknowledged need. Fetish discipline stands for unconditional parental love and devoted parental attention. For the child alter, this dispels the wound of the broken childhood attachment – they are loved and protected.

When we are conflicted about being AB, our resort to these fantasies is guilty and compulsive. We need their unconscious logic to reach sexual arousal and climax but we don't understand much of it. The conflict between our adult host and our child alter can be savage. That can drive us compulsively to the release of sexual climax and ever more extreme fantasies. Typically the B&D themes grow stronger with a greater degree of coercion, humiliation and punishment. That is intrinsically unhealthy. It can represent us punishing ourselves for the existence and real needs of our child alter. And the stronger B&D themes intensify our guilt. It can develop into a negative spiral. The circuit brake is that we exhaust ourselves sexually, physically. But it can still leave us in a dark place at the bottom of the spiral.

After we have genuinely accepted our child alter the absence of the conflict within our psyche drains the energy from compulsive sexual activity. The compulsion disappears. The nappy fetish remains. But the fantasies are less extreme. They still involve submission to a parent/caregiver substitute and some parental like discipline but it doesn't have the hard edge of coercion and humiliation. I believe that when fetish and B&D themes still play a large part in an AB's fantasies or in their self-image, it is a sign of still unresolved conflict about their identity as ABs.

Child Alters and Sex

That brings us to the issue of child alters and sex.

Obviously, people with DID, who may have child alters, have sex with their adult partners. However, the accounts I have read indicate psychologically healthy people with DID take great care not to involve their child alters in sexual activity. Once it is accepted that child alters are subjectively real, it could not be otherwise.

What about ABs? On-line, many ABs seem to have or seek DDLG (Dominant Daddy / Little Girl) relationships – or the gender converse, variously identified as Dominant Mummy or Caregiver / Little Boy, or similar. These relationships commonly include sexual relations and are generally thought of as a fetish, kink, or form of B&D. In these situations, the child self may appear to be involved in sexual activity. In a healthy situation, I believe that is not so.

As we have seen above, sex is the province and the need of an AB's adult host. An AB's child alter wants nappies (only) because they bring emotional comfort and safety. The sexual fetish dimension of nappies and power exchange practices belong to the adult host. In my experience, in sexual activity, my adult host self displaces my child alters.

This does not deny that DDLG or similar relationships can meet the emotional needs of child alters. The DDLG or equivalent relationship pattern can be seen as a potentially positive acceptance of a person's subjective reality of a child alter by their partner. For many people, it is probably the only available model of a relationship which can encompass the needs of imperfectly understood child alters.

However, I believe there are psychological risks in such relationships where there is not an understanding of dissociation and alters. The existence of unidentified and unhealed childhood trauma create a risk of psychological harm where sexual and power exchange behaviours do not respect the boundaries between the adult host and child alters.

A willingness by a multiple to involve their subjectively real child alter in sexual activity may be an indicator of sexual abuse in childhood. The psychiatrists familiar with DID indicate sometimes unhealed dysfunctional alters seek to replicate the abusive and exploitative relationships that caused the original childhood trauma. This can be based on a variety of dysfunctional motivations: an alter that loves the abuser, a desire to confirm the alter is bad and seek punishment or abasement, and so on. These motivations are unconscious but the repetition of the original abusive or and exploitive pattern reinforces the original trauma.

The boundary against involving a child alter in sexual activity must be upheld. The child alter is subjectively real. The same need to protect them (and the whole psyche) from psychological harm applies as for a biological child.

Summary

Sex is complicated for ABs! We have a sexual fetish for nappies. Our alters can switch several times before and after sex. And the erotic target of our sexual fantasies may not be sex with an adult partner, but our transformation into an adorable baby.

17. Self Care for ABs

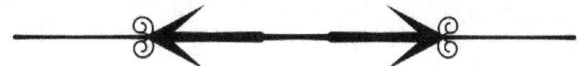

Self-care for ABs extends beyond the inside of our psyches.

We have the example of people with DID to know living with alters can be challenging. Everyone, whether they are singletons or multiples, needs to feel psychologically safe. But for multiples, it is a little more complicated. Alters are there 24/7. *Each* of them processes and sometimes reacts to the stimuli taken in by our senses. *Each* of them needs to feel safe and at ease, for us to go about our lives without disruption.

So self care, and the right self care, is essential. I believe that includes the following –

- a safe physical personal environment;
- a place of sanctuary within our psyche;
- to recognize our need for acceptance by loved ones;
- to recognize our need for fellowship with others like us;
- to have outlets for service and creativity;
- to be cautious about disclosure; and
- to come to terms with childhood trauma.

Each of these is discussed below.

Safe Physical Environment

Everybody needs a safe physical environment. Why that's important is a bit different for people living with alters.

ABs commonly need a somewhat sequestered environment that provides privacy because they have to conceal their lifestyle. The privacy conceals the wearing of nappies and baby clothes, and perhaps baby play. It also commonly conceals a large stock of baby clothes and paraphernalia. But I realized my need for a sequestered environment is not just about physical concealment of an AB lifestyle. Dax, with DID, has a similar need for a controllable environment, and his need has little to do with hiding a lifestyle.

The need relates to living with alters 24/7. It is a need for respite, to minimize stimuli which might trigger alters. Such stimuli include unpredictable interactions with others who are unaware or unaccepting of our alters. Speaking for his 'system' Dax says -

> *"We crave silence always, limit access to TV and rarely listen to music because, noise destroys our ability to focus and hear our thoughts. We like to hear the muffled sounds of each other. We are collectively more balanced and switching is controlled when interactions with people are limited."*

It is also a need not to have to hide - a freedom for alters to be out and express themselves and their needs without fear and inhibition.

A physical environment which meets these needs removes the apprehensions and uncertainty that replicate the symptoms of anxiety. Such an environment remains safe only when it's shared with a partner or others who understand and accept our alters. The form such a safe physical environment takes can vary. At its least, it is likely to involve a room where you can close the door on the outside. At its best, it's a whole dwelling, or even better, a dwelling in a surrounding physical space.

Dax's instinctive affinity for small islands makes perfect sense in this context. His preference is *'the smaller and more isolated the better'*. He explained islands represent safety because in a metaphorical sense they are circles – if you get lost you will end up safely back where you started. Cameron West lives with his wife in a house by the beach. Olga Trujillo lives on a small farm.

Internal sanctuary

A safe physical environment where alters don't have to hide and don't face uncontrolled and unpredictable interactions with others provides a place of respite to re-charge. But if you've got alters you can't live as a hermit. You have to be able to carry a place of psychological safety with you wherever you go.

For Dax and myself, a place of sanctuary within the psyche is very important. Dax describes it as the place where "we [his alters] take our thoughts in times of heightened anxiety and stress. It's a place without walls, it involves water, a never-ending horizon, peace and no people." Again, you can hear the echo of Dax's affinity for small islands in his conception of his internal sanctuary.

Having this internal sanctuary is a technique which is commonly recommended for people with DID. *'Got Parts: An Insiders Guide to Managing Life Successfully with Dissociative Identity Disorder'* says –

> *"Everyone in the System [psyche] needs to work together to create a safe space inside where you all reside. This place is sometimes known as the 'Dome'. This is where parts are when they are not 'out', and is a place to get to know each other better, and to do your healing work individually and together. … Using the creative power of your imaginations, you invent this actual place inside you. It is very important to create the Dome together, and that it is safe. … [it] can take any physical configuration … Examples include a Sphere, or Pyramid, or Lighthouse, or Cathedral, or Log Cabin, or Tepee, or Space Station. It could be a beautiful place in nature, like a serene ocean shoreline or wildflower prairie or lush rainforest …"*

Christine Pattillo describes and even provides a map of the internal share house where her alters and host personality reside when they aren't 'out'. Cameron West has an internal 'comfort room' for his alters.

I have an internal sanctuary. It is described in my book *'The Adult Baby Identity – A Self Help Guide'* -

> *My safe space is a country cottage. It is peaceful but not isolated. The house has a beautiful nursery with white wooden furniture, including a cot, changing table, and nursing chair; and is decorated in pink and soft pastel colours. There are windows and French doors opening onto a broad shady veranda. Beyond is a soft, soft lawn enclosed in a sturdy white open post fence that keeps wandering toddlers safe inside and everything else outside. … In the day it is always barmy, not hot, and at nights it is cuddly cool – perfect for fuzzy, footed sleepers or pyjamas. It is lovely to visit when I am in bed falling sleep. It is where I take Chrissie if she gets frightened.*

I suspect many ABs imagine a fully decked out nursery in their minds. Those who are fortunate to create a nursery in real life are transposing something that already exists in their imaginations.

Acceptance By Loved Ones

I believe ABs and people with DID share a fundamental need - to be believed about our subjective sense of self. Our subjective reality is compelling and fundamental to who we are. But we can't prove it to someone who doubts us. Being believed is an act of empathy which allows us to stop pretending about who we are around others. It lifts the heavy burden of hiding ourselves, and the awful fear of rejection.

For any multiple, once someone accepts our alters are subjectively real, they 'get' us – all our otherwise inexplicable traits and behaviours are completely understandable. (Accepting our subjective reality doesn't compel our loved ones to do anything – they have the same choices as we do in terms of how best to respond to this reality in a way that works for them.)

For ABs, the loving acceptance of a partner also soothes the cognitive dissonance we discussed above. It is powerful because it is an acceptance that is lived out every day, in small unconscious ways. It becomes normal and natural for you and your partner to feel you share your household with a young child.

One of the most challenging situations is for ABs who begin to accept their identities later in life, and who have an established marriage or partnership. There is an awful tension between not wanting to injure or lose a relationship with a beloved and admired life partner, but needing to be true to ourselves and not having to hide a fundamental part of our identity.

As ABs, we know the process of accepting ourselves wasn't easy or fast. Even with the best will of all involved, gaining the acceptance of loved ones, isn't likely to be any different. I suspect most ABs make lots of mistakes in seeking our partner's acceptance – initially we are too desperate and demanding. Compared to our own inner journey we expect our partner to fast track their own processes. We want to dictate what form our partner's acceptance of our subjective reality takes instead of allowing them to choose what is safe for them.

In the hiccups of that process or worst case if we are rejected, we can slip back into shame and denial. In seeking acceptance we can be clumsy and demanding. But we should never reproach ourselves for our need for acceptance. It's normal and healthy.

Fellowship With Like Others

Another important need is for the fellowship of those who share our identity.

The common experience of people with DID and ABs is we are adept at hiding in plain sight. With the prospect of real detriment from broad disclosure, we have to. But if we hide all the time from everyone, that is a road to neurosis. It is not psychologically healthy to go around experiencing ourselves as being the sole outlier in the human experience. No matter how introverted we may be, (like myself) our species are social animals. With that psychology hard-wired in our brains, outlier equals outcast, and outcasts don't live long and happy lives. We need the fellowship of others whose own identity validates ours.

As challenging as it may be, I don't believe there is a tenable longer-term alternative to reaching out to others like ourselves. I am in the early part of this journey so I am not well placed to add much further value on the topic. What I have discovered is, as imperfect as they are, online and social media environments, do provide opportunities for fellowship for those with rare, and misunderstood personal identities.

Service and Creativity

For Dax and myself, service to others in our working life offsets the alienation of having an identity the world doesn't accept. I suspect this is common to many people with minority personal identities. Dax is a gifted teacher for children with learning difficulties. He talks about his lifelong connection to children as a *'strong desire to nurture other children to make them stronger, smarter and less vulnerable than we were.'* I am proud of a career of service to the public good. For both of us, those vocations let us feel good about ourselves – in seeking to be of service to others, we weren't negatively defined by our misunderstood personal identities.

Having an outlet for our personal creativity has also helped us live with our challenging identities. Again, I suspect this is common to many people beyond those with DID, or ABs. Dax is at home in the digital world where his affinity with different media gives him a creative outlet. It is the basis for a successful online consultancy. He relates that success to his DID – which facilitated being able to learn and fulfil a range of roles such as website designer, tech support, service provider, content creator, and more. My creative outlet is writing. To me, writing seems especially suited to exploring and understanding identity, in fiction and non-fiction.

Outlets for service and creativity are important to everyone. They are particularly important for people who feel alienated because of their non-conforming personal identities.

Be Cautious In Disclosure

While accepting our need for the acceptance of our loved ones, and the fellowship of those like us, we also need to recognize general disclosure carries a strong risk of detriment.

Some brave or fortunate multiples do live openly with their identity. Christine Pattillo and Robert Oxnam are examples. Most of us live 'in the closet' because we have a valid fear of harm from the prejudice and misconceptions of others. There are many occupations and employers where your job and your career would be at grave risk if your identity as a multiple were known. Robert Oxnam seems to have had to leave his former career as an international academic when he was 'outed' with DID.

Multiple consciousness scares people. It is equated with dangerous insanity and debilitating dysfunction. That's wrong. It's changing, but slowly. Even when people know multiple consciousness isn't a physical threat, it makes them feel unsafe. It represents the unknown. It is a departure from a unitary view of the psyche whose simplicity is comforting and safe.

I suspect most people are aware their own psyches are anything but simple – consciousness is multi-layered and at times contradictory. But denial is everywhere and it works. The notion of a simple, unitary psyche holds unwelcome questions at bay. Let's face it, if you have DID, or you are AB, we ultimately had to accept our less-than-straight-forward psyches because we had no choice. Other people don't want their option of denial taken away.

Psychiatrist Colin Ross provides the following advice to people with DID who ask 'Should I tell other people about my trauma and dissociation?' –

> *"It really depends. Having a person who understands you is important and helpful. However, there are risks. For instance, the person may not understand, may not believe in what you say, may criticize you, may use this to attack you, or may tell this to others even without your permission. It is necessary to think carefully before you make the decision."*

> *"Another issue that comes up frequently is how much to tell other people about both your trauma and dissociation. Again, it is possible to err in both directions. If you tell too many people too many details too fast, you can drive people away. This isn't proof that you are unloveable. Cancer patients often experience the same thing – many of their 'friends' can't cope with the cancer and disappear. This is when you learn who your true friends are. It's a painful process, but you end up with a smaller collection of true friends who you can focus on."*

> *"For children, overall, the less they are told about your trauma and dissociation, the better. Certainly, you shouldn't explain trauma and dissociation to children under 10."*

> *"For employers, generally, the less they know the better. Sometimes they need to be filled in for leave, disability or other reasons. It's probably better to say you have PTSD, anxiety or depression than to share a DID or OSDD diagnosis. That sets off fewer alarm bells in the outside system. Not telling all the details does not equal lying. It's your business, not theirs. Don't get pressured into telling more than you want to tell."*

For ABs, the fear that some people will conflate our identity with paedophilia is a further risk in disclosure. There has been some progress in public understanding that this is not so, but the risk is still present.

The discussion above applies to simply advising others you are AB /OSDD. That's different from sharing the lifestyle of your very young child alter, their needs and behaviour with others. I believe that is a private matter to be shared only with carefully chosen loved ones. As ABs, we sometimes struggle with doubt and cognitive dissonance about our baby or child alters, even though they are compellingly real to us. It is asking too much of others to deal with that cognitive dissonance. The vast majority will not deal with it well, and will not thank us for asking them to make the attempt. You can't blame them for that.

But I do believe in working towards positive changes in public understanding so ABs can declare without detriment they are 'multiples', functional adults with a young child alter(s).

Come to Terms With Past Trauma

I believe at the source of being AB there is dissociated childhood trauma, together with an insecure childhood attachment. If you have a 'Little' you are a multiple. A Little is an alter. The clear view of contemporary psychology is the source of alters is most likely childhood trauma. It isn't as devastating as that which caused DID, but it's still not good. Just as I believe denial can fuck us up, so can unacknowledged trauma.

Unhealed dissociated childhood trauma is an ongoing risk to our mental health. It predisposes you to anxiety and depression. It subtly warps your perceptions, most notably about yourself, in ways you do not see. It sneaks harmful baggage into the relationships with those you love – baggage you are not fully aware of, but your loved ones most likely are. It can lead you to toy with denying the objective reality you are not a biological child, either physically or psychologically.

Denial is the natural first response to the awareness there might be something bad at the back of the cupboard in our psyche. Don't let it be your last response. Don't be afraid of what is within your psyche. You are already living with it. The choice is between bumping around in the dark or turning on a light to see what needs to be healed. For ABs, dissociated trauma can be healed and that is life-changing. But it needs the help of skilled counsellor. See the appendix 2 on therapy for ABs as an identity on the dissociation spectrum.

Summary

Good self-care is essential for everybody. Living with alters puts a different 'spin' on what good self-care means for a multiple. Good self-care is the difference between living with alters as a gift, and living with alters as a blight.

18. Conclusion

At the start of the book, I talked about how each AB comes to feel their psyche is hard wired differently from those around them.

Well, now we can see it's true. Our psyches were rewired by trauma in our childhood. Dissociation gave us subjectively real child alters. The trauma and the alters were largely repressed in our subconscious for many years.

But not completely, even early on. As biological children, ABs had issues with their continence – toilet training or bedwetting. Years later, the regression to that fixation is the initial point where the repression of our child alter in our subconscious breaks down. Even though the existence of the child alter is at first not understood, they are the source of our craving to wear nappies. The feel of a nappy is a familiar source of comfort to them.

Our daydreams and fantasies are filled with images of being treated like dependent helpless babies and children. Over time, the 'acting out' of our child alter typically expands to other familiar sources of infantile comfort: stuffed toys, pacifiers, child or baby style clothing etcetera. These are a clear signal from our subconscious that we share our psyche with a small child. But typically it takes us many years to accept the blindingly obvious. We can't blame ourselves for that. We were taught to think of alters and multiple consciousness as indications of insanity. We weren't insane, so it must be something else. A fetish? A kink? Those were never good explanations, but they were the distraction our denial required.

But now we understand dissociation. Every person on the dissociation spectrum has a unique 'footprint'. Each different 'footprint' produces a unique experience of self and life. We can recognize DID and being AB are identities on the dissociation spectrum. DID is at the further end of the spectrum, while being AB is 'next door'. With a lifetime of sometimes compulsive infantile behaviours at odds with our adult selves, I believe being AB fits the category of OSDD – *Other Specified Dissociative Disorder*. In the absence of clinically significant distress or impairment, both DID and being AB are minority personal identities, not disorders.

The compelling similarity between DID and being AB is both have subjectively real alters which influence thought, feelings, perceptions and behaviour. For both, alters are present 24/7 and can potentially be triggered at any time. There are striking similarities in the description of child alters between people with DID and ABs.

But DID and being AB are not the same. The defining characteristic of DID is the combination of identity alteration and amnesia. The amnesia causes a devastating fragmentation of the psyche. Being AB is identity alteration without the amnesia. DID represents an unconscious flight from childhood trauma, while being AB is an unconscious attempt to revisit it to change the outcome. There is a family 'likeness' between DID and being AB - but with the important differences, we are like first cousins rather than siblings.

The presence or absence of amnesia produces a different experience of alters between the two identities. For many people with DID, switching means a distinct change between the host personality and an alter, or between alters. Even with co-consciousness, shared memory, if one is 'out', the others are in the background.

It's different for ABs. Typically their host adult personality and their child alter are co-present. That's a term used by Colin Ross, a psychiatrist and authority on trauma and dissociation. When the two are co-present they share the sensations and control over the body. That produces an experience of self which is more like shared consciousness. The change in focus between the host personality and alter is more like 'shifting' than 'switching'. We don't hear distinct voices or dialogue in our heads. It is a more subtle form of alters, consistent with OSDD. That is a key reason why being AB has not been correctly understood by mental health professionals and by ABs themselves.

Okay, we understand being AB is an identity on the dissociation spectrum and we have one or more child alters.

So what now?

It boils down to four things –

1. accept your dual nature;
2. practice good self-care as a multiple;
3. be proud of who you are; and
4. see the gift in who you are.

Each of these is discussed below.

Accept Your Dual Nature

For ABs, denial of *either* our subjective reality, or objective reality, will mess us up. We have a child alter. It is not metaphorical like the inner child of a singleton. A part of our minds *really* does think, feel, perceive and sometimes act like a young child. Through our child alter we have access to innocent joy and contentment, and a feeling of being safe and protected, that most adult singletons don't. They can't be deeply comforted and settled like we can by a soft or wet nappy, or hugging or sleeping with a favourite soft toy. Our child alter's need to be nurtured is real, and must be met for us to live happily. But we are not biological children, either physically or psychologically. We are also adults.

But our dual nature can also be difficult to live with. It brings self-doubt and cognitive dissonance. The latter comes from the contradiction between the real child in our psyche and the visible, objectively real adult we see in the mirror, and experience in our interactions with the outside world.

The doubt and cognitive dissonance can sometimes be painful or tormenting. It can cause us to want to downplay or reject our dual nature in favour of one that embraces just the child. That leads us to flirt in ways that are psychologically unsafe with fantasies of permanent regression and notions of a full-time lifestyle as a child. There is no solution there. Going down that road eventually only makes the cognitive dissonance worse. Taken to an extreme it creates dangerous psychological risks.

To be psychologically healthy, we need to accept our dual nature. Self-acceptance is long, slow, self-disciplined effort. But it does work. It fortifies us against doubt and cognitive dissonance. When we learn to trust the child in our psyche is REAL, we aren't tormented by trying to validate they are objectively real like a biological child.

Good Self Care

We are multiples. The example of people with DID shows us we need to practice good self-care to live happily and safely. As discussed in the last chapter that includes –

- a safe physical personal environment;
- a place of sanctuary within our psyche;
- to recognize our need for acceptance by loved ones;
- to recognize our need for fellowship with others like us;
- to have outlets for service and creativity;
- to be cautious about disclosure; and
- to come to terms with childhood trauma.

Be Proud

As ABs, I believe we are right to be proud of our identity. We can tread the road people of other minority identities have already trodden – from shame to pride.

DID or being AB can be incomprehensible to others. For a time in our lives, our own identities were incomprehensible to us. It is too, too easy to equate different with bad - especially unconsciously.

We cannot judge non-conforming identities by the difficulties or trauma from which they arose, but rather by their success in overcoming those challenges. Those identities can best be understood as the psyche's way of optimizing the chances for 'life, liberty and the pursuit of happiness', even in the face of factors in a person's early life which threatened to diminish or even destroy those chances. Understand the challenges and you will understand the identity. Once you accept the childhood trauma, and the subjective reality of alters, DID and being AB is completely understandable.

ABs show great courage in accepting our child alters, and not turning away from their genuine need for nurturing despite the unconventional way that need presents itself. We have kept faith with our inner child and our true self in the face of persistent public misunderstanding. Many ills of the world would be cured if there was a more general recognition we all have an inner child, and the need for nurturing is a universal need.

I believe just as ABs can learn much from people with DID, ABs also have something to show people with DID. That is the importance of child alters. For any multiple, I believe child alters are central to their healing and their happiness.

See the Gift

There is a gift in being a multiple – whether DID or AB. And that is understanding everyone's life is shaped by their unique subjective reality.

For almost everyone, there will be times in their life when the world does not understand or accept their subjective reality, and that causes pain and alienation. For example, a stranger cannot see we may be in deep grief, yet it shapes our experience of ourselves and life on an hourly and daily basis. In these circumstances, we can all feel very alone.

For all of us, understanding and accepting another's subjective reality about themselves even when that reality seems confronting or incomprehensible is an act of empathy, kindness and love.

People with a non-conforming sense of self are well placed to understand this universal human experience. That is one of the reasons why society as a whole is better for accepting difference. It allows all, to better ask for and receive, the understanding of our own unique experience of ourselves.

Psychiatrist David Yeung says –

> *"There indeed people with DID who have healed. … They do good things in the world and have the capacity to display great empathy towards others." [Engaging Multiple Personalities Volume 3]*

Felix Conrad reached a similar view about the gift in being transgender. He says –

> *"we must forge our own meaning as to why we are the way we are. For me, that meaning lies in the fact that our ever-shifting minds give us an incredible reserve of empathy and understanding for others. That is like a super power. My advice is that you start mining that reserve … and use your super power to change the world." [Quantum Desire: A Sexological Analysis of Crossdreaming]*

I am proud Dax and I are giving that advice, our best shot. I know there are many, many others, either with DID, or who are ABs, who are doing the same.

Appendix 1 – Two Magnetic Resonance Imaging (MRI) Studies of DID

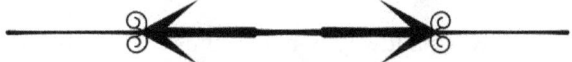

The two studies cited below use MRI to compare the brain structures of people with DID, sub-DID DDNOS, and 'healthy' people.

'Hippocampal and Amygdalar Volumes in Dissociative Identity Disorder' American Journal of Psychiatry. 2006 Apr; 163(4): 630–636. Vermetten, Eric; Schmahl, Christian; Lindner, Sanneke; Loewenstein, Richard J; Bremner, Douglas J.

'Volume of discrete brain structures in complex dissociative disorders: preliminary findings' in Progress in Brain Research, Vol. 167, 2008. Ehling, T; Nijenhius, E.R.S.; Krikke, A.P

The two articles are succinct, readily comprehensible to the lay reader and available free on-line (see the references). Both have useful lists of further references.

The two studies are summarized below.

2006 Study

The study covered 15 patients with a history of severe DID, and 23 healthy subjects without a psychiatric disorder, in Baltimore USA. The DID patients had a history of childhood abuse and had also been diagnosed with PTSD and major depression (both are commonly co-morbid with DID). They had a mean age of 42 years and an average of 16 years of education. All participating subjects were female (this may reflect an intention to remove the issue of age differences in the volume of the hippocampus from the study - unlike men there is no evidence the volume decreases with age in women aged 20 to 50).

Key points –

- Indicates it is the first study to demonstrate differences in key brain structures in people with DID.
- Of prior research, it states – " ... essentially nothing is known about the neurobiology of dissociative identity disorder."
- Hippocampal volume was 19.2% smaller and amygdalar volume was 31.6% smaller in the patients with DID, compared to the healthy subjects.
- Indicates for this area of research generally, it is unclear whether smaller hippocampal volume is caused by trauma, or whether people born with smaller volume are more vulnerable to trauma and dissociation.
- Cites as the key implication of the study – "an understanding of dissociative identity disorder as a trauma-related disorder that involves neural circuitry alterations in brain areas associated with memory that are also affected in PTSD ..".

2008 Study

The study covered 10 DID-patients, 13 DDNOS-patients, 10 DID-patients who completely recovered from DID after lengthy psychotherapy (average duration 4.5 years), and 20 healthy controls. The study was conducted in the Netherlands. All participants were female.

Key points -

- Unlike the 2006 study, this one included a sub-DID DDNOS-1 group. People with DDNOS-1 have either well-developed identity alteration or significant amnesia, but not both (otherwise they would be DID). It is not clear if the people in this group had amnesia (unlike ABs) or identity alteration (like ABs).
- Unlike the 2006 study, this one also measured the volume of the parahippocampal gyrus (PHG) which serves as an interface between the hippocampus and neocortex, and the amygdala.
- Hippocampus volume was 25% smaller in the patients with DID, compared to the healthy subjects.
- Patients with DDNOS were midway between those with DID and the healthy subjects, with 13-14% less hippocampus volume than the latter.
- Otherwise, the DID and DDNOS populations were similar, with both having 19-20% less PHG volume and 10-12% less amygdala volume, than the healthy control group.
- If the two groups with DID are compared, the recovered group had 9 – 18% (left & right respectively) more volume in the hippocampus, but not more PHG volume.
- Hippocampus and PHG volume were also strongly correlated with reported exposure to potentially traumatizing events.

Appendix 2 - Thoughts on Therapy for ABs as an Identity on the Dissociation Spectrum

The following discussion is intended to assist ABs to find the therapist and the therapy which will meet their needs. It is also intended to inform the treatment options of mental health professionals.

We now understand that being an AB is an identity on the dissociation spectrum. ABs have subjectively real child alters which originated in dissociated childhood trauma. The latter also produces symptoms such as anxiety, depression and eating disorders which can persist through life. It is often a lifetime habit to deny and minimize the impact of distressing feelings and experiences in childhood. It was for me. But if you are AB and you have distress and impairment which seems disproportionate to the objective circumstances of your life, I believe those dysfunctions will not heal without addressing the root cause of childhood trauma. Psychotherapy with a skilled psychotherapist works.

When trauma and a broken childhood attachment are addressed, being an AB can be a healthy personal identity. But when there is distress or impairment, being AB fits with the category of Other Specified Dissociative Disorder (OSDD). That is next door to Dissociative Identity Disorder (DID) on the dissociation spectrum.

This following discusses effective therapy for AB / OSDD. You will be better able to find a suitable therapist if you have some idea of the kind of therapy that you are seeking - and the kind that you are not.

For people with DID, there is already a substantial body of knowledge on effective treatment and therapy, developed by skilled and empathic mental health professionals. (I recommend the books by Psychiatrists David Yeung and Colin Ross cited in the references.) There is no similar body of knowledge for ABs.

I reiterate I have no qualifications in psychology. It might be perceived as presumptuous for me to provide any thoughts on therapy. I believe it is justified by the present lack of insight into ABs amongst mental health professionals. I am guided by my own experience of therapy for dissociated trauma and alters some four years ago. I have also drawn on the books of three psychiatrists who understand dissociation and multiples (see their experience cited in Chapter 3). Take what you find useful from this discussion and leave the rest behind.

I am guided by the view of psychiatrist Colin Ross that the treatment for OSDD follows a similar pattern as for DID. He states-

"I tell patients that it doesn't really matter where they are on the dissociation spectrum – from no dissociative disorder to full DID – as long as it is clear that they are at least 2/3 or 3/4 of the way out to DID. If that is so, the treatment is pretty much the same, whether they have OSDD or DID. This is important to understand because it interrupts unproductive obsessing about whether the person really has DID or not."

A similar view is stated by the International Society for the Study of Trauma and Dissociation's (ISSTD) 2010 Guidelines -

"In terms of treatment, however, the expert consensus is that DDNOS-1 [the DSM-IV TR label for OSDD] cases—whether they are as-yet-undiagnosed DID or almost-DID—benefit from many of the treatments that have been designed for DID."

I have quoted extensively from the three psychiatrists. When reading the quotations you may find it helpful to substitute the terms OSDD for DID, and Little or Little(s) for alters.

Diagnosis

As with anyone, the effectiveness of the assistance depends on an accurate diagnosis. That raises a concern. There is a strong prospect being AB will not be understood to be an identity on the dissociation spectrum. In turn, that creates a high risk that a response by a mental health professional will be premised on an inaccurate diagnosis and therefore be ineffective.

The problem starts with the fact dissociation is not well understood by most mental health professionals. The ISSTD's 2010 Guidelines state -

> *"The difficulties in diagnosing DID result primarily from lack of education among clinicians about dissociation, dissociative disorders, and the effects of psychological trauma, as well as from clinician bias. This leads to limited clinical suspicion about dissociative disorders and misconceptions about their clinical presentation."*

This is despite DID or MPD being listed in the DSM since 1980. It is common for people with DID to spend 5 to 10 years being misdiagnosed. Dr Yeung indicates even when he wrote in 2018, many of his colleagues denied DID was real. They preferred other, pathological explanations, and persist in misdiagnosing people with DID.

I suspect a key reason why many mental health professionals don't accept DID is they fear engaging with such a seemingly outlandish condition would diminish their standing as medical scientists. They are afraid of being seen as quacks by skeptical peers or the public.

How much more difficult will it be for ABs to get a valid diagnosis? Firstly, the population of ABs is much smaller than people with DID and hence will be unfamiliar to most therapists. Secondly, being AB is associated in the minds of most mental health professionals with sexual fetishism. That's how it is incorrectly categorized in the DSM, the authoritative catalogue of mental disorders.

This state of affairs is likely to produce -

- a focus on treating the symptoms of dissociation, like depression, anxiety and bulimia, to the exclusion and perhaps to the detriment of the treatment of the primary issue, dissociated trauma; and
- misdiagnoses of distressed or impaired ABs, likely with Borderline Personality Disorder (BPD) or Bi-Polar Affective Disorder or similar.

The problem is that dissociated childhood trauma can produce a complex and confusing array of symptoms. Dr Ross indicates –

> *"The common comorbid diagnoses in DID include – depression; PTSD; panic disorder; OCD; substance abuse; borderline personality disorder; eating disorders; somatic symptom disorders."*

On failing to treat dissociation as the primary issue psychiatrist David Yeung says –

> *"Treating depression in a DID patient as the primary mood disorder without dealing with the underlying trauma, is like treating a fever with aspirin while ignoring the underlying infection."*

He discusses the high probability of misdiagnoses where distress or impairment comes from dissociated trauma-

The Adult Baby – An Identity on the Dissociation Spectrum

"In psychiatry, unlike other branches of medicine, diagnosis relies mostly on clinical descriptions, as few laboratory tests are available. In both Bipolar Affective Disorder and Borderline Personality Disorder, for example, one finds abnormal mood changes. When DID is ignored or missed, one of these two diagnoses is invariably dragged in as the explanation for what appears to be cycling between different mood states.

There is a common misunderstanding which causes this confusion. The switching of affect in in Borderline Personality Disorder (or Bipolar Disorder) is based on the emotional instability of a unitary personality. The apparent switching of affect in MPD [Multiple Personality Disorder / DID] is based on the appearance of different alters. ...

DID often presents as depression and other mood disorders and is commonly misdiagnosed as Borderline Personality Disorder, Bipolar Disorder and Treatment Resistant Depression. If the clinician is not wary, it can be confused with Schizophrenia as well. These misdiagnoses are based on an inappropriately low level of suspicion for DID. The confusion is compounded by exclusively biological view of mental illness and the unfortunate over-reliance on pharmacological approaches to treatment. The resulting ongoing, under-reporting of DID leads to a misperception that DID is extremely rare."

"The misdiagnoses of DID patients are the result of misunderstanding the etiology of changing emotional presentations. There are four basic target symptoms in psycho-pharmacology: mood fluctuation, psychosis, anxiety, and depression. Psychiatrists who are trained to look primarily for these target symptoms will seize the symptom(s) and prescribe medication accordingly, rather than look deeper into the roots of the symptomology." [Engaging Multiple Personalities Volume 2]

If the mental health professional is not sufficiently knowledgeable or skilled, dissociated childhood trauma will not be diagnosed. It will continue to drive symptoms of distress or impairment which are then labelled as treatment-resistant.

It takes a skilled mental health professional to see beyond individual symptoms and recognize the underlying cause common to each of them. Dr Ross describes the perspective required -

"Another motto of Trauma Model Therapy is the problem is not the problem. This means that the presenting symptom, behavior, addiction, social role, or diagnosis is not the problem: it is the solution to a problem in the background. This doesn't mean that the problem is not a problem, or can be ignored. It means that the symptom or behavior occurs in a context, has a meaning and function, is a survival strategy, and can best be understood in the context of the person's life story. The symptom is not just the brain on the fritz or a symptom of neurotransmitter imbalance.

The therapist's job is to figure out the function or purpose of the behavior and the problem in the background it is meant to solve. The treatment goal is then to help the person find a better way to solve the problem in the background, so she can let go of the unhealthy coping strategy."

The categorization of being AB as a sexual fetish in the DSM is an example of the failure described above – mistaking a symptom for the cause of the condition.

To be fair, ABs have probably contributed to some of the dismal history of their reception by mental health professionals. I suspect many ABs seeking treatment for symptoms such as anxiety, depression or bulimia do not realize this has any relationship to their being AB (ie. comes from the same source). Or they have an undefined fear it does but are too scared of being harshly judged to disclose being AB. I suspect it is rare for ABs to disclose the full extent of the tormenting conflicts of the 'binge and purge' cycle; the involuntary triggering; or the extent of the identification in their fantasies with being a helpless, dependent baby. The fear behind this non-disclosure is perfectly valid. Most mental health professionals have no understanding of ABs and many would quickly label these symptoms as a pathological psycho-sexual disorder as per the DSM. But it's a vicious cycle. Without this knowledge, there are no indications which might point the more insightful therapists to the real origin of being AB in dissociated childhood trauma.

Over time, things will get better. The awareness of dissociation is growing, albeit from a low base. Chapter 3 cited studies which suggest around 10 per cent of the population has substantial symptoms of dissociation. That makes dissociation as prevalent as mood disorders such as depression and anxiety. It took decades, but awareness of these mood disorders has grown amongst the public and mental health professionals. That has reduced their stigma and increased the prospect of receiving appropriate treatment. In time it is likely the awareness of dissociation will follow the same trajectory.

That's not much help right now.

Finding a Therapist

The current situation places an onus on ABs, and those who love them, to insist on an accurate diagnosis and appropriate treatment, and to find a mental health professional capable of providing both. Treating dissociation is a specialist branch of psychotherapy. (For guidance on selecting a mental health professional see the appendix in my book *'The Adult Baby Identity – A Self Help Guide'*).

An AB needs to find a therapist who –

- accepts the existence of subjectively real alters created in childhood trauma (as per the DSM), AND
- believes in an outcome where alters and the host work as a team or family, rather than requiring the alters to fuse with the host to create a unitary psyche (as discussed in Chapter 14).

The first point needs a therapist who can see beyond the nappies et al to the dissociated child alters and trauma behind it. It's good if they have some experience with treating dissociation, but even if they don't but are willing to learn it's a good start. The mental health professionals who successfully treated Christine Pattillo and Robert Oxnam didn't have a lot of experience with DID when they first started treating Christine and Robert.

The second point needs a therapist who adheres to humanistic psychology that respects the self-determination of the client, rather than believing they know better what is good for the client.

So the therapist you are looking for is likely to combine an unusual level of empathy, an open mind and professional courage.

What to Look For In Treatment/Therapy

I believe if you an AB / OSDD the most effective therapy would reflect the following: –

1. psychotherapy is likely to be more helpful than medication or hypnosis;
2. effective psychotherapy for multiples is based on working with alters;
3. psychotherapy does not require reliving the original trauma;
4. much of the healing is self-directed;
5. the support of loved ones, especially a loving partner, is invaluable;
6. if you have a consoling faith, don't be afraid to draw on it;
7. you define what the end goal of therapy means for you; and
8. it's okay to provisionally self-diagnose to provide a starting point for therapy.

Each of these is discussed below.

Psychotherapy is Likely to be More Useful Than Medication or Hypnosis

Several of the psychiatrists cited in the book indicate dissociation generally does not respond to drug treatment. Medication may be used to address symptoms such as depression, anxiety or sleep disturbances to allow an interval for the treatment of the underlying cause, dissociated trauma. But medication is unlikely to heal the causes of those symptoms.

Psychiatrist Dr Colin Ross says –

> *"In some cases, medications can be very helpful in managing some presenting symptoms (eg. depression, insomnia). Some medications may have small positive impacts on certain post-traumatic symptoms. However, until now, there is no evidence that medications can help a person process and integrate his/her trauma or dissociated parts of the personality. It is also important to be aware of the potential side effects of medications. In the literature, it has been reported that some medications may worsen certain dissociative symptoms. Different dissociated personality states of the same person may respond to medications differently. Psychosocial interventions (eg. psychotherapy) are primary treatments for post traumatic mental disorders."*
> *[Be a Teammate With Yourself: Understanding Trauma and Dissociation]*

The appropriate treatment for dissociated childhood trauma is psychotherapy – 'the talking cure'. The good news is with an accurate diagnosis, psychotherapy is effective. For example, the greater majority of people with DID who receive psychotherapy have positive life outcomes.

Dr Ross says–

> *"The main conclusion [of studies], though, is that the psychotherapy of dissociative disorders is evidence-based and effective."*

Hypnosis has value only as an ancillary to psychotherapy. Careful therapists like Dr Steinberg see a role for hypnosis in relaxation techniques and the like. However, the use of hypnosis to 'call out' secretive or reluctant alters, or to elicit memories of childhood abuse is dangerous and potentially harmful. Therapists who use these practices should be avoided.

In the 1990s, in the first stage of treating DID at least one leading authority (Richard Kluft) promoted the use of hypnosis as central to treatment. In more recent times both psychiatrists David Yeung and Jeffrey Smith did not favour hypnosis. Jeffrey Smith states –

> *"… hypnosis seemed controlling and manipulative, and multiples have already had enough of this type of experience for a lifetime. It seemed to place the doctor too much in charge. My experience of treatment is much more as a partnership in which the patient brings knowledge about his or her inner life and I contribute my understanding of people and my personal reactions. Together, we pool our information and work on healing."*

Effective Psychotherapy for Multiplies is Based on Working with Alters

The central fact about being a 'multiple' is you have subjectively real alters. Recognizing and accepting this, for both you and your therapist, is the key to effective psychotherapy. The three psychiatrists agree on that.

Don't be afraid of your alters. They may have scared you at times with their unexpected power to influence your thoughts, feelings and actions. But you have the power to heal and change wounded or dysfunctional alters. Finding out you have a subjectively real child alter doesn't mean you have to hand your whole life and psyche over to them. Nor does it mean your partner or your therapist have to acquiesce to all the demands of a hurt and angry alter. You can learn to live together happily, without disruption or dysfunction. In therapy and healing, you and your therapist respond compassionately but firmly to a demanding or dysfunctional child alter just as you would to a distressed and angry small biological child.

Psychiatrist Dr David Yeung says –

"The heart of DID therapy is engaging alters on their own terms."

"Treating a person with DID means developing an attitude of compassion and respect towards the alters whenever and however they emerge, whether it be shyly, boldly, flirtatiously or aggressively. Successful treatment of the alters does not mean eradication of them or their functions."

"Common courtesy – and the necessity of establishing a therapeutic bond – dictates that a therapist speak to each alter as if he or she is an individual. This requires a willingness on the part of the therapist to engage the dissociation in therapy. Many therapists may be unable to do this for personal or philosophical reasons.

Therapists may be stuck in the paradigm that alters are pathological manifestations and therefore they should neither be acknowledged for spoken to. In treating patients with schizophrenic hallucinations, psychiatrists try to persuade them to ignore the voices that they hear. In DID therapy, to the contrary, communication between the therapist and an alter, as well as among alters, is fundamental to successful therapy."

… a key principle of MPD treatment; to treat each single MPD patient as if I was conducting group therapy. Knowing they [the alters] are all listening, one can start talking to them as a group."

The ISSTD's 2010 Guidelines state -

"Helping the identities to be aware of one another as legitimate parts of the self and to negotiate and resolve their conflicts is at the very core of the therapeutic process. It is countertherapeutic for the therapist to treat any alternate identity as if it were more "real" or more important than any other. The therapist should not "play favorites" among the alternate identities or exclude apparently unlikable or disruptive ones from the therapy … The therapist should foster the idea that all alternate identities represent adaptive attempts to cope or to master problems that the patient has faced. Thus, it is countertherapeutic to tell patients to ignore or "get rid" of identities … "

I have had successful therapy which recognized and worked with my child alters. If you are self-conscious and inhibited like I am, you do not have to speak as an alter. Dr Ross says-

"Talking through means that you talk to an alter in the background while another part – usually the host – is in executive control. The part then answers inside the person's head and the host passes on that by saying it out loud. Not uncommonly, after a few questions and answers, the alter emerges spontaneously. If this happens, I acknowledge the switch, confirm who I'm talking to, and carry on with the conversation. …"

Effective psychotherapy does not require a detailed biography of every alter. Dr Yeung advises mental health professionals –

"As a general rule, resist the temptation to try and find out more about these alters. Once their function is clear – such as holding an emotional aspect of a traumatic experience – that is all that is needed for therapy. Knowing their function enables the therapist to acknowledge and work with whatever the alter is holding. This is a far more important task than exploring the

personality specifics, the storyline, of each individual alter." [Engaging Multiple Personalities Volume 2]

Dr Yeung's comments point to the difference in perspective between a mental health professional treating distress and impairment, and a person who sees being a 'multiple' as their personal identity. It isn't necessary for a therapist to know the 'life story' of each alter to provide effective therapy. But for ABs, I believe it is psychologically healthy to get to know your alter(s). But that is part of the normal process of human growth and discovery which everyone does for themselves.

Colin Ross emphasizes in working with alters, neither the AB, nor the therapist can lose sight of the 'whole person' -

> *"Treat the person who has the DID, not the DID. This will involve working with the DID, but while you're working with the parts, keep a firm grip on the whole person perspective. This is a single person with human problems that are fragmented into parts. You have to work with the parts to help the single parts; but there is only one person there ..."*

Healing trauma and building cooperation with alters are the two key objectives of therapy for 'multiples'. Dr Smith says –

> *"... there are just two therapeutic goals. The first is to process and detoxify the buried memories of trauma and the second is to help the long-separated parts come to know, respect, and ultimately love one another. As these are accomplished, continuing to remain a multiple will no longer be a necessity but a choice."*

All the psychiatrists accept these two objectives. But there can be differences between them in terms of which is more important. Dr Yeung emphasizes the primary importance of healing trauma whereas Dr Colin Ross emphasizes the healthy functioning of alters. Dr Ross says -

> *"In any case, trauma memories are only one topic in DID therapy – I don't think they are the main one. A lot of the work involves learning grounding and self-soothing skills, and self-regulation, saying 'no' to addictions, correcting cognitive errors, forming healthy relationships and other tasks that aren't 'memory work' as such. In DID, additional tasks include: orienting alters to the body and the present; building inter-personality communication and cooperation – building a team; building co-consciousness and co-presence; reducing host resistance; and other tasks which are not directly connected to memories as such."*

Psychotherapy Does Not Require Re-living the Original Trauma

I suspect a key reason for denying or minimizing distressing experiences in childhood is we fear 'touching that hotplate again' – reliving something very painful. Effective psychotherapy does <u>not</u> require people with dissociated trauma remember and relive every frightening detail.

Contemporary treatment of dissociated trauma emphasizes several purposes –

1. to initially stablise a person by allowing them to recognize the distressing sensations belong to past events and they are safe in the present; and
2. subsequently, to build a 'trauma narrative' which allows the person sufficient understanding of what happened to make sense of their response.

Of the first point, Dr Yeung says –

> *"Patients must learn to know when they are ready to venture inward and explore more deeply. They need to be taught and actually experience the key fact that processing the trauma in*

order to gain some sense of mastery over it is <u>not</u> the same as reliving it. It is also not the same as just talking about it. It is about touching the wound lightly, experiencing and recognizing the discrepancy between one's heightened arousal and the actual situation happening right now in a safe place, where there is no threat."

The memory of trauma has a special character. People can accurately recall the subjective sensations caused by trauma – the emotions, thoughts and physical sensations. The memory of objective detail – where, when, who – can be more difficult and unreliable. There are well-understood reasons for these differences in recall in terms of how the brain functions (see the discussion in Chapter 3). The point is, the validity of a person's recall of their subjective experience does not depend on forensically accurate recall of objective details. Creating a trauma narrative is about reconstructing a sufficient understanding of what happened long ago to make sense of it, without needing it to satisfy some forensic or legal requirement.

Dr Smith helpfully distinguishes the two healing mechanisms at work in the therapeutic recall of past trauma.

"The first is the mechanism by which painful experiences are detoxified. … I will refer to this by its original name catharsis. The second is the process by which negative values, attitudes, and attachments derived from abusers are modified. I will refer to this healing mechanism as internalization. Both mechanisms may be involved in any phase of therapeutic work.

It is important to note that internalization works differently with multiples than it does with others. What is internalized belongs to one alter, not to the whole. … Some alters become the embodiments of destructive and self-negating attitudes so that others can be spared. This naturally leads to tensions among alters, rather than ambivalence within oneself, as is the case with other trauma survivors. In fact, it is the healing of these tensions that constitutes the major therapeutic goal along with the healing of painful experiences. Thus, internalization is the key therapeutic goal of bringing alters together, while catharsis is the process most closely allied to working with traumatic memories."

The internalization of negative messages can happen in other forms of trauma than abuse. The experience of not being protected or able to turn to a parent figure for help, can make a child feel unloved and unloveable. And as with abuse, instead of laying that feeling with an adult on whom they are dependent, the child's unconscious invents reasons why they were unloveable.

Most of the Healing is Self-Directed

Based on the published material it is common for people with DID to be in therapy for many years. This lengthy treatment was due to the depth and harm of the childhood abuse, and the strength of the denial of being a multiple.

If the estimates people with DID represent one per cent of the population are valid, then the published accounts may not be representative. For every person who can find and afford a therapist to be in treatment for many years, there must be many others who have to, or chose to, take a different road. There simply aren't the number of skilled therapists around to treat everyone for that length of time.

The numbers suggest there must be many people with substantial dissociative symptoms who have more positive outcomes but who have to rely more on their own psychological resources. There is a pointer towards this even in the published cases of lengthy treatment. Two of the psychiatrists emphasize even in those latter contexts much of the healing is self-directed.

Dr Smith says –

"Multiples seem to have their own blueprint for healing, and one of the main contributions a therapist can make is to recognize and value the patient's inner direction."

Dr Yeung says –

> *"I firmly believe that all therapy contains a large measure of self healing. DID patients need to develop the confidence to take up a measure of self-directed therapy. It is necessary for the alters to cooperate and work as a team. The therapist must encourage the patient's to do this."*

I suspect for most people who are AB / OSDD the level of childhood trauma is less than for people with DID. This makes it both possible, and likely, their healing will be largely self-directed and will not require the kind of lengthy therapy found in published accounts of people with DID. In my case, the therapy took months rather than years.

Much of this healing will be concerned less with trauma, and more with the broken bond in childhood with the AB's mother/primary caregiver. The latter is called an insecure attachment (see Chapter 11) and is common amongst the broader population. See Jasmin Lee Cori's excellent book *'The Emotionally Absent Mother: How to Recognize and Heal the Invisible Effects of Childhood Emotional Neglect'* for self-directed healing of an insecure childhood attachment.

Support of A Loving Partner

I believe over the long run, the most important sources of healing for someone with AB / OSDD are themselves, the support of a loving partner, and the assistance of a skilled therapist, in that order.

In the healing process, the acceptance of a partner relieves someone with AB / OSDD of the burden of having to fight denial by themselves. In everyday life, the acceptance of a partner means we are not alone with our doubt and cognitive dissonance.

Dr Yeung gives the inspiring example in his casebook of 'Joan' whose husband was an indispensable partner in his wife's healing and full recovery from fragmented DID (*'Engaging Multiple Personalities Volume 1'* Chapter 1). Joan's husband's level of participation in her therapy was unusual, but it is a pointer to the obvious fact your partner is a far more constant and significant presence in your life than any therapist, and their empathy is powerful. That is affirmed in Christine Pattillo's account of her husband Christopher's support through her diagnosis and treatment, and Cameron West's account of his wife Rikki's support.

Consoling Faith

If you have a consoling faith in God or a higher power, don't be afraid to call on it. Dr Yeung, who treated around one hundred people with DID over his career, welcomed such faith and saw it as a source of resilience. In his book *'Engaging Multiple Personalities Volume 1'* (Chapter 5) he gives a case history for 'Ruth', a young woman who persistently pursued successful healing in the face of great obstacles, because of the strength she drew from her faith.

If you are a multiple, your dissociation and alters are not beyond your faith. God loves all of you, including your alters. The therapist I saw about my childhood trauma and my alters worked with my faith in the therapy. I found that made therapy easier and more effective.

You Define the End Goal of Therapy

There are two expert views about the intended outcome of therapy for multiples (as discussed in Chapter 14). One is to fuse alters with the host to create a unitary psyche – in essence, to stop being a multiple. The other is continue being a multiple and for the alters to work as a cooperative team or family.

Those who favour fusion see it in the following terms. The alters merge with the host and the positive capabilities and traits of the alters are not lost but become available to the whole psyche. The damage and the pain originally held by the alters from the original trauma(s) is resolved in therapy before fusion and is not carried forward. The person now has a unitary psyche. There are no 'fault lines' remaining in the psyche which might again fracture in the face of future stresses or crises. To effect fusion requires years of intensive weekly therapy.

Those who favour cooperation see it in the following terms. The alters are like a family, each loving and respecting the others and their different roles within the psyche. There is no amnesia and all the alters are co-conscious. Shifting is more common than switching. The alters may be co-present.

The key point is, it's your choice about which outcome you want. You need to find a therapist who respects your self-determination and doesn't have a hidden agenda to push you towards their favoured option.

Provisional Self Diagnosis is Okay

After researching this book one of the questions I had for myself was what do I do if I need to seek therapy again in the future? Do I declare to a psychotherapist what I now understand about ABs being on the dissociation spectrum? My concern is they will be dis-believing and pissed off I am usurping their professional skills to make a diagnosis. It's tough enough talking about being AB without making the initial interview any harder. And we live in the age of Dr Google and Dr Wikipedia which I am sure pisses off many mental health professionals.

I was comforted to read the following from psychiatrist Colin Ross, an authority on dissociation -

> *"A person with DID that hasn't yet been officially diagnosed may or may not already know they have DID. Some people have done reading and research, are aware of having blank spells, know some of their parts by name and age, and really only need confirmation of the diagnosis."*

So, if I do seek therapy in the future, I will declare what I understand about my AB identity. To do otherwise would seem like wasting time and money in dancing around the bushes. My understanding of myself is going to have to be 'on the table' sooner or later. I will try and hold my views lightly and respect that a skilled psychotherapist is going to bring knowledge and insights 'to the table' that I don't have. Effective therapy is a collaboration between the client and the therapist. It works best when each respects what the other brings to the collaboration.

Glossary

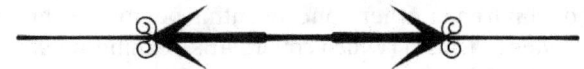

The book uses the following terms.

See also the discussion at the beginning of Chapter 4 on terminology relevant to DID and 'multiples'.

AB	Adult Baby – adolescents or adults or wear diapers/nappies and are attracted to the trappings and fantasy of infancy
alter	alternative personality
B&D	bondage and discipline
cognitive dissonance	the mental discomfort (psychological stress) experienced by a person who holds two or more contradictory beliefs, ideas, or values
DDNOS	Dissociative Disorder Not Otherwise Specified – the category below DID on the dissociation spectrum – introduced in the DSM-IV TR, the penultimate version of the DSM
DID	Dissociative Identity Disorder – previously known as Multiple Personality Disorder (MPD)
differential diagnosis	A systematic diagnostic method used to identify a condition where multiple alternatives are possible. It is akin to the process of elimination and involves matching symptoms with the attributes of alternative conditions to find which condition best explains all the symptoms.
DL	Diaper Lover – adolescents or adults who wear diapers/nappies but do not acknowledge any other attraction to the trappings of infancy
DSM	Diagnostic and Statistical Manual of Mental Disorders - the standard diagnostic tool published by the American Psychiatric Association. The latest version, the DSM-5 was published in 2013. The DSM is one of two classification systems for mental disorders. The other is the ICD (International Classification of Diseases)-10 Classification of Mental and Behavioural Disorders, produced by the World Health Organization. The DSM is generally used in the US (and Australia?), while the ICD is used more widely in Europe and other parts of the world. For a discussion of the treatment of dissociative disorders in the DSM and ICD, see Rob Spring's blog 'DSM-5: what's new in the criteria for dissociative disorders?' (cited in the references).

fetish	The clinical term for fetish is a paraphilia. The penultimate version of the DSM, the DSM-IV-TR, describes paraphilias as "recurrent, intense sexually arousing fantasies, sexual urges or behaviors generally involving nonhuman objects, the suffering or humiliation of oneself or one's partner, or children or other nonconsenting persons that occur over a period of six months." It includes fetishism (which covers ABs), exhibitionism (flashing), frotteurism (groping), pedophilia (child molesting), voyeurism (peeping toms), and transvestism (cross dressing). The inclusion of consenting and non-consenting (coercive, illegal) behaviours under the same definition is unhelpful and unnecessarily stigmatizing (for the former).
host	the alternative personality who is out in front most of the time
ISSTD	International Society for the Study of Trauma and Dissociation
Little	The term AB's often use for the child part of their psyche. For the purposes of this book it is construed as referring to a child alter.
mental health professionals	Psychiatrists, psychologists, therapists and counsellors
MPD	Multiple Personality Disorder – the old term for Dissociative Identity Disorder
multiple	A person with alternative personalities
OSDD	Other Specified Dissociative Disorder – the category below DID on the dissociation spectrum - replaces DDNOS in the DSM-5, the latest version of the DSM
singleton	A person with no alternative personalities
trigger	A sensory input (sight, sound, smell etc) that causes a change (switch) in the alter which is in executive control of a multiple's body.

Annotated List of References

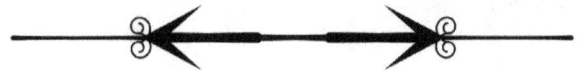

Books on DID and Dissociation

There is a vast literature on dissociation and Dissociative Identity Disorder (DID), including autobiographies of people with DID, and material by mental health professionals. A search on Amazon will produce a large selection. I chose amongst the material that was accessible and affordable and seemed insightful in the case of autobiographies, and authoritative in the case of the non-fiction material.

There is a good reading list of authors with DID, writing about DID at –

http://www.zoramquynh.com/a-did-book-list/

Ehling, T; Nijenhius, E.R.S.; Krikke, A.P	'Volume of discrete brain structures in complex dissociative disorders: preliminary findings' in Progress in Brain Research, Vol. 167, 2008, E.R. de Kloet, M.S. Oitzl & E. Vermetten (Eds.) Succinct and readily comprehensible to the lay reader. Useful list of references. Available free on-line at – https://s3.amazonaws.com/academia.edu.documents/45354174/Volume_of_discrete_brain_structures_in_c20160504-793-1b98uyu.pdf?response-content
International Society for the Study of Trauma and Dissociation	Guidelines for Treating Dissociative Identity Disorder in Adults, Third Revision Succinct and useful. Imbued with the adverse, 'fusionist' view of alters. Includes abreaction & hypnosis in treatment options. Has a comprehensive list of authoritative references as at 2010. Can be accessed at – https://www.isst-d.org/wp-content/uploads/2019/02/GUIDELINES_REVISED2011.pdf
Kate, Mary-Anne, Jamieson, Graham & Hopgood, Tanya	The prevalence of Dissociative Disorders and dissociative experiences in college populations: a meta-analysis of 98 studies. Journal of Trauma & Dissociation Can be accessed at - https://www.researchgate.net/profile/Mary_Anne_Kate A statistical meta-analysis (a study of studies) testing whether dissociative disorders are linked to trauma or suggestable fantasy. The article affirms the former and finds an incidence across countries of dissociative disorders of the magnitude of 10% of the population. Dry and technical.

Oxnam, Robert B.	A Fractured Mind: My Life With Multiple Personality Disorder (2013) (digital and hardcopy: Amazon). The author was a prominent US academic. Shows his treatment journey from the inside. Includes an insightful essay on the nature and treatment of DID by the author's psychiatrist Jeffrey Smith.
Pattillo, Christine, and the Gang	I Am We: Living With Multiple Personalities (2014) (digital and hardcopy: Amazon) This remarkable account has the voice of the host, each alter, and the host's husband and mother. She lives openly as a 'multiple' and her husband embraces her alters as his family. Shows compelling courage and warmth. Highly recommended. Digitial copies are inexpensive. Search on 'Christine Pattillo' for her clips on YouTube
Ross, Colin A.	Treatment of Dissociative Identity Disorder: Techniques and Strategies for Stabilisation (2018) (digital and hardcopy: Amazon) A practical, pragmatic and concise guide to life with alters. The author is an authority on trauma and dissociation and has written a key textbook on DID. Highly recommended.
	Dissociative Identity Disorder: Diagnosis, Clinical Features, and Treatment of Multiple Personality. Second Edition (1997). Available in hardcopy only, second hand only (try abebooks) An update of the original 1989 text on DID. Authoritative in its comprehensive scope and detail. The author's views can be respected without agreeing with them.
Ross, Colin A.	Be A Teammate With Yourself: Understanding Trauma and Dissociation (2019) (digital and hardcopy: Amazon) Useful coverage of the topics. I prefer the author's other recent work 'Treatment of Dissociative Identity Disorder'.
Spring, Rob	'DSM-5: what's new in the criteria for dissociative disorders?' PODS (Positive Outcomes for Dissociative Survivors) Website. Posted 9 January 2013

	A useful description of the treatment of dissociative disorders in the latest version of the DSM. Can be accessed at - https://information.pods-online.org.uk/dsm-5-whats-new-in-the-criteria-for-dissociative-disorders/
	'DID or DDNOS: does it matter?' PODS (Positive Outcomes for Dissociative Survivors) Website. Posted 1 May 2013 An insightful article exploring the sub-DID part of the dissociation spectrum. Highly recommended. Can be accessed at - https://information.pods-online.org.uk/did-or-ddnos-does-it-matter/
Steele, Kathy; Boon, Suzette; van der Hart, Onno.	Treating Trauma Related Dissociation: A Practical Integrative Approach. (2016) (digital and hard copy: Amazon). A text for therapists. Notable for its pejorative treatment of alters. Promotes manipulative, ethically doubtful intransigence by therapists working with DID clients. The approach appears to have been inappropriately transferred from DBT therapy with PTSD & BPD. Expensive. Not recommended.
Steinberg, Marlene	The Stranger in the Mirror: Dissociation The Hidden Epidemic (2010) (hardcopy: Harper Collins. Digital: Amazon). Excellent at explaining dissociation. The author is the psychiatrist who developed the leading diagnostic questionnaire for identifying dissociative disorders. Highly recommended.
Trujillo, Olga	The Sum of My Parts: A Survivor's Story of Dissociative Identity Disorder (2011) (digital & paperback: Amazon) A story of great courage surviving severe abuse. The first half is concerned with the abuse (v. confronting), and the second with treatment based on the first-generation understanding of DID. The author was a high powered Justice Department lawyer.
Vermetten, Eric; Schmahl,	'Hippocampal and Amygdalar Volumes in Dissociative Identity Disorder'

Christian; Lindner, Sanneke; Loewenstein, Richard J; Bremner, Douglas J	American Journal of Psychiatry. 2006 Apr; 163(4): 630–636. Succinct and readily comprehensible to the lay reader. Claims to be the first study to demonstrate different brain structures in DID. Useful list of references. Available free on-line at – https://www.ncbi.nlm.nih.gov/pmc/articles/PMC3233754/
W, A.T.	Got Parts: An Insider's Guide to Managing Life Successfully with Dissociative Identity Disorder. (2005) (digital & paperback: amazon) A good self help book, recommended to me by a family member with DID (Dax). It is relevant to anyone with multiplicity of consciousness. Digital copies are inexpensive.
Walker, Herschel	Breaking Free: My Life with Dissociative Identity Disorder. (2008) (Digital: Amazon. Hardcopy: Touchstone) The author is a highly successful NFL player. His DID did not originate with sexual abuse but principally from prolonged bullying.
West, Cameron	First Person Plural: My Life As a Multiple (2013 edition) (Digital: Amazon) Has powerful insights into denial, treatment, & DID in a loving marriage. He and his wife embraced his alters. Highly recommended.
Wikipedia	Amygdala Dissociation (psychology) Dissociative Disorder Not Otherwise Specified Dissociative Identity Disorder * Herschel Walker Hippocampus * The article on DID has some useful material. However it conveys a misleading view of the validity of DID. It gives equal credence to the view DID is the product of fantasy/false memory. This is false equivalence. It is the same as an article on the Earth giving equal credence to the 'flat earth theory', and on this basis declaring the Earth being round is a 'controversial' theory.

Yeung, David	Engaging Multiple Personalities (Volume 1): Contextual Case Histories (2018) (Digitial & hardcopy: Amazon). 14 case histories of people with DID from the practice of a retired psychiatrist. Shows the unique character of each, and differing outcomes. Compelling and insightful. Highly recommended. Digital copies are inexpensive.
	Engaging Multiple Personalities (Volume 2): Therapeutic Guidelines (2018) (Digitial & hardcopy: Amazon) Intended to guide and encourage other mental health professionals to treat people with DID. Consolidates the insights from Volume 1. I prefer the latter as the case histories are notably insightful.
	Engaging Multiple Personalities (Volume 3): Living in Multiplicity (2018) (Digital: Amazon). A guide for people with DID written by a retired psychiatrist who had many DID clients. Written as a question-and-answer format between the author and an imagined recently diagnosed client with DID. Repetitive but insightful.

Books on ABs and Other Topics

By contrast to DID the non-fiction literature on adult babies is sparse. That includes life histories/autobiographies, self help material, and empathic and insightful material by mental health professionals. Most of this is cited in the annotated references to my book *'The Adult Baby Identity – Coming Out As An Adult Baby'*, and most of it is published by abdiscovery.com.au and available from there or Amazon.

Bader, Michael	Arousal: The Secret Logic of Sexual Fantasies (2003) (Virgin Books) (ISBN 0 7535 0739 0) Paperback only. No digital copy. Highly recommended for anyone wanting to understand troubling sexual fantasies. Finds the emotional meaning of fantasies with compassion and insight. The author is a gifted intuitive psychotherapist.
Bent, Michael	Being an Adult Baby: Articles and Essays on Being an Adult Baby. (2016) (Amazon & Abdiscovery.com.au)

	A collection of insightful and thought provoking articles on the AB identity. Notably – 'Identity Confusion in the Adult Baby', 'Finding Balance Between the Baby and the Adult', and 'Binge and Purge'.'
Bent, Rosalie	There's Still A Baby in My Bed: Learning To Live Happily With the Adult Baby in Your Relationship. (2015) (Amazon & Abdiscovery.com.au) A revised version of the ground breaking 2012 book that first articulated being an AB was a personal identity, not just a fetish. Written by the wife of an AB. Evergreen.
	'When it all goes wrong' Rosalie Bent's on-line blog entry for 26 March 2013 See – https://rosaliebent.wordpress.com/
Conrad, Felix	Transgender: Fact or Fetish (2016) (Digital: Amazon) Takes issue with sexologists view of transgender as a fetish. There is a parallel between this and AB's issue with their identity being similarly categorized. Insightful. Includes the insight the target of erotic fantasies may not be sex with a partner, but transformation of the self to the desired form (the desired gender for transgender people). Recommended. See Conrad's blogs at – https://novagirl.net/latest-articles-2
	How to Jedi Mind Trick Your Gender Dysphoria (2016) (Digital: Amazon) The intended audience are people who identify as transgender but decided not to transition. Iconoclastic and insightful.
	Quantum Desire: A Sexological Analysis of Crossdreaming (2016) (Digital: Amazon) Makes the case for an inclusive definition of transgender which includes those who identify as crossdressers or with a sissy fetish. There is a parallel between the author's view of the transgender identity and my view of the AB identity.
Cori, Jasmin Lee	The Emotionally Absent Mother: How to Recognize and Heal the Invisible Effects of Childhood Emotional Neglect (Second Edition) (2017) (digital & paperback: Amazon)

	A brilliantly written discussion of insecure attachments in childhood and their effects. Makes Attachment Theory, Bowlby and Winnicott accessible to the lay reader. Highly recommended and inexpensive.
Joyce, Maggie	The Full Time Permanent Adult Infant (2019) (Amazon & Abdiscovery.com.au) An account of an AB living a 24/7 AB lifestyle by their wife, and the mother of their 'Little'. I disagree with the author on key points, but it is a work of courageous honesty.
Lewis, Dylan	The Adult Baby Identity – Healing Childhood Wounds (2019) (Amazon & Abdiscovery.com.au) Explores the origins of the identity in an insecure attachment and trauma in childhood. References John Bowlby and Attachment Theory, and Donald Winnicott.
	The Adult Baby Identity – A Self Help Guide (2019) (Amazon & Abdiscovery.com.au) Focuses on self acceptance and resolving the internal conflict between the Inner Child, Inner Parent and Adult.
	The Adult Baby Identity – Coming Out as an Adult Baby (2019) (Amazon & Abdiscovery.com.au) Makes the case being AB is a minority personal identity and considers the stages by which the identity is formed.
	Living With Chrissie: My Life As An Adult Baby (2018) (Amazon & Abdiscovery.com.au My account of my life as a very late bloomer as an AB ('better late than never').
Wikipedia	Cognitive dissonance Regression (psychology)
Winnicott, Donald W.	'Transitional Objects and Transitional Phenomena—A Study of the First Not-Me Possession' (1953) International Journal of Psycho-Analysis, 34:89-97

	Winnicott's ground breaking original exposition on the subject. Includes concise statement of Winnicott's view of infant psychological development. Available free, on-line at – https://pdfs.semanticscholar.org/a56f/ba056a21039574e5b2371f4ad01728b54366.pdf
	'Playing and Reality' (1971) Tavistock Publications. (hardcopy only, no digital copy) Recommended for those with a keen interest in Winnicott. Written for psychotherapists. Best read after reading some secondary sources, or Winnicott's books for laypeople. A seminal book published in the last year of Winnicott's life.

Now that you have read this book you might be interested in more of Dylan Lewis' books. Go to https://abdiscovery.com.au/dylan-lewis/ **to find more of his work. You will also find our complete collection of AB fiction and non-fiction.**

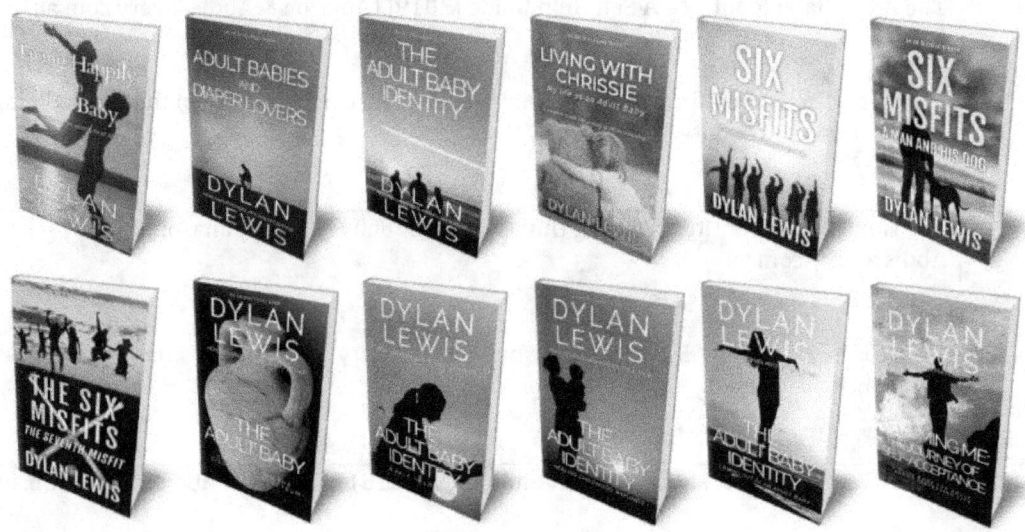